Nutrition Therapy

by

Kathy King, RD, LD

Private Practitioner, Author, Speaker, Publisher
Lake Dallas, TX

Bridget Klawitter, PhD, RD, FADA

Manager, Department of Clinical Dietetics,
All Saints Healthcare System, Racine, WI

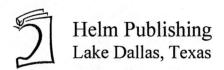

Helm Publishing
Lake Dallas, Texas

*I dedicate this book to my daughters, Savannah, Cherokee, and Peggy Leslie,
the flowers in my garden of life and God's gifts.   KK*

*One's future is built upon those who color the rainbow around us and give meaning to all
our endeavors. Without the strength and determination I have learned from my husband,
Kurt, and the support and encouragement of my parents, Joe and Patracia Swik, this project
would have seemed overwhelming. It is with much love and gratitude I dedicate this work to
them and God, for the inspirations, faith, love, and hope that have made my rainbow shine
through the most difficult times. BK*

Nutrition Therapy: Advanced Counseling Skills, Second edition

Cover design: The Mark Wyatt Group and Southwestern Colorgraphics
Printing: Pro Printing, Dallas, Texas
Copy editor: Dollie Parsons

Copyright 1995 First edition
Copyright 2003 Second edition

For information on ordering books and self-study courses or handouts, call, fax, write, or go online:
Helm Publishing
213 Main Street
P.O. Box 2105
Lake Dallas, TX 75065
phone 940-497-3558   toll free 877-560-6025   fax 940-497-2927
www.helmpublishing.com

ISBN 0-9631033-7-7

TABLE OF CONTENTS

Preface

Our Professional Imperative as Nutrition Experts
Sue Rodwell Williams, PhD, MPH, RD

When I was asked to contribute my views on how we can best collectively and individually advance our profession, I happily accepted, using the above title as a starting point. During my career in nutrition, covering over four decades of experience as a clinical nutritionist, teacher, and writer, I have had the pleasure of witnessing and participating in the wonderful and dramatic growth of our profession.

We have come a long way, and can justifiably feel pride in our profession. But what now? Look again at the above title. Two key questions immediately confront us: Collectively, where does our profession need to be in these challenging times? Individually, as nutrition experts, how must we conduct our practice? For answers to these questions, I look to my own career experiences.

Through my years of practice as a clinical nutrition specialist in four different states—the Carolinas, Arizona, and finally in California—I have learned a great deal about my chosen profession. I learned about people from my clients and patients with varied cultural backgrounds and needs. I learned about team care from the group of medical specialists with whom I worked as the nutrition authority. Here in California, I had the good fortune to come in on the pioneer beginnings of what was to become one of the largest Health Maintenance Organizations (HMO) in the United States, with a growing group practice of medical specialists who viewed me as a peer specialist. With them I was able to build and head a clinical nutrition division, establish clinical training for dietetic interns and Public Health fieldwork, and participate in research. But mostly through these years, I learned more about myself, my love for my work and my thirst to know more, not just through two earned graduate degrees but daily on the job. All of my experiences in clinical work, teaching, and writing have taught me that with the rapid advance of scientific knowledge, the true professional never stops learning. The excitement is to be always on the "cutting edge."

My purpose here is to encourage you, whatever your working situation, to be *proactive,* ahead of the trend. Return to our title and consider the meanings of three key words:

Profession. This word comes from the Latin verb *profiteri,* which means to declare or avow publicly. A true profession is a vocation based on knowledge of a specific area of learning or science that requires advanced education and training and involves intellectual skills. Thus, as nutrition professionals, we must not only possess this high standard of knowledge and skills, but also be committed personally to the profession's ideals and values. Public professional registration and state laws of certification or license govern and protect our practice. We, through our professional organization, control our own practice and conduct. This is a wonderful profession for people who love what they do and are totally committed to it.

Imperative. This word, from the Latin verb *imperare* meaning to command, conveys two meanings: (1) authority or power and (2) urgency, absolute necessity. Thus, as professional nutrition authorities, we are compelled and entitled to maintain our high standards of practice in our own right, and to carry individual responsibility for these high standards.

Expert. Two interesting Latin roots form this key word: (1) the prefix *ex,* meaning from, and *(2) periri,* meaning peril, danger, harm, or injury. Thus, as the nutrition expert, we use our professional knowledge and skills to promote the health of our clients and patients and help protect them from harm or illness.

My second purpose here is to inspire you, if you truly desire to be proactive rather than merely reactive to someone else, to develop consistent client-centered work habits based on your professional knowledge, skills, and personal concerns for quality care.

In my own clinical experience, three basic professional actions in some form have become imperative:

♦ *Search* for all possible information and clues to help identify individual needs. Develop communication skills, especially learn to *listen,* not only for what is said but also for what is often unsaid. Try to see the situation through the client's personal and social lens. This is the person-centered base of our work.

♦ *Research* the problems presented through every available resource. Check the person's clinical chart. Communicate with other medical team members. Use any medical and university sources at hand for current scientific and practice information about the medical problem. Here in my office, for example, my computers can access the statewide University of California library system, through my personal account, to review any journal source and receive any desired printouts. Beyond that, the worldwide databases and professional forums of the Internet are available. This is the growing knowledge base of our work.

♦ *Develop a working plan* based on your initial search and research. Then constantly update the plan with client feedback, new knowledge, and ongoing medical team communications; this is the action base.

Some of my personal clinical experiences serve as illustrations of this type of nutritional practice:

Nutritional care plan. In my years of clinical work at the large HMO, our health plan physicians simply referred their patients to me with their clinical data records. It was my responsibility to establish the nutritional care plan, based on these data and my own interview and history, to monitor the person's progress, and to adjust the care plan as needed. For example, in our Northern California regional metabolic newborn screening program, as soon as initial testing and medical examination identified the genetic disease, the parents were immediately referred to me for ongoing nutritional care, since that constituted the basic treatment. Following our team protocol, I was then responsible for selecting and calculating the initial special formula, for immediately giving phone instructions to the parents in various areas of Northern California. I also was responsible for monitoring blood levels of the involved nutrient or metabolite, for recalculating formula needs according to the infant's growth rate, and for calling parents with the adjusted formula. I also made home visits and held periodic outreach nutrition clinics with our team nurse coordinator. Metabolic clinics for patients and parents at our central medical center, morning clinic visits with each family and child and afternoon case conferences involved all members of the regional metabolic disease team: pediatrician specialists in genetics and endocrinology, clinical nutritionist, nurse coordinator, and pediatric social worker.

In my private practice, I continued this special metabolic work under a personal consultant contract. Other clients have come to me by referral or on their own. In either case, I follow the same procedure, sending a copy of my findings, nutritional care plan, and periodic progress notes to the physicians involved, who often respond with additional referrals.

Charting. In the clinic, as well as when these patients were hospitalized, it was always my practice and responsibility as the clinical nutrition specialist to enter my patient care activity in the patient's chart. Nutrition charting has also come a long way. In the beginning, the usual practice in our hospital was to place nutritionist chart entries in the section of the patient chart reserved for miscellaneous nursing comments. But that changed after one dramatic high-risk patient incident. In that case, our specialist team had carefully managed the high-risk pregnancy of one of our clients with insulin-dependent diabetes mellitus (IDDM) that she developed in early childhood. She had suffered two prior stillbirths. In this pregnancy, she was hospitalized early to prepare for the obstetrician's carefully planned delivery. But one day, before term for this pregnancy, I discovered to my astonishment that the patient's blood sugar control had been dangerously compromised and mishandled. My previous nutrition charting was ignored, staff resident physicians had given wrong routine diet orders, and my specifically ordered interval foods had not only *not* been served to the patient, but had actually been eaten by night staff who thought it was just leftovers to be discarded! After exploding my outrage and anger in all directions, I immediately charted my findings, this time in the physician's notes section of her medical record, outlining and documenting in full my nutritional care plan to meet her diabetes and pregnancy needs. During her remaining hospital days, all medical and nursing staff followed my nutrition care plan notes to the letter, and our patient was able for the first time to deliver a healthy baby.

After that incident, I always placed my charting notes and instructions in the same section of the chart as that used by the attending physician, and made sure that my instructions, as the clinical nutrition specialist, were known and followed. All the nutritionists who have followed me in that position have continued that same practice.

Laboratory tests. As part of my clinical nutrition work at a large HMO health care center, I always ensured that appropriate laboratory tests were specifically written into the protocol for each nutrition-related program. In some instances I helped to write the initial protocol itself. Periodically, as part of team management, each program physician and I reviewed the protocols and added or revised appropriate tests for nutrition assessment. In private practice, this same function of ordering lab tests requires that the practitioner must be recognized as a clinical nutrition specialist by the medical community, with similar protocols written jointly by the clinical nutritionist and a physician, and filed with a nearby reputable clinical laboratory.

So what is our answer to the initial question of nutrition imperatives? Where must our profession be focused? Essentially, in our changing world we must stretch our boundaries of the past. We must continue to shed any lingering subservient attitudes and roles. We must work with physicians as nutrition specialists in our own right, viewing them as team peers, not patrons--but we must earn that right individually. It is past time that we accept full ethical, moral, and legal responsibility for our own practice as full professionals. We must collaborate with all other health professionals, physicians and nonphysicians, as team partners with common goals of patient/client care, provide expert nutritional care, and demonstrate a high level of skill and competence. Nothing less is acceptable professional behavior.

Our professional imperative flows from the inner drive and dedication of each of us. Our profession can advance in responsibility and stature and value only as far as we advance as individual nutrition experts.

Introduction

As Nutrition Therapists, we make our living because what to eat is not a simple choice for many people. Factors such as taste preferences, family and cultural habits, psychological relationships to food, disease processes, the affordability and availability of food, and a person's ability to chew, digest, and absorb food affect what he or she eats.

Today's health care marketplace and competitive environment demand that our counseling skills evolve at a fast pace. The days of the "one session miracle" should be a thing of the past, except when the client only needs basic nutrition survival skills or until the client can return for a more extensive consultation. Basic nutrition information and lists of foods to avoid are readily available to both the public and for use by other health professionals. As clinical dietitians our job is not just the dissemination of information. If that's all we do, a floppy disk, on-line service, preprinted food list, or a health educator can replace us. We must advance our clinical practice through becoming highly qualified and effective nutrition therapists in counseling. We must learn how to diagnose nutritional deficiencies and toxicities, and interpret biochemical and genetic nutrition assessments of the human body.

We must produce successful outcomes in a larger proportion of our client populations, and we must market our successes! No one else will do this for us; it is our responsibility.

Origin of this Book

When co-author, Bridget Klawitter, and I acted as content experts for The American Dietetic Association's "Counseling" self-assessment module, developed by Pennsylvania State University, we were awed by the enormity of the project. What counseling theories? What counseling skills? What body of knowledge or book would most practitioners agree is the state-of-the-art in nutrition counseling? What questions could we ask that would "stretch" but not fail the majority of practitioners? Our committee had to write four "typical" counseling scenarios with subtle counseling "mistakes" interspersed in conversations with over 400 rationales on why each answer was best or incorrect. It took two and a half years, extensive input from Penn State's staff and consultants, review by over 100 registered dietitians, and untold hours to produce the final product.

This book is an outgrowth of the above process. While we worked on the module, I telephoned across the country talking to and interviewing dietitians on what they were doing with their patients or clients. I also conducted surveys at state dietetic meetings and at other group meetings of dietitians to see how often they saw patients, on their counseling skills, and perceived barriers to success. I wanted to know what a "typical" interview entailed. Many shared their counseling resources, their strategies, and their client protocols.

I found highly successful practitioners in acute care settings as well as outpatient clinics, and of course, private practice. Most had evolved to more comprehensive skills by observing what worked in their practice or through training in advanced degrees in counseling. Some had been practicing that way for over 20 years. Many of these people are now authors of chapters, case studies, or sidebars in this book.

My questionnaire and informal surveys found that too many dietitians spent too little time actually working with clients to help them achieve the necessary benefits. For example, the majority of hospital-based practitioners usually only saw their patients once and often for less than 30 minutes. They reported they seldom referred patients to an outpatient department unless the hospital had an on-going diabetes group or in-house cardiac rehabilitation program. They also rarely referred patients to a private practice or managed care dietitian for follow-up at home.

Nutrition Therapy

Many highly qualified practitioners share their practical skills and years of knowledge in the pages of this book. We do not presume to have all of the answers, we struggle at times like everyone else but we have learned through trial and error what works most of the time with our client populations. Contributing authors give many examples of counseling strategies and business skills they learned from their own efforts, and from books, published research, and other professionals.

This book is meant to challenge readers to try new "helping" and counseling skills, as well as give role models for nutrition "therapy." What do you talk about after you review the food record and patient's weight? How often should you see a patient? How do you help a patient in denial or sliding into relapse? How can you attract patients back for revisits? When should a patient be referred for psychotherapy? How do you work with other counselors for the benefit of the client?

Since obesity is the number one malnutrition problem in the U.S., we have added many examples of the different approaches used to manage this problem. As you will see, not all of them agree in approach or philosophy, but there are many common threads. This book also includes many examples from the prevention, chronic care, and outpatient settings since we believe that the market is moving in those directions. For that reason and the fact that in outpatient settings a nutritionist usually sees far more overweight women as clients, a chapter has been included on feminist counseling.

It is hoped that as you read the pages, they will validate what you presently do, while stretching you to conquer new or traditional areas of practice with renewed excitement.

This book is intended to help readers reduce the time spent developing the necessary skills to become an effective nutrition therapist in any setting. However, each counselor must generate his or her own philosophy and style in the nutrition therapy process.

It is understood that even with the best of knowledge and skills, some work situations are not easily changed to the ideal. Our contributing authors started in similar situations, but they did what was necessary to make their counseling more conducive to "positive patient outcomes." That also will be your strongest argument as you negotiate for better counseling space, more time to conduct counseling sessions, and sufficient well-trained staff. *Positive patient outcomes* should be the motivating factor for your professional efforts in counseling.

Kathy King, RD, LD, Publisher

We want to thank all of the people, especially the contributing authors, who helped bring this project to fruition and provided input into its content and philosophies.

Section I

The People Involved

Chapter 1

The Nutrition Therapist

Kathy King, RD, LD

After reading this chapter, the reader will be able to:
 ♦ Identify the helping skills and their role in nutrition therapy.
 ♦ Define transference and list two examples in the nutrition counseling setting.
 ♦ List five ethical guidelines for the counseling of clients on nutrition.
 ♦ Identify three core conditions for building counseling relationships.
 ♦ Identify the basic themes underlying five common counseling theories.

THE EVOLUTION OF COUNSELING IN DIETETICS

Nutrition counseling skills began evolving for the profession as a whole more than twenty-five years go when people decided to take responsibility for their own health and seek nutrition care outside the acute care hospital setting. These clients had to make the effort to walk into the outpatient or private practice dietitian's office and pay for the visit themselves with little hope of being reimbursed by insurance or government funding.

The clients' high expectations for change and their willingness to return and pay for revisits quickly changed the expectations of the providers of care: the consulting dietitians. This was a new revelation. However, it soon became apparent to nutrition counselors that what they had been trained to do in counseling only took one or two visits to cover at most. Counseling skills that appeared to work in the hospital setting only scratched the surface in outpatient counseling.

To help improve their skills, these budding nutrition therapists started reading about counseling in other fields, attending conferences, joining individual and group therapy sessions for their own personal growth, and observing other counselors in action. They hired psychologists and exercise specialists to speak at their group weight loss programs. They also listened to their clients. As is often the case, these early therapists were taught how to address clients' needs and work with them personally based upon simple comments like, "You know what you said that really worked for me?" or "You are trying to push me too fast; I'm not ready for that yet."

Trial and error taught clients and therapists what worked and what didn't work for that client. Soon the therapist started seeing commonalties between certain types of problems and therapies. This body of experience helped the therapist become more effective in working with each new challenging person who walked through the door for help. The client played a very active role in the entire process. Therapists and clients found psychological needs often exerted more influence on food habits than logic. (1) It also became clear that the interaction, mutual respect, and genuine caring shared between the client and the counselor were as therapeutic as the printed diet.

Research Supports Evolution
In the 1970's the first significant body of research on the "helping" skills emerged (new strategies for counseling). (2,3,4,5,6,7) They were in response to disputed conclusions from the 1960's that traditional psychotherapy and counseling skills only produced favorable outcomes in a small percentage of clients. Researchers concluded that "helping" is simply a learning or relearning process leading to change or gain in the behavior of the client. (2)

Leaders in the helping skills concept also supported the philosophy that many professionals (police, teachers, dietitians, nurses, and so on) in the course of their normal jobs are in the position to psychologically interact with people and enter into caring relationships with them for the benefit of that

1

person. To facilitate the helping process, communication and interactive skills were identified so the process was not left to random whims that might do more harm than good. In fact, active, caring listening skills form the basis for "helping." Often just talking about a problem with another person will help someone find solutions. This new, broader philosophy of therapy supported the nutrition therapist as he or she stretched formerly accepted practice boundaries.

BALLARD STREET by Jerry Van Amerongen

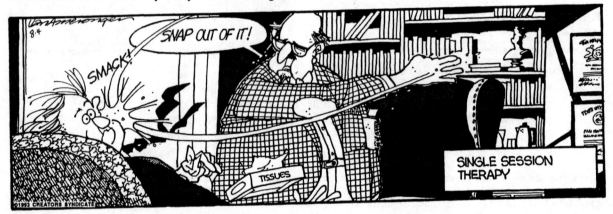

Used with permission. Jerry Van Amerongen and Creators Syndicate

In the 1980's, nutrition research and literature broadened the generally accepted scope of nutrition counseling practice, even more to include a strong emphasis on behavior modification. (8,9,10) However, after a time, it was agreed that dietitians should not only ask about someone's eating behaviors and other lifestyle habits, but they should also encourage their clients to come to new awareness about their food habits. This included food-related issues when they were growing up, their recent normal and not so normal eating habits, their inability to handle stress and interpersonal relationships without misusing food, and others. Dietitians began helping clients find coping strategies. new behaviors, and new ways of thinking. This level of counseling was practiced by many of dietetics pioneer nutrition therapists.

Advancing beyond the understanding of nutrition science to understanding human nature brings new growth and stature to dietetic practice.

In the 1990's, dietetics was in a transition, where many of these new helping and psychotherapy skills were being integrated into all counseling settings. Coupled with this, health care was changing at an alarming pace and more patient education was being transferred to outpatient clinics, private practices, Health Maintenance Organizations (HMOs), physicians' offices, long-term care settings and patients' homes. Disordered eating, a new term covering a variety of weight related eating habits, was growing in interest and concern among nutrition professionals.

> **Definition:** Disordered Eating is characterized by eating without regard to internal hunger and satiety cues or physical needs. Restrained eating, repeated dieting, diet-induced obesity, compulsive eating, bulimia nervosa and anorexia are included in this category.
>
> Karin Kratina, PhD, MPE, RD

Holding Nutrition Counselors to the Light

According to Donna Israel, PhD, RD, licensed counselor, "There is another developmental stage that our dietetic profession needs to embrace along with more education in counseling, and that is professional supervision of our skills. Just like any other counseling profession, we need to 'hold ourselves up to the light.' In other words, we must begin to feel comfortable with having other mental health professionals or nutrition therapists with more skill and practical experience than ourselves, look over our shoulders and evaluate how we work with our clients."

Not only our skills need to be evaluated, but also our "baggage": the biases, "blind spots" and underdeveloped emotional growth of our own (called *countertransference* issues). As a counselor, you have the responsibility to identify and control your countertransference issues and try to keep them out of your clients' therapy sessions. You can also help clients identify and work through their issues, so that together you can establish better rapport and facilitate collaboration. *Transference* refers to feelings and thoughts the client has toward the counselor. (11) Sometimes without realizing it, either the client or the counselor sabotages the effectiveness of the counseling efforts.

Supervision: Developing a Psychotherapeutic Style of Counseling
Karin Kratina, PhD, MPE, RD

A psychiatrist, psychologist, psychiatric social worker, licensed counselor, or a dietitian skilled in the psychotherapeutic model can act as a supervisor. It allows feedback around treatment interventions, as well as provides an opportunity to discuss limits and boundaries. This will help you understand and deal with the denial, manipulation, power struggles, transference, countertransference and other issues that may arise. In long-term work with clients, dietitians are more likely to come across negative emotions, such as anger, hostility, and reluctance. The client may also be overly compliant or defensive. Dealing with these emotions effectively has not been part of our training. Often, dietitians attempt to make their clients feel good, placate them, or at least get them to a place of neutrality. In other words, rather than dealing with these feelings, we try to change them, avoid them, or re-direct them.

Supervision can be accomplished one-on-one or in groups. One-on-one supervision allows more time to explore individual cases, or to assess personal issues. Many dietitians feel it is invaluable to experience the counselor/ client relationship first hand. To do this, locate a respected therapist and together assess your own relationship with food, weight, exercise, body image, and size acceptance. (13) Discover what techniques, approaches, and counseling styles you prefer. Keep a personal journal and learn to identify, talk about, write about and express your feelings. (14)

Group supervision is where several dietitians meet together to discuss cases, often facilitated by a skilled therapist. Another option is meeting with therapists at work. The fee a therapist or dietitian will charge for supervision is usually similar to the fee charged for other clients.

Examples of issues that you can explore include:
What kind of clients will you take and how many?
How do you decide if a client is too difficult or complex to work with?
What kind of contracts, if any, do you set with your clients?
What are the consequences for broken contracts? How do you enforce them?
How do you identify the limits of your competency?
What is appropriate limit setting? What is intrusive limit setting?
How aware are you of your own comfort level with personal limits and boundaries?
How much of yourself do you share in session?
What are your personal limits regarding physical contact, extra sessions, contact with client's
  family members, fees, and grounds for termination, etc.?

NUTRITION THERAPY
Experience has shown us that handing out lists of foods and meticulously calculated diets will not guarantee compliance nor motivate clients to change their behaviors. It is not that simple. At best it will produce "first order change," removal of the symptoms. (15) People are intertwined with their food and eating habits. Human nature, a person's will, and mental health can play major roles in the change process. The goal is to produce "second order change," which means to address and change the causes of the problem. (15)

Clients are often "stuck" in ways of thinking and acting around food. A counselor can help them "explore" new ways of thinking, try new actions, respond to stimuli differently, choose foods based on new criteria, handle stress without turning to food, and take more responsibility for their lifestyle choices.

Curry states, "Nutrition counseling involves a process, a sequence of events, and the interpersonal relationship between the counselor and client. The most important aspect of counseling is the interpersonal relationship. It is also the most difficult to understand and master." (1)

The traditional medical model is fast, short-term intervention primarily of a content-oriented educational nature with minimal relationship development or input by the client, little or no follow-up, and a standardized plan of action. *We know what's best for them and it's their problem or lack of motivation if they don't follow it! This approach works when the client makes the effort to read, learn and apply the content.* Dietitians can't take much of the credit except for teaching the content. Advanced counseling skills and the psychodynamic model of therapy empower the dietitian to become an active facilitator in the therapy process enabling a larger percentage of clients to successfully make and sustain lifestyle choices that will improve their health, and possibly, longevity and quality of life.

Table 1.1 Comparison of Nutrition Education and Psychotherapeutic Counseling

Nutrition Education	Psychotherapeutic Counseling
1. Short-term	Open-ended
2. Content-based	Process (continuous series of interdependent events)
3. Goal-oriented	Relationship-oriented
4. Improve knowledge & skills	Resolution of issues & barriers that inhibit a person from making healthy choices
5. Work on behaviors	Work on thoughts, feelings, behaviors
6. Address cognitive deficits	Addresses motivation, denial, resistance
7. Success measured objectively (e.g. knowledge, behavior change, or health parameters)	Success measured subjectively (e.g., happiness, mood shift, movement, relationships)

Adapted from (c) 1993, Johanna H. Roth, RD, LD, CHES, CAS, Bethesda, MD. Used with permission. (16,17)

Advanced counseling skills include:

- **Relationship building skills: empathy, warmth and genuineness**
- **Helping skills: attending, helping a client explore, active listening responses**
- **Ability to gain collaboration and empower the client**
- **Sensitivity to multicultural and other client-specific uniqueness**
- **Ability to sustain a long-term counseling relationship**
- **Ability to assess and teach developmental skills**

All of these skills can be taught to counselors. However, a therapist's own personality and ability to work with clients determines his or her effectiveness as a counselor more than years of dietetic experience.

The client has the right and responsibility to make choices about his or her own health care. The nutrition therapist's role is to *facilitate* the process by which patients or clients more clearly identify where they are, where they want to be, what they need to learn to get there. You help identify the pros and cons of the various options, and step-by-step guidance on how to get to where they want to be.

To accomplish the "facilitator" role, the therapist must become a *trainer* (one who facilitates growth and change in the patient or client through guidance and practice) instead of a teacher who only discusses content (diet lists, exchange system, etc.) and checks understanding of the content. See how to become a National Certified Counselor and Licensed Psychotherapist in Appendix 1-A.

Ethics and Responsibility
The core of ethical responsibility is to *do nothing that will harm the client, allow the clients to make their own decisions based on good information, be fair and just, and keep your work with them confidential.* (6) As the counselor, you carry the responsibility to be professional, knowledgeable, and skilled. The client is more vulnerable and is coming to you for help and assistance. Go to The American Dietetic Association's web site (www.eatright.org) to read its Code of Ethics. Following are the most important ethical guidelines: (6,8,11)

1. ***Maintain confidentiality.*** The client trusts that what he or she tells you will be held in confidence. You have the responsibility to not disclose information shared by the client or about the client's therapy without the client's permission. If you are a student, you do not have legal confidentiality, and your clients should be made aware of this. (6) See Appendix 1-B for a sample confidentiality statement.

2. ***Recognize your limitations.*** It is important that you talk to your clients about the process you want to use to help them improve their nutritional intake and give them the option of stopping at any time. Know your limitations, as described in this book, in the areas of counseling and exercise recommendations. Nutrition therapy deals with what a person eats or doesn't eat, weight and body image issues, the availability of adequate wholesome, safe food and the behaviors, thoughts, and feelings that affect a client's decisions in these areas. With training it can include other health related lifestyle choices, such as adding physical activity, stress management, and smoking cessation. It is about helping others, not examining and delving into their lives. (6)

3. ***Seek consultation.*** Counseling is very private. Hold yourself to the light in order to grow personally and improve your skills. Review ethical standards frequently.

4. ***Treat the client, as you would like to be treated.*** Every person deserves to be treated with respect, dignity, kindness, and honesty. (6) *Informed consent* means the patient voluntarily gives permission to have therapy after a thorough explanation has been given of the proposed therapy. Some practitioners have patients or clients sign an Informed Consent form (see sample in Appendix 1-C).

5. ***Be aware of individual differences.*** One diet does not fit all just because the diagnosis is the same!

6. **Be aware, respectful, and sensitive to cultural and ethnic differences.**

The Goals of Counseling

Many sources identify what they believe are the goals of nutrition counseling or therapy. These goals help the client or patient to: (17,18)

- Increase self-awareness and decrease denial that nutritional problems exist, and that these problems can be resolved.
- Become aware of inner strengths so the person can function independently and challenge old beliefs about how to eat or change weight.
- Increase feeling responsible for his or her feelings, thoughts, behaviors, and relationships instead of staying in the "victim" role.
- Learn to take risks like being more flexible and more tolerant of incongruities.
- Trust more and give new behaviors and thoughts a chance before discounting them.
- Become more conscious of alternative choices when responding to stress and other stimuli, or choosing foods based on new criteria.
- "Have a functional lifestyle where his values (what he believes to be true) and his behaviors (what he does) are consistent; there is a good level of self-acceptance. He is doing what he believes he should be doing, and feels good about it," states Beckley. (18)

Table 1.2   Functional vs. Dysfunctional Lifestyles (18)

Functional:	(Self-acceptance)
	Values are consistent with behaviors
	Values are semi-flexible
	Behaviors are moderate
Dysfunctional:	(Denial, low self-esteem, depression, anger)
	Values conflict with behaviors
	Values are rigid
	Behaviors are extreme

Used with permission. Copyright, Lisa Beckley, RD and Nutrition Dimensions,
in *Diet, Addiction and Recovery* (4th ed.) 2002. (18)

Core Conditions and Skills for Building Relationships

In the context of therapy, client growth is associated with high levels of three core, or facilitative, relationship conditions: empathy (accurate understanding), respect or warmth (positive regard), and genuineness (congruence). (6,19,20) When these conditions exist in a counseling relationship, positive change often takes place irrespective of the philosophical orientation of the counselor. Successful clients in behavior therapy and psychotherapy rate their personal interaction with the therapist as the single most important part of treatment. (6) If these conditions are absent, clients may not only fail to grow, they may deteriorate. (2,21) In recent years, researchers like Carkhuff, Egan, Gazda, and Ivey have developed concrete, teachable skills that have made it possible for people to learn how to communicate these core conditions to clients. (2,4,5,21,22)

Empathy means the counselor truly tries to understand what the patient feels from his/her frame of reference, and responds accurately to that person's concerns and problems. For example, if a client says, "I have really tried to eat differently, but by the time I get home I'm too starved and I overeat," an empathetic response would be something like "You feel if you cut calories earlier in the day, you don't have control that evening." In contrast, if you say something like "You ought to try harder," you are responding from your frame of reference, not the client's.

Empathy serves the following purposes: it builds rapport, elicits information by showing understanding, and fosters client self-exploration through conveying that the environment is safe and confidential. You can convey empathy to clients through certain verbal and nonverbal messages.

Verbally, you can show a desire to comprehend by asking for clarification about the client's experiences and feelings. You can discuss what is important to the client and respond with statements that show you understand the client's concerns. Refer to the client's feelings or add to implicit client messages. (6,18) For example, you might say, "Food seems to mean love and anger to you. Love because it reminds you of the special foods your grandmother baked for you, and anger because at times when you binge, you are angry at the food and your attraction to it. Is that right?"

Attentive nonverbal behavior also conveys empathy. Such things as direct eye contact (but not staring), a forward-leaning body position (at times), facing the client, and an open-arm position all show interest in the other person. (6,8,19) See Table 1.3 on nonverbal cues of warmth and coldness.

Table 1.3 Nonverbal Cues of Warmth and Coldness (U.S. Anglo)

Nonverbal cue	Warmth	Coldness
Tone of voice	Soft, soothing	Callous, reserved, abrupt
Facial expression	Smiling, interested	Poker-faced, frowning
Posture	Relaxed, leaning toward the other person	Tense, lean away
Eye contact	Looking into the other person's eyes (intermittently)	Avoiding eye contact
Touching	Touching the other softly and discreetly	Avoiding all touching
Gestures	Open, welcoming	Closed, guarded
Physical proximity	Close (arm's length)	Distant

Adapted from *Reaching Out: Interpersonal Effectiveness and Self-Actualization* (3rd ed.), by D.W. Johnson. Copyright 1986 by Printice-Hall. Reprinted with permission.

Genuineness means being yourself without being phony or playing a role. The counselor is honest and straightforward with the client. You act human and collaborate with the client, which reduces the emotional distance between you and the client. There are at least five components of genuineness: (6,19)

- **Nonverbal behaviors** (mentioned in Table 1.3);
- **Honest interest in helping people** (not just a role to play for the moment);
- **Congruence** (your words, actions, and feelings match and are consistent); for example, if you become uncomfortable about something that is being said or how the client handles a situation in a violent manner, you tactfully address it instead of feigning comfort;

- **Spontaneity** (the capacity to express yourself naturally without deliberating about everything);
- **Openness and self-disclosure** (the ability to be open, to share yourself, and to disclose certain information about yourself when it is appropriate).

Self-disclosure is any information you share about yourself with the client. The information may be general in nature like the fact that you also have children or what college you went to, or it can be personal in nature and either positive or negative. For example, a positive self-disclosure is, "I used to eat whether I was hungry or not. Now I eat according to my appetite, and you can too." Negative self-disclosure provides information about personal limitations, unsuccessful or inappropriate behaviors and situations, and experiences dissimilar to the client's. (6) For example, "I also have a hard time telling people 'no' and taking time for myself."

Self-disclosure can increase the client's level of disclosure, close the distance between you and the client, and bring about changes in the client's perception of his/her behavior. On the negative side, too much talk about you can take too much time away from working with the client's needs, it may appear you lack discretion, or need therapy as much as the client. (6)

The best rule of thumb until you have more experience in this area is to make your self-disclosure brief, and at the same depth as the information shared with you by your client. (6,19) Clients who are white professionals in America usually are very open about sharing intimate facts, but other cultures take more time to get to know someone. Self-disclosure too early in the counseling relationship can be a problem.

Respect or warmth or positive regard means the ability to prize or value the client as a person with worth and dignity. (23) The four components of positive regard are: (6)

- **Openness and self-disclosure** (This is the ability to be open, to share yourself, and to disclose certain information about yourself when it is appropriate.)
- **Commitment** (You are interested in working with the client and show up on time, reserve private quiet time for the appointment.)
- **Understanding** (You act interested by using techniques mentioned earlier, and by using specific listening responses such as paraphrasing and reflecting client messages.)
- **Nonjudgmental attitude** (You suspend judgment of the client's motives and actions to avoid condemning or condoning the client's thoughts, feelings, or actions. **You are able to remain objective and not become involved in the client's personal affairs.** If a female client discloses that she hates her husband when he makes derogatory comments about her weight, you might answer something like "You feel hurt when your husband isn't sensitive about your weight.")
- **Warmth** (Most clients, even hostile ones, usually respond with warmth if you offer it first.) Without verbal and nonverbal warmth many helping strategies are therapeutically impotent. (24)

As a poor example of nutrition care, a friend was in a hospital several years ago and was throwing up in the sink when the dietitian walked in to give a low-fat diet instruction. Upon seeing the ill woman, the dietitian proceeded to introduce herself, discuss the purpose of the diet, and briefly explain the sample menu and lists of foods to avoid. The patient asked the dietitian to return at another time since she would be in the hospital another day or two, but the dietitian said this was her best time. The consult resulted in an $80 charge for the 10-15 minutes, and an angry instead of impressed patient. This was not good nutrition therapy; there was no empathy, no rapport, no positive interaction, no concern for where the patient was coming from, and no assessment to adapt the information to the patient's lifestyle. Ethically, the charge was questionable.

COUNSELING THEORIES
It is estimated there are over 40 different therapy models or theories with seven or so being the most commonly used: (6,8,19)

- **Psychodynamic theory** is primarily associated with its founder, Sigmund Freud. This long-term therapy works by getting to the unconscious roots of present behavior. Today, derivatives of this theory such as attachment theory (how securely an infant or child was attached to his or her mother), object relations theory (our relationships with key people in our lives), and ego psychology (helping people balance between their id (unconscious rebellion) and their superego (conscious rules that give the person more power to control his or her own life), have the most immediate impact on practice. Free association of words or ideas (say whatever comes to mind), regression (clients return to past traumatic experiences) and dream analysis are commonly used strategies. (25) A major drawback to this type of therapy is that the client is not typically oriented to transfer learning from the therapy into daily life and present day problems. That may happen as a result of therapy, but it often takes extended periods of time to make breakthroughs.

- **Existential-humanistic** is best known through Carl Rogers' and Viktor Frankl's work (also includes Gestalt). Frankl holds that the critical issue for humankind is not what happens, but how one views or thinks about what happens (cognitive change), but he also believes in taking action. From his concentration camp experience during World War II, he learned to help people who are faced with problems that cannot be solved, like rape or AIDS, and to find love and meaning in their lives.

  Rogers is the listening or attending therapist. He is the founder of **person-centered therapy** that focuses on each person's worth and dignity, and accepts that the person's perceptions are reality. The emphasis is on the ability to direct one's own life and move toward self-actualization, growth and health. (26, 27)

  Gestalt was developed by Frederick (Fritz) Perls. Counselors want to operate in the "here and now" instead of retelling stories from the past. The client may be asked to close his or her eyes and describe a typical incident that needs work. The client may retell a recent conversation and then be asked to create a more suitable ending to the problem. The client may be asked to rehearse messages to an empty chair so that it will be easier to say them to others. The goal is for clients to take responsibility for change. (28)

- **Cognitive-behavioral** (includes rational-emotive and psychoeducational therapy) is the evolution of cognitive (what a person thinks) along with behavioral (what a person does) therapy that made therapy "brief" in comparison to the long-term commitment of psychoanalysis. Once problem behaviors or irrational beliefs are identified, strategies for change can be made more quickly. It helps clients define their problems and promote cognitive, emotional and behavioral changes, and prevent relapse. (See Chapter 9.)

  Psychoeducational therapy "implies a process of learning about oneself (one's physical and mental impulses, instincts, and/or patterns of behavior), gaining new knowledge (i.e., the number of grams of fat in a teaspoon of butter), and learning to regulate one's behavior in accordance with some standard" (definition by Murray, EdD, RD see Chapter 9 for more detail). Guerney, Stollak, and Guerney (29) developed this technique as a method, not focused on "curing," but rather, on "managing" physical and mental impulses appropriately. Nutrition therapists help clients integrate individualized nutrition knowledge through cognitive and behavioral change.

  Rational-Emotive Therapy (RET), developed by Albert Ellis, believes irrational ideas and negative self-talk can cause emotion-related difficulties. Emotion must be present along with logic and rational thought in order for change to likely occur. In other words, you may know that your serum cholesterol is too high but unless you feel emotion (fear, anxiety, etc.), change may never occur.(30)

- **Multicultural therapy (MCT)** recognizes that traditional theories of helping, developed in a predominantly white male Northern European and North American context, have gender and cultural limitations when working with clients from other cultures, and women and minorities in the US, and they give little consideration to family issues. MCT draws upon the above therapies but tries to respect multiple perspectives and give culturally appropriate treatment.(19)

  Feminist Therapy is eclectic, endorsing theoretical positions, which encourage empowerment and self-growth, but also recognizing woman's more interdependent way of living and relating.

- **Family counseling** recognizes that the family of origin is where the client's culture manifests most clearly. For clients with problems related to their relationship or function in the family, working within the family context helps clients have fewer relapses and quicker improvement than when treated individually. (19) This type of therapy has proven to be the only consistently successful mode of therapy in adolescent obesity.

Today, psychoeducational, family counseling, and multi-cultural counseling are growing in popularity as more therapists become aware of and trained in these methods. Empowerment and self-growth are being integrated in many other therapy styles. We come from different perspectives and biases. To be successful as a counselor, we must learn to be flexible, tolerant, and accepting of others' points of view. To illustrate how we see things differently, look at the picture below and answer: Do you see a young woman or an old woman? Ask other people and recognize that others may not see what you see so clearly.

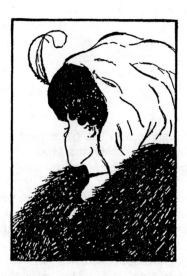

Figure 1.1 Dual Figure Source: Originally drawn by W.E. Hill and published in *Puck*, Nov. 6, 1905. First used for psychological purposes by E. G. Boring, "A New Ambiguous Figure," *American Journal of Psychology*, 1930.

NUTRITION COUNSELING APPROACHES

As you can see by the overlap in theories, and from your experience with clients and their problems, no one therapy or model holds all the answers for each client. The counselor's personal and professional judgment is crucial to the outcome of the therapy. (1) For more consistent success in counseling, Gilliland (31) suggests a flexible, client-centered problem-solving approach that merges the best ideas from the most popular models. The assumptions of this eclectic approach to counseling include: (31)

- No two clients or client situations are alike.
- Each client and counselor is in a constant state of change and flux—no person or situation in counseling is or can ever be static.
- The effective counselor exhibits a flexible repertoire of activity on a continuum from directive (telling the client what to do) to nondirective.
- The client is the world's greatest expert on his or her own problems.
- The counselor uses all the available personal and professional resources in the helping situation, but is fully human in the relationship and cannot ultimately be responsible for the client.
- Counselors and the counseling process are fallible and cannot expect to observe overt or immediate success in every counseling or client situation.
- Competent counselors are aware of their own personal professional qualifications and deficits and take responsibility for ensuring that the counseling process is handled ethically and in the best interest of the client and public.

- Client safety takes precedence over need fulfillment of the counselor.
- Probably there is no one best approach or strategy in dealing with each problem.
- Many problems in the human dilemma appear insolvable, but there are always a variety of alternatives, and some alternatives are better for the client than others.
- Generally, effective counseling is a process that is done *with* the client rather than *to* or *for* the client.
- For most people requiring changes that are basic to their lifestyle, three months is probably a minimum and six months should not be considered too long a time for counseling. Weight control can often take years to accomplish, and it is time that the need for long-term attention to this problem is recognized. (1)
- When the client and therapist believe it is time to stop therapy, the client should identify his or her "red flags" that will signal a need to return to therapy, and the door should be left open for future informal contact by either party.

It is most valuable when a client is able to take new insights or information out of a session and apply it in daily life. A criticism of the psychodynamic approach is its constant emphasis on insight, which produces a client who is diligently searching the past while still having problems in the present. (19) When you first assess a client, note how the client is treating you during the interview. The ways clients treat you provide clues to: 1) their developmental history in their family, 2) the nature of their current interpersonal relationships, and 3) function in their work environment. (19)

The Helping Model
One of the first and best-known researchers in the helping-type therapy movement was Robert R. Carkhuff. Many have adopted his model to explain the process. There are four phases in Carkhuff's Helping Model that identify the interpersonal stages of a counseling relationship: (32)

Pre-Helping Attending: The counselor "attends" to the needs of the client or patient by giving undivided attention, listening, observing, and physically showing interest through positive body language. This helps the client become interested and involved in the process.

Responding: The client's apparent interest triggers the counselor to respond with empathy, respect, and sometimes concreteness (the opposite of vagueness) in focusing the client's attention on experiences. As the client becomes comfortable, the counselor can help him or her *explore* experiences and develop insight. Exploring is a pre-condition of understanding, giving both counselor and client an opportunity to get to know where the client is in the world. Exploration is a self-diagnostic process for the client. Exploration is an art under the control of the counselor and in part under the control of the client. *High-level functioning clients explore themselves independent of the level of interpersonal skills offered by the counselor while moderate to low-level functioning clients are dependent upon the counselor's skills for their level of exploration.*

Personalizing: These skills involve filtering the client's experiences through the counselor's experiences, which serves to facilitate client understanding. Clients go from *exploring* where they are in relation to their experience to *understanding* where they are in relation to where they want or need to be. The basic foundation for understanding rests with insights, which reveal the client's own deficits and role in the situation. This may increase the probability that related behaviors will occur. Unfortunately, action does not always follow insight.

Initiating: This phase involves developing a course of action to resolve the client's problems. It emphasizes the action-oriented counseling dimensions of honest assessments, self-disclosure (the counselor sharing personal revelations), specific problem solving and program development, and under some conditions, confrontation of discrepancies in client's behaviors.

It must be said here that not all client or patient situations call for extensive interaction and problem solving, especially when the person is motivated and is already somewhat knowledgeable about the content. When the person is not ready or willing to hear the content or to become more involved, that is his or her right, and does not reflect poorly on the therapist if concerted effort is made to give the person or the family as much information and support as desired.

Using Psychology
Nutrition therapy should contribute to a client's good mental health, not sacrifice it. Psychiatrist, Scott Peck, author of *The Road Less Traveled,* writes, "Mental health is an ongoing process of dedication to reality at all costs. *Giving up is the most painful of human experiences...* giving up personality traits, well-established patterns of behavior, ideologies, and even whole lifestyles."(33) Think how often in the past we nutritionists asked clients to change *all* of those factors at once!

Peck goes on to explain that it is easier to work with patients who have neurotic tendencies (they take too much responsibility for what happens) than patients with character disorders (they take no responsibility for what happens and blame it on someone or something else). (33) That is one explanation why some clients are so much more difficult to work with than others.

In their article on "Incorporating Psychological Principles into Nutrition Counseling," Stuart and Simko clearly outline how psychology can be used in nutrition counseling: (34)

It is very important to encourage self-help and self-responsibility, thereby putting the client or patient in control. Having a sense of control is an essential component of self-esteem. Clients will exhibit less self-destructive behavior and think about themselves as responsible and able to care for themselves (and follow dietary guidelines better).

The nutrition counselor briefly helps the client define problems, accepts the client's feelings, gives permission for normal responses, expects the client to handle the problems, and suggests specific follow-up assignments and tasks. By giving permission and information that normalizes the client's reactions, providing specific suggestions, and making a contract to continue to work on the problem, the counselor is creating highly therapeutic conditions. Providing supportive psychotherapy in this manner can only benefit a client.

BOUNDARIES BETWEEN NUTRITION TREATMENT AND PSYCHOTHERAPY

Saloff-Coste, Hamburg and Herzog give examples of practice boundaries in their article, "Nutrition and Psychotherapy: Collaborative treatment of patients with eating disorders." (35)

In general, the dietitian's territory properly includes almost any issue related to food, weight, eating patterns, and body image. So, for example, if a patient with anorexia nervosa who has achieved a safe, stable weight laments that she will never be happy because she is not tall and beautiful like her sister, it is well within the nutritionist's domain to challenge the patient's underlying notion that happiness depends on physical appearance. The nutritionist may also remind the patient that she possesses other qualities that impart value to her life.

It may also be appropriate for the dietitian to challenge a patient's view of herself and the world when it specifically perpetuates inappropriate eating patterns. In this instance, the nutritionist's non-nutrition interventions serve to provide necessary room for discussions concerning improved eating behavior.

When to Make Referrals to Other Mental Health Professionals
Referral to other mental health professionals is indicated when the patient or client discloses information such as suicidal tendencies, physical abuse, severe marital difficulties, feelings of depression, past unresolved sexual abuse, recurring self-destructive behaviors, eating disorders, and other severe problems that are beyond the scope of nutrition practice.

The patient or client may or may not choose to see a mental health professional or abuse counselor. If they go to see another therapist, you may continue to see them concurrently or you may wait until the other issues are resolved. If they choose *not* to seek other help, your options are to continue seeing the person for his or her nutrition-related problems that you can work with (in hopes that you will be able to influence the person to seek help at some future date), or to explain that you must terminate your nutrition therapy until the larger issues are handled (and risk alienating the patient). If the situation is very severe and urgent (like for threatened suicide), you may have to be more forceful and seek help for patients or clients *with their permission* as they sit in your office. Either call their physician or therapist or refer the unstable patient to an emergency psychiatric service. (35)

Establishing a Relationship with a Therapist or Treatment Team

Karin Kratina, PHD, MPE, RD (12)

Continuing collaboration with therapists or becoming part of a treatment team will increase your effectiveness with clients. Legal and ethical standards require a signed release from your patient in order to communicate with others about his or her case in a private practice setting.

To begin collaboration, make contact with the patient's therapist to schedule an appointment in person or on the telephone. Discuss philosophy of treatment, length of expected therapy, expectations of treatment, and assessment tools used such as body fat analysis and computer diet analysis. Determine the therapist's expectations of nutrition counseling: A one time visit and meal plan? On-going nutrition counseling? Exploration of feelings behind the food and weight related behavior by the dietitian? (13)

Establish boundaries with the therapist. Determine mutual responsibilities of treatment. Who will weigh the client? What happens when the client asks the therapist a nutrition-related question? When working as a treatment team there is potential for "splitting," a situation in which the client pits one member of the team against another. Effective communication helps avert this. If a client tells you that she doesn't like the therapist or is not listening well, encourage the client to bring up her feelings at the next visit with her therapist. Don't take sides. Listen but let the client take action. **Let a problem between the therapist and client remain a problem between just the two of them.** It is ethical, however, to encourage the client to seek help from another therapist if he or she is unhappy.

While you are seeing a client who also sees a therapist on issues that may relate to nutrition, maintain contact with the therapist, in person or by phone, with brief progress notes, or by leaving a message on the therapist's voice mail (make sure it is a confidential line). If you are seeing several of a therapist's clients, you may want to set up a standing lunch meeting. (13)

THE COUNSELOR OR THERAPIST

The terms counselor or therapist are used interchangeably in this book just as they are by other members of the counseling profession. The term therapist is also consistent with other allied health professionals, such as physical therapist and occupational therapist.

The nutrition counselor or therapist takes on a large responsibility when he or she decides to help other people with their problems and needs. The managerial skills that make a dietitian good at running and managing a food service are not usually the skills that make a dietitian good at counseling patients. Collaboration and patience are necessary to be a counselor. Also, some people like working with other people and their problems while others find it depressing and tedious. Not every dietitian that likes nutrition education will be good at or interested in counseling. Our profession and institutions need to do a better job of identifying and training dietitians who show interest and skill in counseling.

Whether we intend it or not, patients and clients look to nutrition therapists as role models. It is therefore important that the nutrition counselor be mature and emotionally stable, and obviously, eat healthy. Each therapist should look at his or her own abilities to appropriately cope with stress, to successfully handle interpersonal relationships, and to relate with others. Many counselors have found invaluable assistance with personal problems, which may impact their ability to counsel others, by seeking help from a psychiatric social worker, psychologist, or psychiatrist.

It is imperative that each counselor be familiar with his or her patient populations, their common needs and nutrition-related problems, their usual food supplies, and customs. It is the counselor's responsibility to adapt educational materials and nutrition counseling to the patient, not the patient's responsibility to interpret what the counselor probably meant.

A good counselor uses power appropriately and does not dominate patients or clients, is able to give and receive love, is willing to admit mistakes, uses humor, and is not afraid to seek counsel and supervision from other qualified professionals. The next time you go to a lecture on a topic of interest to you, think about how many details you remember the next day, or the next week. Compare that to how much more you retain from a session where you freely interact, summarize the key points, and identify what you will work on for the next visit. That is what a good counseling session can do for a client.

HERMAN by Jim Unger

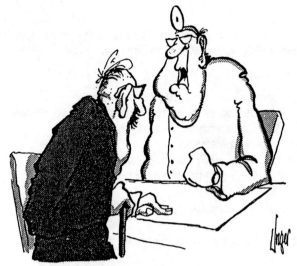

"I'm well aware you're only 28 years old. That's
why I'm telling you to take better care
of yourself."

Reiff and Reiff summarized what qualities people with eating disorders want in a nutrition therapist; the list is adapted for nutrition problems in general: (11)

- Patient, caring, and nonjudgmental
- Flexible, not a perfectionist
- Sensitive comments
- Realistic expectations
- A pace the client can handle
- Experienced with the problems the clients face
- Understands fears about food and weight
- Optimistic and hopeful
- Works in a collaborative manner

Learning New Counseling Skills

Danish suggests from his experience with teaching dietitians new counseling skills that the best way to learn skills is in a situation like a two-day seminar or a course where skills can be taught, modeled, practiced, evaluated, and refined. Afterward, the practitioners must use them upon returning to work and incorporate them into daily counseling sessions. He gives four steps that must occur to learn a new counseling skill: (36)

1. Name and describe the skill
2. Understand the rationale for the skill
3. Demonstrate the skill—what it should be and what it should not be
4. Practice extensively under supervision

To further improve your counseling style, read books on assertiveness, boundaries, and getting in touch with feelings. Take a psychology class that is beyond the basics to learn about personality disorders, cognitive-behavioral interventions, family systems theory, and different counseling styles. Attend conferences like those on disordered eating that usually explore counseling and psychological issues. (13)

The need for nutrition counseling skills in dietetic practice is being widely recognized. Two different groups have formed in The American Dietetic Association to promote and support practitioners with the desire for increased expertise in counseling. They are the Nutrition Therapists subgroup of the Nutrition Entrepreneurs (NE) Dietetic Practice Group and the Disordered Eating Networking Group within the Sports and Cardiovascular Nutritionists (SCAN) Practice Group. Their purposes are to lead, support, and train practitioners to be high-level therapists. You can find out more information or join the DPG groups by calling ADA at 1-800-877-1600 or going to www.eatright.org.

Five Significant Barriers to Becoming an Effective Counselor
Dietitians have identified their biggest barriers to becoming effective counselors in questionnaires passed out at dietetic meetings. (37) Those barriers have included:

- Patients don't keep initial appointments
- Patients don't return for follow-up appointments
- Physicians convey to patients that the "diet probably won't help"
- Patients not motivated
- Patients do not receive insurance reimbursement

Each one of these barriers will be discussed in detail in the pages of this book through case studies and chapters.

Although these barriers seem universal to counseling, many therapists' counseling strategies and business skills are so effective *they do not have these problems.* For example, Philomena Koulbanis, RD, was in private practice in Mystic, CT for seven years before she retired, and in those years, she reports only having four "no-shows" for appointments. In a busy clinic it's not unusual to have that many people who do not show for appointments before noon some days.

Appendix 1-D "Outpatient Counseling Peer Review Criteria" was developed by Bridget Klawitter to help dietetic students and members of her staff improve their counseling skills. See Appendix 1-E "Becoming a Certified Lactation Consultant."

Just Starting to Counsel?
Kim Reiff, psychologist, gives very good suggestions on what to do if you are just starting to counsel: (16)

- understand that it's normal to have anxiety—confidence builds with experience;
- no one expects you to be perfect;
- set limits on your time and accessibility, and maintain a good quality of life for yourself;
- one therapist may not cultivate a patient's whole healing process—the person may need to see several different therapists;
- it is a mistake to think that advice (telling the person what to do) is counseling;
- results may come slowly—don't get frustrated;
- accept that you won't succeed with every patient; and
- it is painful for every therapist when patients don't return.

CONCLUSION

For the dietetic profession and for practitioners looking for new career avenues, nutrition counseling or therapy is potentially an enormous area of growth. With the current emphasis on prevention, functional medicine, obesity, genetic testing for disease markers, and nutritional assessment of the whole human body, nutrition counseling will only grow in importance to the health care system and to the public.

With organized, supervised training and experience, we can elevate the clinical counseling practice of dietetics and bring more practitioners to the therapist level. It is not too soon for practitioners to think about supporting the move to create a certification as a Nutrition Therapist.

Following is an article about how students learn counseling skills best. (38)

How Students Learn Counseling Skills Best

Connie Vickery, PhD, RD, and Nancy Cotugna, PhD, RD, Department of Nutrition and Dietetics, University of Delaware
Adapted from *Nutrition Therapy, 1st edition*

Classroom Practice Versus Modeling Practitioners

Nutrition counseling is an integral part of a clinical dietitian's responsibility. The techniques of interviewing and counseling are both knowledge and performance requirements of dietetic education programs. (1) The typical training for dietetic counseling skills includes "modeling" where students observe practitioners in action and imitate their behaviors. *This is an acceptable method of training if the student is observing a role model with adequate counseling skills.* However, observations of practicing dietitians counseling surrogate patients (2,3) and of those in actual clinical practice (4,5) have underscored the poor instructional quality used by many of these health professionals.

Counseling skill techniques have improved dramatically in the last years. However, research has suggested that practicing dietitians need supplemental training to learn the new skills and improve the quality of their patient education. (5) Many dietitians do not routinely use the techniques known to help patients learn and use information better. With this in mind, we designed a project to evaluate the effectiveness of a counseling course versus role modeling with practicing dietitians. We compared the counseling skills of students who had only classroom lecture and simulation experiences with those in a coordinated program who had little classroom training but actual practice of skills learned primarily through modeling practitioners in healthcare settings.

Results

Results showed that students who completed the nutrition counseling course that included technique modeling and skills identification presented via videotapes or live demonstration by a skilled instructor, practice and evaluation, performed significantly better than coordinated students in all counseling skills evaluated. This included areas of establishing relationships with clients, needs assessment, communication techniques, and behavior change strategies.

Students in both groups demonstrated respect for their clients, which is in agreement with research noting that dietitians do have effective interpersonal skills. (4,5) However, our study detected significant differences in the use of behavior change strategies between the groups. Students who had taken the course demonstrated effective use of contracting, cue elimination, reflective listening, relanguaging, and visualization. The students who modeled their behavior on practitioner observations were more likely to develop instructional plans with little input from their clients. Students who completed the course were more likely to encourage client participation and assess commitment to change, while coordinated students typically queried, "Do you think you will be able to do this?" or "Do you have any questions?" failing to recognize or acknowledge signs of doubt or concern expressed by the client.

Components of an Effective Course

We agree with others who recommend that a course in nutrition counseling is a necessary addition to dietetics curriculum and should be recommended for practicing dietitians along with supervision. (6,7) Many universities are starting to offer courses on helping skills and effective patient education. In our nutrition counseling course, (8) we found it most effective to combine lecture and discussion with modeling, role-playing, and evaluation. As part of the introduction to basic components of a nutrition assessment, the instructor models the skill of conducting a dietary history as the counselor with a willing student serving as the client. Roles are then reversed. As students become comfortable, they are invited to assume these roles with the remainder of the class evaluating their performance by reinforcing positive attributes and identifying negative practices.

Videotapes of counseling sessions are useful in helping the class analyze the needs of the client and identify potential obstacles to making necessary lifestyle changes. In class scenarios, the "counselor" must interview the "client" using appropriate strategies. Then the "counselor" identifies whether the problem is related to a knowledge or skill deficit, lack of social support, competing activities, treatment costs, or stress.

Communication techniques are demonstrated throughout the course. Such behavioral strategies as relanguaging, reflective listening, reinforcement, and self-esteem building are practiced.

Students learn to conduct a cost-benefit ratio and to develop a contract. Negotiation strategies, also an essential component of the nutrition counseling course, are illustrated using videotaped counseling sessions with appropriate and inappropriate scenarios. Throughout the course we stress there is not one correct way to counsel per se. Repeated videotaping allows students to see themselves as others see them and to become comfortable with evaluation. Near the end of the course, each student is videotaped conducting a session from start to finish. *The student's grade is based on a self-evaluation of the counseling scenario rather than on the actual performance.*

REFERENCES (for this discussion)
1. *Accreditation/Approval Manual for Dietetic Education Programs.* 2nd ed. Chicago, IL: The American Dietetic Association; 1991.
2. Danish SJ, Ginsberg MR, Terrell A, Hammond MI, Adams S. The anatomy of a dietetic counseling interview. *J Am Diet Assoc.* 1979; 75: 626-630.
3. Snetselaar LG, Schrott HG, Albanese M, IasielloVailas L, Smith K, Anthony SL. Model workshop on nutrition counseling for dietitians. *J Am Diet Assoc.* 1981; 79: 678-682.
4. Roach RR, Pichert JW, Stetson BA, Lorenz RA, Boswell EJ, Schlundt DG. Improving dietitians' teaching skills. *J Am Diet Assoc.* 1992; 92:1466-1473.
5. Stetson BA, Pichert JW, Roach RR, Lorenz RA, Boswell EJ, Schlundt DG. Registered dietitians' teaching and adherence promotion skills during routine patient education. *Patient Educ Couns.* 1992; 19: 273-280.
6. Isselmann MC, Deubner LS, Hartman M. A nutrition counseling workshop: Integrating counseling psychology into nutrition practice. *J Am Diet Assoc.* 1993; 93: 324-326.
7. Lewis NM, Hay AL, Fox HM. Evaluation of a workshop model for teaching counseling skills to nutrition students. *J Am Diet Assoc.* 1987; 87: 1554-1557.

Learning Activities

1. With a colleague, discuss your personal limits and boundaries in regards to nutrition therapy, using the sample questions/ issues listed on page 4.

2. In a nutrition counseling session in which you function as an observer, identify at least six nonverbal and verbal cues that convey empathy.

3. Demonstrate the effective use of nonverbal behavior in a role-play medical nutrition therapy counseling session.

4. Identify attitudes or behaviors about yourself that may facilitate or interfere with establishing a successful counseling relationship (hold yourself "to the light").

5. Using the Peer Review Counseling Tool in Appendix 1-D, observe at least two medical nutrition therapy counseling sessions (or role plays) and note positive counseling behaviors exhibited as well as those behaviors that could be enhanced. Share your observations with the counselor.

References
1. Curry KR, Jaffe A. *Nutrition Counseling and Communication Skills.* Philadelphia: W.B. Saunders; 1998.
2. Carkhuff RR. *Helping and Human Relations.* Vol. 1. New York: Holt, Rinehart & Winston; 1969.
3. Danish S, Hauer A. *Helping Skills: A Basic Training Program.* New York: Behavioral Publications; 1973.
4. Egan G. *The Skilled Helper.* Monterey, CA: Brooks/Cole; 1975.
5. Ivey A, Authier J. *Microcounseling.* 2nd ed. Springfield, IL: Charles C. Thomas; 1971, 1978.
6. Cormier WH, Cormier LS. *Interviewing Strategies for Helpers,* 3rd ed. Pacific Grove, CA: Brooks/Cole; 1979, 1985, 1991.
7. D'Augelli A, D'Augelli J, Danish S. *Helping Others.* Pacific Grove, CA: Brooks/Cole; 1981.
8. Snetselaar L. *Nutrition Counseling Skills: Assessment, Treatment, and Evaluation,* 3rd ed. Gaithersburg, MD: Aspen Pub; 1997.
9. Pace PW, Russell ML, Probstfield JL, Insull W. Intervention specialist: New role for dietitians' counseling skills. *J Am Diet Assoc.* 1984; 84: 1357.
10. Brammer LM. *The Helping Relationship: Process and Skills,* 8th ed. Boston: Allyn & Bacon; 2002.
11. Reiff D, Reiff K. *Eating Disorders: Nutrition Therapy in the Recovery Process.* Life Enterprises; 1997.

11. Reiff D, Reiff K. *Eating Disorders: Nutrition Therapy in the Recovery Process.* Life Enterprises; 1997.
12. Kratina K, Albers M, Meyer R. Treatment of Eating Disorders. Chapter in The Florida Dietetic Association Diet Manual: *Manual of Clinical Dietetics.* Tallahassee, FL: FDA; 1995.
13. Kratina K. In: King K, Klawitter B. *Nutrition Therapy, 1ˢᵗ ed.* Lake Dallas: Helm Publishing; 1995.
14. King N, Kratina K. *Student Fact Sheet Series: The Disordered Eating Fact Sheet.* Chicago, IL: Amer. Dietetic Assn.; Sports, Cardiovascular and Wellness Nutritionists, 1996.
15. Carl Greenberg, MS, Behavior Science Faculty, Family Medicine, University of Washington, Seattle, Phone interview January 1995.
16. Reiff K, Reiff D. *Advanced Counseling,* Workshop, Amer.Dietetic Assn., Orlando, FL, October 17, 1994.
17. Johanna H. Roth, RD, LD, CHES, CAS, Bethesda, MD. Adapted from: Reiff D, Reiff KL. *Eating Disorders: Nutrition in the Recovery Process.* Gaithersburg, MD: Aspen Pub, Inc.; 1992.
18. Beckley L. *Diet, Addition and Recovery,* (4th ed.) San Marcos, CA: Nutrition Dimension; 2002.
19. Ivey AE, Ivey MB, Simek-Morgan L. *Theories of Counseling and Psychotherapy: A Multicultural Perspective.* (5th ed.) Boston: Allyn and Bacon; 2001.
20. Truax CB, Carkhuff RR. *Toward Effective Counseling and Psychotherapy.* Chicago, IL: Aldine; 1967.
21. Carkhuff, RR. *Helping and Human Relations.* Vol. 2. New York: Holt, Rinehart and Winston; 1969b.
22. Gazda GM, Asbury FS, Balzer FJ, Childers WC, Walters RP. *Human Relations Development.* (2nd ed.). Boston: Allyn & Bacon; 1977.
23. Ivey AE, Ivey MB, Simek-Downing L. *Counseling and Psychotherapy: Integrating Skills, Theory and Practice,* Englewood Cliffs, NJ: Prentice-Hall; 2002.
24. Goldstein AP. Relationship-Enhancement Methods. In Kanfer FH, Goldstein AP (Eds.), *Helping People Change* (3rd ed.). Boston: Allyn & Bacon; 1991.
25. Freud S. *A General Introduction to Psychoanalysis.* New York: Washington Square Press; 1952. (original work published in 1900.)
26. Rogers C. *Client-centered Therapy.* Boston: Houghton-Mifflin; 1951.
27. Rosal MC, Ebbeling CB, Lofgren I, Ockene JK, Ockene IS, Hebert JR. Facilitating dietary change: The patient-centered counseling model. *J Am Diet Assoc.* 2001;101:323-338,341.
28. Perls FS. *The Gestalt Approach and Eyewitness to Therapy.* Palo Alto, CA: Science and Behavior Books; 1973.
29. Guerney B, Stollak L, Guerney L. The practicing psychologist as educator: An alternative to the medical practitioner model. *Professional Psychologist.* 1971; 2: 276-282.
30. Ellis A. *Reason and Emotion in Psychotherapy.* New York: Lyle Stuart; 1962.
31. Gilliland BE, James RK, Roberts GR, Bowman JT. *Theories and Strategies in Counseling and Psychotherapy.* Englewood Cliffs, NJ: Prentice-Hall; 1984.
32. Carkhuff R. *The Art of Helping,* 8th ed. Amherst, MA: Human Resource Development Press; 2000.
33. Peck MS. *The Road Less Traveled, 25ᵗʰ Anniversary.* Touchstone Books; 2003.
34. Stuart M, Simko M. A technique for incorporating psychological principles into the nutrition counseling of clients. *Topics in Clinical Nutrition.* 1991; vol. 6: 4; 32-39.
35. Saloff-Coste C, Hamburg P, Herzog D. Nutrition and psychotherapy: Collaborative treatment of patients with eating disorders. *Bulletin of the Menninger Clinic.* Fall 1993; 57: 4: 504-516.
36. Danish S. *Advanced Counseling Skills.* Presentations at American Dietetic Assn. Convention, Orlando, FL, October, 1994.
37. Unpublished surveys of *Counseling Habits and Barriers* taken at various state and regional dietetic meetings in 1993-94 by Kathy King, RD.
38. Vickery CE, Cotugna N, Hodges PAM. Comparing counseling skills of dietetic students: A model for skill enhancement. *J Am Diet Assoc.* 1995;95 (8): 912-913.

Chapter 2

Counseling: *Child, Adolescent, and Family*
Bridget Klawitter, PhD, RD, FADA

After reading this chapter, the reader will be able to:
- ♦ Identify basic differences in learning for children and adolescents.
- ♦ List at least six developmental skills that should be considered when counseling adolescents.
- ♦ Identify the role of family in the nutrition counseling process.
- ♦ Apply learning principles in various child and adolescent counseling environments.

Our challenge as nutrition therapists is to adapt our counseling style, language, and information to different individuals of various ages. Children learn differently from adolescents, who learn differently from adults at different ages. If we, as nutrition therapists, understand how people learn, we may be better able to predict when and how learning is facilitated and arrange for its occurrence. The initial formal education of children is referred to as pedagogy, and androgogy is defined as "the art and science of helping adults learn." (1)

Pedagogy is often used as a synonym for teaching and in the pedagogic model, "teachers assume responsibility for making decisions about what will be learned, how it will be learned, and when it will be learned. It can be simply called *teacher-focused education*. Learning can be defined as the act, process, or experience of gaining knowledge or skills. Remarkably, we learn from the moment of birth, however, learning can, and should be, a lifelong process." (2)

CONSIDERATIONS SPECIFIC TO CHILDREN

The eating behavior of infants is controlled by innate preferences and dislikes as well as by biological self-regulation. (3) These innate processes become modified by the learning process. Children learn a new skill or body of knowledge when they are physically and mentally mature enough to do so. That is why it can be frustrating for a parent to watch a small child learn to run without falling or to catch a ball. Throughout childhood, academic learning is traditionally organized around certain fundamental subjects (i.e., math, reading, writing). The child accumulates facts and has a subject-centered focus on learning, quite different than the problem-focused learning of the adult.

Children in different developmental age groups and different cultures perceive the world in different ways.(4) The goal is full mastery of whatever a child is doing, whether it's making a mud pie or memorizing a song on the piano. The child can experience mastery through personal accomplishments and interaction with peers. They also need love, guidance, and emotional support to develop a sense of worth and to understand themselves.

Parents and Family

Parents and family should serve many functions in the life of a child: as sources of unconditional love and acceptance, morale boosters, and role models. They should teach and mold the child with lessons such as delayed gratification, discipline, problem-solving techniques, and traditional values. Providing a safe environment with adequate food, shelter, and clothing is expected.

Parents influence their child's meal patterns and food preferences through the foods they make available, the family food habits, and their own eating behaviors. (5-7) The Framingham Children's Study demonstrated that parents' eating habits have a significant effect on the nutritional intake of their preschool children, particularly for saturated fat, total fat, and cholesterol. (8) Counseling interventions should involve the family and actively engage the child and parent(s) in adopting healthy lifestyle habits.

Unfortunately, these positive things that "should" happen do not always occur. Although children are not always aware that their home environments are less than ideal, they often carry "baggage" from those formative years for the rest of their lives. Specific to food and lifestyle choices, the child may learn by example to console himself with food when he is sad or frustrated; he may learn to "pig out" on the holidays and at other family gatherings; he may crave or avoid certain foods that remind him of home. Many children are greatly influenced by how they see their parents reacting to life's problems and stresses. Others see, recognize, and vow never to repeat inappropriate behavior they see in their parents.

Today, family counselors report an increase in the number of children growing up without good role models or adequate guidance due to the increase in single parent households, or overly tired or guilty working parents. In these circumstances the parent(s) abdicates the parent role to become a peer to the child providing little or no guidance or rules. On the other end of the spectrum are the inflexible families (that have been around forever) with rigid rules and roles that often produce children who are not ready for responsibility or decision-making. (9)

The Foundation Of Good Mental Health

As Peck states in his book, *The Road Less Traveled*, (10) *"Life is a series of problems. Do we want to moan about them or solve them? Discipline is the basic set of tools we require* (beginning in childhood) *to solve life's problems. What makes life difficult is that the process of confronting and solving problems is a painful one. Problems, depending upon their nature, evoke in us frustration or grief or sadness or loneliness or guilt or regret or anger or fear or anxiety or anguish or despair. Yet it is in this whole process of meeting and solving problems that life has its meaning. It is only because of problems that we grow mentally and spiritually.*

Fearing the pain involved, almost all of us, to a greater or lesser degree, attempt to avoid problems. We procrastinate, hoping that they will go away. We ignore them, forget them, and pretend they do not exist. This tendency to avoid problems and the emotional suffering inherent in them is the primary basis of all human mental illness. Since most of us have this tendency to a greater or lesser degree, most of us are mentally ill to a greater or lesser degree, lacking complete mental health. Some of us will go to quite extraordinary lengths to avoid our problems and the suffering they cause, proceeding far afield from all that is clearly good and sensible in order to try to find an easy way out, building the most elaborate fantasies in which to live, sometimes to the total exclusion of reality."

The use of defense mechanisms like denial (deny reality) or distortion (reject or change the perceived reality) often occurs when a person has difficulty dealing with the reality of an experience. Often these responses are at an unconscious level and they help the person feel better by avoiding reality. Dietitians may see these kinds of responses in people with new diagnoses of chronic conditions such as diabetes, cancer, or eating disorders. Other commonly seen defense mechanisms are fixation and regression where the person stays at the present stage of development or returns to an earlier stage, respectively, that seemed safer. Some young women will choose to be very thin and young looking, or very overweight in order to avoid facing growing up and being sexually attractive. Rationalization is where the person makes excuses instead of facing reality. For example, a male client may blame his increased blood lipid levels and weight gain on his wife's cooking instead of on his hearty appetite.

> *A mentally well person works through, confronts, forgives, forgets, or reinterprets things that bother him or her instead of letting them fester and become wounds.*

The way out of this fog is to face reality and work through the problems. If the layers of self-deception are severe, the person may need psychotherapy in order to identify and "unpeel" the layers and face the reality and possible suffering. The nutrition therapist can help other more typical clients by helping them learn life-skills like assertiveness and setting boundaries that were never fully developed while growing up (perhaps due to lack of good role models), but which effect how they take care of their health. You can help the person confront irrational dieting and self-perceptions like, "It's not fair that I can't eat as much as my sister, the marathon runner. I walk, sometimes." or "I can only lose weight on 500 calories per day, that's the way I lost the other three times." You will see many clients who want results, but since childhood they have never been able to delay gratification. They want it NOW!

Nutrition therapy can serve as a reality check for clients and their lifelong beliefs and habits. That is why cognitive (thoughts), behavioral (habits), and psychoeducational therapies (applying psychological or helping skills to learning a body of knowledge) are so important to nutrition counseling. Albert Ellis teaches through his Rational-Emotive Therapy that, it is too bad if something awful happened to you as a child, but it is worse if as an adult, you do nothing about it.(11) A mentally well person works through, confronts, forgives, forgets, or reinterprets things that bother him or her instead of letting them fester and become wounds.

When A Child Needs Nutrition Counseling

Clients of all ages may have difficulty in accepting and adjusting to health or lifestyle changes. Children, because of a limited reasoning ability, may have an even harder time. Children do not always understand the reasons why they must change habits or perform certain tasks. Allowing children to have some part in the planning of their care may assist them in feeling they have control over the situation.

Previous hospital experiences can also modify a child's behavior. Children are especially influenced by how they were cared for during prior hospitalizations. Children particularly remember in great detail the attitudes of those who took care of them, especially related to truthfulness. (12) A child's sense of trust is largely influenced by any past relationships with adults. Any previous experiences with a nutrition counselor can influence the child's expectations. A child, just like an adult, fears the unknown and the experienced pediatric nutrition counselor can alleviate these fears through telling a little about yourself or your children, and by asking about the child and his family to first establish rapport.

Most children are quick to express their feelings. It becomes very important to listen to these feelings and discern their meanings in the situation at hand. All behaviors have meaning, but when a child speaks very little, it is more of a challenge to decipher. Is the child shy, totally satisfied, angry, or ready to go?

Some techniques are more effective than others in changing specific behaviors. Many strategies for teaching young children center on play, the primary way in which children learn. Cognitive behavioral play therapy (CBPT) typically uses role modeling to demonstrate adaptive coping skills.(13) Through play, cognitive changes are communicated indirectly and more adaptive behaviors are introduced. Play in the therapeutic setting, even with a minimum of verbalization and interpretation, can be a powerful impact on development.(14) A child may be motivated to learn by playing games, reading books, or using dolls and puppets. When a child, even as young as five years old, understands and "buys-into" solving a nutritional problem, he or she may actually prove to be more disciplined than the parents. Some children take "rules" very seriously, so be sure to assess the child and choose your words carefully so that "guidelines" don't become "rigid rules" unless they are meant to be.

Also, it has happened that one parent, sometimes unknowingly, will sabotage the efforts of a child and the other parent through offering trips to the ice cream store as reward for good grades, to show love, or for any other reason. The counselor must then work to help that parent (who often will not come in) to find other ways to show love and share special times with the child without turning to high calorie foods.

In some instances, a child, adolescent, or adult client may place the counselor in the position of role model or surrogate parent. Coaches of youngsters on athletic teams often serve the same function. It is important that the counselor recognize the potential influence he or she may have in the child's life and do no harm, while modeling mature, rational, caring behavior.

Parent/Child Considerations

It is important to take into consideration the relationship between a child and his or her parents, as well as the parental expectations of the counseling experience. You should also learn as much as possible about a child from the parents, especially facts about feeding and toilet habits, and social environment.

Throughout the counseling experience, you should seize opportunities to observe the child-parent interaction and gather information relative to the child's learning needs, any cultural factors that may impact interventions, interaction patterns within the family, the child's level of development, and the parents' level of understanding and coping capabilities. (15) Counseling in the pediatric setting also entails an understanding of adult learning principles to work with the parents and to solidify the entire family-counselor relationship. See Appendix 2-A Working with a Child with a Feeding Disability.

The major goal in counseling parents is to help them increase their competence and confidence in meeting the needs of their child. Consequently, you must establish rapport and trust in the relationship with the parents. Hornby (16) proposes a three-stage counseling model, which can be used with children and adults in a wide variety of settings. The problem-solving approach involves three stages: listening, understanding, and action planning. The rationale for using the model is based on the premise that any problem or concern parents bring to counseling can be dealt with by going through the three stages and determining the solution that best suits the family unit.

Ivey and Matthews (17) describe a five-stage decisional framework to facilitate counseling. They argue that effective counseling and therapy tend to cover these five points over the time span of the counseling experience. Table 2.1 lists the general guidelines for counseling children using the five-stage model.

Table 2.1 Interviewing Children Using the Five-Stage Model

Stage 1 Establish rapport
> Establish rapport in your own way: use facial expressions (i.e. smile, laugh), share stories, play activities, or draw.

Stage 2 Data gathering emphasizing strengths
> Paraphrase, reflect child's feelings, summarize frequently. Keep questions and concepts concrete, and avoid abstract talk. Identify positive aspects.

Stage 3 Determine goals
> Ask what the child wants to happen. Accept a child's goals but focus on the concrete short-term goals. Allow a child to explore the ideal world and discover fantasies and desires.

Stage 4 Generate alternative solutions and actions
> Utilize creative brainstorming techniques. Try small groups with children having similar problems. Imagine the future and explore various alternatives.

Stage 5 Generalize
> Maintain concrete goals day to day. Homework assignments are useful. Observe behavior and interactions with others.

Adapted from Ivey AE, Ivey MB, Simek-Morgan L. *Counseling and Psychotherapy: A Multicultural Perspective, 3rd ed.* Boston: Allyn and Bacon; 1993. Used with permission.

Lipkin and Cohen outline potential approaches and helpful tips for working with pediatric clients in the health care setting: (12)

- ***Establish a friendly relationship with the child.*** Take time to talk to the child without the parents present. Respect the child's unique feelings and needs and show an interest in his or her interests. Be open to the child's way of doing things if it does not interfere with the goals of therapy.
- ***Help the child deal with problems as they arise.*** Provide information in simple terms and honestly.
- ***Do not overwhelm the child with facts and explanations.*** Encourage discussion using drawings, pictures, or food models to help the child understand basic concepts. Answer questions as they are asked, simply and concisely.

- *Recognize that children may view any limitation (such as food or fluids) as punishment.* Limitations may be met with anger or resentment. Continue to approach the child with gentle kindness and genuine concern.
- *Provide outlets for a child's anger or hostile feelings.* Encourage the child to draw pictures or act out feelings with dolls or puppets.
- *Give a child choices, but only if you can respect their decisions as part of the counseling experience.* Build trust by acting on the child's decisions and providing for some control over the situation.
- *Encourage the parents to ask questions.* Provide factual explanations that assist parents in support of the counseling experience.
- *Be flexible.* Flexibility is particularly important when working with children. Short-term goals that can be accomplished easily are vital as the counseling relationship develops.

CONSIDERATIONS SPECIFIC TO ADOLESCENTS

Developmental Skills

The extent to which developmental tasks (4) are completed or resolved successfully influence the adolescent's success in finding an identity. Developmental skills that should be learned are: (See Chapter 12 for more discussion on seven of the list below.)

- **Identifying needs** (What makes him or her feel stable, happy, secure, and loved?)
- **Active listening** (This is focused, involved listening that enhances communication and relationship building.)
- **Assertiveness** (This is the ability to stand up and be proactive; it means you believe your opinions have merit.)
- **Separation** (You see yourself as an individual with needs and wants that are valid but possibly different from parents, siblings, and peers; you have the ability to function alone.)
- **Limit setting** (You have the ability to set boundaries to your actions and those actions you allow in others that involves you.)
- **Decision making** (You have the ability to look at the facts and draw your own conclusions and you commit yourself to timelines, appointments, and other responsibilities.)
- **Organization** (You can prioritize and structure random information and commitments in order to manage time or complete tasks better.)
- **Appropriate pacing** (You can manage your time and physical and mental capabilities to promote good health and productive work output.)
- **Support systems** (You acknowledge that other people are very important to you. Your happiness and productivity are often highly influenced by the people you *choose* to be around and whether they positively support you.)
- **Delegation** (You can manage your time and energy better by asking or allowing other people to share some of the responsibility by doing tasks they do best.)

Adolescence is characterized by dramatic biological, cognitive, and sociocultural change. (18) It is a period where health behaviors are most vulnerable. Adolescents can be most challenging as they struggle to emerge from the role of dependent child to that of independent adult. Through their peers, adolescents learn about life beyond the family unit. Peer groups offer the adolescent the opportunity to try new roles, different identities, and behaviors not experienced at home. Children progress from a strong conformity to what parents mandate, to an equally strong conformity to their peers, and eventually move to their own identity with the maturity and independence of adulthood.

The central task of adolescence is the establishment of identity, with the primary risk being identity confusion, which means the adolescent wants to be like someone else (a movie star, favorite friend, or popular kid in school). (4) An adolescent feels the need to establish a personal identity, but with this desire comes increased assertiveness. Adolescents increasingly feel able to make decisions regarding well being including the choice of food, activity, clothes and friends.

Psychological influences on health decisions are ultimately related to developmental processes. Four influential factors on adolescent eating behaviors have been described:(19) individual or intrapersonal (e.g., psychosocial, biological), social environmental or interpersonal (e.g., family or peers), physical environmental or community (e.g., schools, fast food places, stores), and societal (e.g., mass media and marketing, social and cultural norms).

The relationship between the diets of adolescents and chronic disease risk is based on the assumption that eating behaviors are learned and solidified during childhood and adolescence and are maintained into adulthood. (20) It is important to identify the health concerns of adolescents independent of health knowledge, beliefs and behaviors in order to be an effective counselor. Adolescents often understand the whole notion of health differently than adults do. Health compromising behavior decisions like riding a motorcycle or drinking alcohol can represent a way of controlling the environment or testing one's independence from family or peers. Advice about reducing health-compromising behavior, like cutting down on candy bars, may be viewed as adult methods to limit the adolescent's independence and freedom of choice.

Adolescent Autonomy

Two aspects of adolescent autonomy have been distinguished: mutuality (perception of parents encouraging independence) and conflictual dependence (negative perception of "self-in-relation-to-parent" and related feelings of anger and shame). (21) Adolescents establish autonomy when they search for avenues to express their free will. They will often use food choices as a way to establish independence. (22)The adolescent needs to feel autonomous and have a true sense of commitment to any proposed lifestyle changes. Adolescents tend to be concerned about their physical development, appearance, and emotions. In terms of cognitive development, early adolescents think in the concrete here and now. Abstract or long-range consequences of health behaviors are difficult for adolescents to comprehend. Emphasis for counseling adolescents must be on the immediate, concrete, personal impact of health-compromising behaviors. An emphasis on restrictions and negatives are counterproductive; effective health promotion messages emphasize personal power and control by the adolescent.

> Emphasis for counseling adolescents must be on the immediate, concrete, personal impact of health-compromising behaviors. An emphasis on restrictions and negatives are counterproductive; effective health promotion messages emphasize personal power and control by the adolescent.

Specific counseling strategies for those dietetic practitioners working with adolescents have been outlined. (23) Lipkin and Cohen outlined potential approaches to the adolescent client in the health care setting.(12) Several can be adapted and applied directly to nutrition counseling practice:

- *Understand the adolescent's need to mature.* It is important to include an adolescent in decisions and goal setting, as well as keeping him or her informed about progress during therapy.
- *Do not impose your value and belief system (counter-transference issue on your part).* Allow the adolescent to verbalize his opinions and feelings and agree or disagree without you becoming judgmental.
- *Recognize that adolescent problems usually involve family interaction issues.* Assist adolescents in evaluating their surroundings, and praise and encourage them when they make independent decisions.
- *Treat the adolescent with dignity and respect.* Stress positive aspects and allow adolescents to express their ideas and concerns openly without criticism.
- *Set limits that are fair, and enforce them consistently.* Recognize the adolescent's individual needs and set goals realistically.
- *Do not work with adolescents unless you genuinely like and care about them.*

Adolescents are going through many conflicts (physically, emotionally, and psychologically), and need assistance in guiding them through this difficult period. Adolescents need to feel secure in any relationship and guided by individuals they can trust.

CONSIDERATIONS SPECIFIC TO FAMILIES AND NETWORKS

Traditional counseling in North America centers on the individual, and too little on his or her family and network of friends or significant others like a work group. Many times a spouse, friend, or peers at work play significant roles in whether a client is able to make and sustain eating behavior changes. In some cultures it is most appropriate to work through the family to facilitate changes. In some types of cases such as adolescent obesity counseling, if the family dynamics, rigid rules, or alcoholic parent are the major problem creating stress for the child, working with just the child will not necessarily make the child's life more comfortable. In such cases, nutrition counseling is often not the type of counseling that needs to be instituted first!

The family unit is both affected by an ill member and it has an impact on that family member. (24) For example, having a child with diabetes or PKU usually affects parents' entire lives, and how the parents respond to the child and his needs will have an important bearing on the child's behavior and coping skills. Another example might be having an older parent with several diet limitations come to live with a family, requiring more time being spent on meal planning and preparation, and more money being spent on special foods. In these instances, nutrition counseling for parents or other family members is intended to help normally functioning individuals better cope with the additional demands of living with a family member struggling with a health alteration. If the nutritionist perceives that family members are not coping, it is appropriate and ethically responsible to suggest a referral to a family counselor skilled in this area.

It is important to consider the effects of an alteration in health status or behavior changes on the family unit as a whole. The social as well as potential economic impact must be recognized and dealt with. An understanding of the process by which family members adapt to change is essential. It is also important to understand the ways in which the family unit typically functions.

A client's readiness to learn can be enhanced by identifying and utilizing the client's support system to assist the individual in coping with change. Family counseling has been shown to be the most effective therapy for treating adolescent obesity. (25) The nutrition counselor can encourage family and friends to create a supportive environment in which the child works to make lifestyle changes. If they will not agree to that, try to have them agree that they will not sabotage the child's efforts. Studies indicate that a child's support system is helpful in long-term adherence to diet regimens. (26,27)

Practitioners can promote acceptance of feeding changes by involving parents and children in making the changes, helping everyone involved to be as comfortable as possible with the feeding decisions, and by being open to suggestion. (28) People will best follow advice that makes sense to them. If the practitioner senses their advice is not being accepted, encourage the child or family to ask questions. ***"Help me to understand why you feel this is the best choice,"*** is a good phrase to teach any child or family. The practitioner may want to ask ***"This seems to me to be the best choice, but will this work for you?"*** This phrase can help bring out perceived disadvantages that the parent may otherwise be reluctant to share. Be alert to signs that parents or kids do not truly buy into the nutrition care plan. Children are frequently taught not to disagree with adults and may be reluctant to indicate a suggestion is not workable.

In practice, you may work in a clinic or on a team with a family counselor, or you may refer children and their families to a private practicing family counselor. Trained family counselors come from many disciplines, i.e., psychiatry, psychology, psychotherapy, and psychiatric social worker. They all must have a minimum of a master's in counseling with special emphasis and supervision in family dynamics and counseling. (9) It is not an easy job to step into the emotional dynamics of a family that has been functioning only marginally for many years. Without proper training, a nutrition therapist should not attempt it. It is appropriate, however, to work with a client and his supportive family members on nutrition-related issues if the child wants the help.

Learning Activities

1. Observe a family nutrition counseling session. What role does each family member play in the counseling session? What interactions between family members do you observe? What impact does the nutrition problem being addressed play on the family unit as a whole?

2. Counsel (or observe a counseling session) for a child under age eight. What counseling strategies are utilized? How does the child respond to each strategy identified? What changes would you recommend if the session were to be repeated based on your observations?

3. Counsel (or observe a counseling session) for an adolescent between age 10 and 16 years. What counseling strategies are utilized? How does the adolescent respond to each strategy identified? What changes would you recommend if the session were repeated based on your observations?

4. Look at the photo of the counseling session below. Critique the session and describe what elements of the interaction are consistent with good body language and building rapport. What could you change to improve the counseling setting?

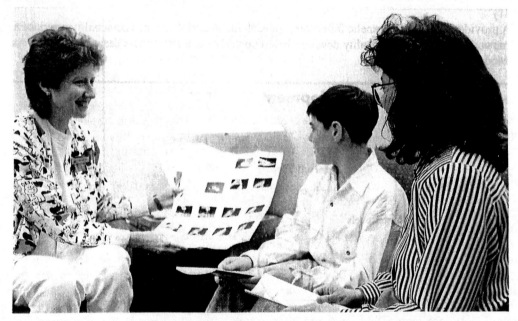

Photo: Mark Albertini, All Saints Healthcare System, Inc., Racine, WI

5. Review each of the following case studies and outline/discuss applications of counseling principles as discussed in this chapter.

Case studies: *Courtesy of Lillis Ling, MS, RD, CDE, Director, Department of Nutrition Services, Children's Mercy Hospital, Kansas City, MO (28)*

Case Study #1
Many times the health beliefs of the parents and extended family affect feeding practices employed and the acceptance of nutrition information from health care providers. These practices may not be initially apparent but can be discovered by taking time to do an indepth nutrition history. Maria was seen at the age of 5 months in the outpatient cranio-facial clinic for absent muscles in the left side of her face. She had gained 11.1 grams per day. The expected gain is 16.1 grams per day. The growth grid for linear growth was also beginning to flatten. Initially the mother reported the infant was taking 46 ounces of Enfamil with iron every three to four hours. She reported adding cereal to the bottle over the past month. Although Maria initially had difficulty drinking from a bottle she was doing well with a

Haberman bottle, as long as she was allowed to drink with her neck hyperextended or lying flat on her right side. When the dietitian observed the baby feeding, she noticed the liquid in the bottle looked more like breastmilk than formula. When the parents were asked about the formula, they explained the feeding was a Mexican health drink made from dry milk, cinnamon, sugar, and rice water. Since the parents believed this to be a health promoting supplement and baby preferred this to formula they had been using it for two feedings per day. The nutritionist acknowledged the taste preference and comfort value of traditional ethnic foods, but explained why the feeding was inappropriate for a child this age. The growth grid was reviewed with the parents with an accompanying discussion of appropriate types of protein and the potential dangers of using the rice water mixture for a child of this age. The parents' beliefs that only traditional foods promoted "health" were not initially evident but were affecting the growth and development of this child.

Case Study #2

Parents of children with a major medical problem or chronic illness may resist change, especially if the child is currently doing well. Robert was born with a cleft palate and significant cardiac anomalies. He grew very little until after his cardiac surgery was performed at the age of 3 months. He was discharged on a 30 calorie per ounce formula at a volume calculated to promote catch up growth. Robert grew and gained well and started to develop some subcutaneous fat stores, especially in his extremities. His feeding of infant formula with macrolipid was delivered via gastrostomy feeding tube. When the child was seen in cleft palate clinic at the age of 11 months, the dietitian advised an increase in the volume of the feeding to enable the child to continue to grow. Solid foods were reported to cause gagging and were deferred until a swallow study could be performed. The mother was very reluctant to change the volume of the feeding, as the child was doing so well. The cardiologist cautioned her about the dangers of obesity. In order to get this mother to accept the change in formula, she needed to be reassured that she was right to be concerned about obesity and that the dietitian recognized the development of subcutaneous fat stores significantly changed her child's appearance. This was inconsistent with the mother's perception of her child's body image. The mother verbally acknowledged that she herself was very thin and that although she knew her son's face remained very thin and that he was still less than 50% weight for height, she still feared the added weight would put undue stress on her child's heart. By contacting the cardiac dietitian the mother had seen previously for affirmation that the formula change was indeed appropriate, reviewing and explaining the child's growth on the growth grid, and encouraging the parent to voice her concerns, the change in formula was accepted.

Case Study #3

In working with children, it is very important to make the child the focus of attention. Even as early as four years of age, a child knows what he or she wants to eat. Shannon is a six-year-old who has had insulin-dependent diabetes mellitus since she was 16 months old. As early as four years of age, she came to the clinic with her own list of questions about diet. Of course, her parents encouraged her to participate in the clinic visit by helping her remember the questions that had occurred since the previous visit. It is important to remember that sometimes a child wants to assume responsibility for his or her disease and at other times the child wants to have help. Asking the child if there are any changes to be made in the meal plan lets the child feel more in control of his or her care. Quite often the parent has never asked the child this question and can't answer for the child. If the child doesn't want to answer, he or she will defer to the parent.

Case Study #4

Charlie, age 12 years, was diagnosed with hypercalcuria and the physician prescribed a diet with low-protein, low-sodium, the RDA for calcium and high potassium. With so many nutrients being modified, it was important to get Charlie involved in the decision-making process early. A diet history and a list of favorite foods was obtained with the reassurance that he could help decide what changes would be made. To start on a positive note, he was given a list of potassium-rich foods and asked which ones he was willing to add to his regular food intake. Because he was using the school breakfast and lunch program, his grandmother was asked to secure the appropriate school menus and to alert the cafeteria manager of Charlie's diet recommendations. In a follow-up conversation with the cafeteria manager, she was very willing to make additional fruits and lower-sodium cereals available.

Charlie wanted to be able to eat pizza when it was on the school menu and to have canned beef stew weekly. With a 1200 mg sodium limit, he learned to eat low-sodium foods at the other meals. Fortunately, he became fascinated and challenged with reading labels and figuring out which food selections worked for him. He wasn't happy changing from canned to frozen vegetables until he realized how many more food choices he could have. A computer printout gave him more information about the nutrients in foods. Because he was bright, open to change, involved in developing new skills and had support from his grandmother and the school, he did well with his diet restrictions.

Case Study #5

Adolescence is a time of variable acceptance of advice from adults and of follow-through on the part of the child. Developing rapport may take time and an accepting attitude on the part of the nutritionist. Jackie is a child with spina bifida who has always had to consume a diet lower in calories than her peers to remain at an appropriate body weight. As she entered adolescence she started to gain too quickly and was counseled by a nutritionist. Jackie was able to make enough lifestyle changes to lose weight and receive praise from the medical team. At a later follow up appointment she was surprised to learn she had regained her lost weight and more. A different nutritionist saw her at this appointment, as the previous practitioner had moved. Initially, Jackie did not want to engage in conversation of any kind. Her grandmother answered for the teen at first but the dietitian continued to talk directly to Jackie, accepting all information without judgment, and acknowledging how common it is for people to slip back into previous eating habits. The teen continued to give little or no response until the grandmother made a statement with which she strongly disagreed. At this point, Jackie started to converse with the nutritionist and several mutually acceptable strategies were identified to help her get back on track again. What started out as an uncomfortable meeting evolved into a positive problem solving session with the teen as the leader and the grandparent and nutritionist taking supportive roles. The grandparents were able to change some established food preparation methods and work on portion control, which in turn assisted the adolescent in meeting her goals.

References
1. Knowles MS. *The Modern Practice of Adult Education.* Chicago: Follett Publishing Company; 1970.
2. Conner ML. *Learning: The Critical Technology, 2nd ed.* St. Louis MO: Wave Technologies International, Inc. 1996.
3. Westenhoefer J. Establishing good dietary habits: capturing the minds of children. *Public Health Nutr.* 2001;4(1A):125-129.
4. Erickson EH. *Childhood and Society.* New York: Norton; 1963.
5. Birch LL. Psychological influences on the childhood diet. *J Nutr.* 1998; 128:S407-S410.
6. Hill AJ, Hill AJ. Developmental issues in attitudes to food and diet. *Proc Nutr Soc.* 2002; 61(2): 259-266.
7. Skinner JD, Carruth BR, Bounds W, Zeigler PJ. Children's food preferences: a longitudinal analysis. *J Am Diet Assoc.* 2002; 102;1638-1647.
8. Oliveria SA, Ellison RC, Moore LL, Gillman MW, Garrahie EJ, Singer MR. Parent-child relationships in nutrient intake: the Framingham Children's Study. *Am J Clin Nutr.* 1992;56: 593-598.
9. Phone interview with Carl Greenberg, MS. Behavior Science Faculty, Family Medicine, U of Washington, Seattle, WA, January 1995.
10. Peck MS. *The Road Less Traveled.* London, England: Arrow; 1990.
11. Ellis A. Rational-emotive psychotherapy. In: Arbuckel D, ed. *Counseling and Psychotherapy.* New York: McGraw-Hill; 1967.
12. Lipkin GB, Cohen RG. *Effective Approaches to Patient's Behavior.* New York: Springer Publishing Company; 1980.
13. Knell SM. Cognitive-behavioral play therapy. *J Clin Child Psych.* 1998; 27(1):28-33.
14. Ablon SL. The therapeutic action of play: clinical perspective. *J Amer Acad Child Adol Psych.* 1996; 35(4): 545-547.
15. Sedlacek KK. Patient Teaching in a pediatric unit. In: Bille DA, ed. *Practical Approaches to Patient Teaching.* Boston: Little, Brown and Company; 1981.
16. Hornby G. *Counselling in Child Disability: Skills for Working with Parents.* London: Chapman and Hall; 1994.
17. Ivey AE, Ivey MB, Simek-Morgan L. *Counseling and Psychotherapy: A Multicultural Perspective.* 3rd ed. Boston: Allyn and Bacon; 1993.
18. Perry CL. Lifecycle III: preadolescent and adolescent influences on health. *The Institute of medicine Symposium, "Capitalizing on Social Science and Behavioral Research to Improve the Public's Health".* Atlanta GA: National Academy of Sciences Press, 2000.
19. Story M, Neumark-Sztainer D, French S. Individual and environmental influences on adolescent eating behaviors. *J Am Diet Assoc.* 2002; 102(3): S40-S51.
20. Lytle LA. Nutritional issues for adolescents. *J Am Diet Assoc.* 2002; 102(3): S8-S12.
21. Frank SJ, Schettini AM, Lower RJ. The role of separation-individuation experiences and personality in predicting externalizing and internalizing dimensions of functional impairment in a rural pre-adolescent and adolescent sample. *J Clin Child Adol Psych.* 2002; 31(4): 431-442.

22. Neumark-Sztainer D, Story M, Perry C, Casey M. Factors influencing food choices of adolescents: findings from focus-group discussions with adolescents. *J Am Diet Assoc.* 1999; 99(8): 929-937.
23. Sigman-Grant M. Strategies for counseling adolescents. *J Am Diet Assoc.* 2002; 102(3): S32-S39.
24. Mink IT, Nahira K. Directions of effects: Family lifestyles and behavior of TMR children. *Am J of Mental Deficiency.* 1991; 91 (11): 1418-1422.
25. Mellin L. Child and adolescent obesity: The nurse practitioner's use of the SHAPEDOWN method. *J Ped Health Care.* 1992; 6: (4): 187-193.
26. Morton A, Ringles S, Christakis G. Social factors affecting participation in a study diet and coronary heart disease. *J Health and Social Behavior.* 1967; 8: 22-31.
27. Andrew GM, Oldridge NB, Parker JO, Cunningham DA, Rechnitzer PA, Jones NL, Buck C, Kavanaugh T, Shepard RJ, Sutton JR, McDonald W. Reasons for dropout from exercise programs for post-coronary patients. *Medicine and Science in Sports and Exercise.* 1981; 13: 164-168.
28. Ling L. Counseling the pediatric client. In: Helm KK and Klawitter BK, ed. *Nutrition Therapy: Advanced Counseling Skills.* Lake Dallas TX: Helm Seminars; 1995.
29. Cloud HH. Dietitian as team leader in caring for a child with a feeding disability. In: Helm KK and Klawitter BK, ed. *Nutrition Therapy: Advanced Counseling Skills.* Lake Dallas TX: Helm Seminars; 1995.

Additional Reading

1. Satter E. *How to Get Your Kid to Eat...But Not Too Much.* Palo Alto, CA: Bull Publishing Co.; 1991.
2. Satter E. *Child of Mine: Feeding with Love and Good Sense.* Palo Alto, CA: Bull Publishing Co.; 2000.
3. Lane SJ, Cloud HH. Feeding problems and intervention: an interdisciplinary approach. *Topics Clin Nutr.* 1988; 3:23-32.
4. Lichtnwalter I, Freeman R, Lee M, Cialone J. Providing nutrition services to children with special needs in a community setting. *Top Clin Nutr.* 1993; 4:75-78.
5. Ekvall SM, ed. *Pediatric Nutrition in Chronic Diseases and Developmental Disorders. Prevention, Assessment, and Treatment.* New York, NY: Oxford University Press; 1993.

Chapter 3

Counseling: The Adult Learner

Bridget Klawitter, PhD, RD, FADA

After reading this chapter, the reader will be able to:
- ♦ Identify basic principles of learning for adults.
- ♦ List at least four counseling strategies that should be considered when counseling adults.
- ♦ Identify literacy considerations in the nutrition counseling process.
- ♦ Apply learning principles in various adult-counseling environments.
- ♦ Identify four evaluation methods and their application in nutrition counseling.

OVERVIEW OF ADULT LEARNING CONCEPTS

The field of adult learning has grown and expanded as the need for lifelong learning became more widely recognized. It wasn't until the late 1960's that attitudes about teaching adults began to change. Andragogy was initially defined by Knowles (1) as "the art and science of helping adults learn," but has taken on a broader meaning since his original work. Those involved in education began to see an important difference between the initial formal education of children and how adults learn. The term refers to learner-focused education for individuals of all ages, particularly adults. The andragogic model asserts five considerations for those involved in adult learning: (2)

1. Let the learner know why something is important to learn.
2. Show the learner how to get through the information.
3. Relate the topic to the learners' experiences.
4. The learner will not learn until ready and motivated to learn.
5. Help the learners overcome inhibitions, behaviors, and beliefs about learning.

The commonly recognized principles of adult learning are: (3)
- Adults like to determine their own learning experiences.
- Adults want to have efficient use of their time.
- Adults are more motivated to learn if they see a purpose or need.
- Adults can learn from the experiences of others as well as their own.
- Adults desire practical solutions to problems they encounter.
- Adults like physical surroundings conducive to their comfort.
- Adults operate from a problem-solving mode.
- Adults want to be active participants in their learning experiences.
- Adults draw on their own experiences when evaluating a learning environment.
- Adults do not like to be treated like children.
- Adult learning is an active and continuous process.
- Adults learn at different rates and in different ways.
- Adults like to know whether progress is being made.

These assumptions have many implications for the planning, implementation, and evaluation of nutrition counseling interventions. See Table 3.1 on Adult Learning Concepts and Nutrition Counseling.

Table 3.1 Adult Learning Concepts and Nutrition Counseling

CONCEPT	COUNSELING STRATEGY
Clients want to be treated as adults.	Do not reprimand or talk down to clients.
Every client is an individual.	Individualize a teaching plan for each client's situation. Avoid "standardized" materials unless they can be individualized.
Most adults prefer objectivity and a business-like approach.	Use of titles or surnames is appropriate unless the client mentions otherwise. Treat the client with respect.
Clients have difficulty with change.	Explain that change will minimize threat rather than insist on change.
Some clients lack confidence.	Lack of education, fear of failure, distrust of the medical community may be barriers. Patience, answering questions, and realistic goals may help promote a sense of confidence.
Some clients are overconfident.	It is important to set realistic goals.
Adults need positive reinforcement and feedback.	This assists in overcoming fear and anxiety; may improve compliance.

Used by permission. Dietitians in General Clinical Practice, 1992. In: Klawitter B. The Dietetic Practitioner as Adult Educator: An Overview. *DGCP Newsletter.* 1992; 9; 4: 4-9.

Self Concept and Learning

As individuals mature, independence develops as adults take control of their lives. Adults in our society develop a deep psychological need to be perceived by others as being self-directing. Therefore, in situations that do not allow them to be self-directing, adults experience tension between the situation and their self-concept. Their reactions are tainted by resentment and resistance to change. Adults "tend to avoid, resist and resent being placed in situations in which they feel they are treated like children---told what to do and what not to do, talked down to, embarrassed, punished and judged." (3)

Clients who discover nutrition "truths" on their own are more likely to accept, integrate, and apply these concepts. (4) The level of learning may also be related to the level of trust and rapport that exists between the counselor and the client. This process includes collaboration with the counselor in decision-making in regards to the client's nutritional needs. Nutrition therapists must involve the client in selecting what to learn, how to present the information, and how to evaluate whether goals were met.

> Clients who discover nutrition "truths" on their own are more likely to accept, integrate, and apply these concepts.

Evaluation can evoke anxiety in many adult clients. The best evaluative methods are those that are not intimidating, and allow for determination of what is learned. For example, having the client verbally list basic concepts, or tell how newly learned information will be incorporated into daily activities (selecting foods from a sample restaurant menu). Individuals need to participate in choosing the methods used to assess their learning and see their own progress towards established goals and objectives.

Life Experience

The past experiences of adults have a tremendous impact, positively and negatively, on learning. Previous counseling experiences, interactions with dietitians, or prior knowledge on the subject can affect the counseling process. In andragogy, there is less emphasis on the transmittal techniques found in traditional educational settings like lectures, canned audiovisual presentations and extensive reading, and an increased emphasis on experiential techniques to tap the experience of adult learners and involve them in analyzing their experiences. Examples include discussion, simulation, practice sessions, graphic aids like food models and clogged arteries, and other action-learning techniques like cooking classes or a variety of several techniques.

Due to the fact that individuals learn and process information in different ways, it is important that content be presented in a variety of formats. Some clients are visual learners and prefer to see what they are learning while auditory learners prefer spoken messages. Kinesthetic learners want to sense learning, while tactile learners want to touch. (2) Some clients prefer to read information, for example, while others learn best through audio or visual media or communication. Table 3.2 lists some general points to consider when selecting printed or audiovisual materials for adult learners. Table 3.3 gives teaching strategies for individuals with limited literacy skills.

Table 3.2   Media Considerations for the Adult Learner

Printed materials	Is content written at an appropriate level for clientele?
	Is content clear and concise?
	Is material organized in a logical sequence?
	Is important information highlighted?
	Are visuals attractive, and do they contribute to understanding?
	Are the print and type easy to read?
	Is the content accurate?
	Does the material allow for patient participation/ interaction?
Nonprint materials	Are they appropriate for the topic?
	Are they accurate yet appealing?
	Are important points easy to identify?
	Can opportunities for cognitive practice be provided?
	Are the sounds and /or colors acceptable?

Used by permission. Dietitians in General Clinical Practice, 1992. In: Klawitter B. The Dietetic Practitioner as Adult Educator: An Overview. *DGCP Newsletter.* 1992; 9; 4: 4-9.

In their initial assessments, nutrition counselors need to determine the clients' feelings and experiences related to the counseling process they are about to be involved in. For example you might ask, "Have you attempted to make any of these changes before?" The counseling plan must incorporate this knowledge and be built on positive experiences in order to overcome any negatives that may block learning or change.

Some literature indicates adults prefer one-on-one interventions that allow for individualized counseling strategies and content based on the individual's limitations and barriers. If a counseling strategy is unfamiliar to a client, like the exchange system or keeping extensive behavioral records, evaluate whether the client has difficulty using it or is bored with it, since trying to master content and learn a new skill at the same time might inhibit learning and change.

Group education has become more common for adult learning. One of the benefits of groups is the increased social integration and sharing of experiences that happens. Social integration has been shown to have a significant positive effect on retention of information. (5) The social environment may also facilitate learning by aiding adult learners to persist through difficult concepts. (6) The group counselor should explore additional training on group facilitation methods to make this strategy most advantageous to learners.

Table 3.3   Limited Literacy Teaching Strategies

Needs of People with Limited Literacy	How to Meet Those Needs
Use of relevant material	Base materials on learner needs and interests. Link information to learner's experience.
Flexible learning pace	Allow individuals the time they need. Keep sessions short & amounts of information small. Avoid sudden surprises or changes.
Involvement in learning process	Encourage clients to set goals & discover resources. Promote client's responsibility for learning. Use discovery techniques (hands-on experience).
Organized, useful materials	Encourage group problem-solving & simulation. Use information & materials with practical meaning.
Evaluate efforts	Recognize achievements. Minimize chances of failure. Provide regular feedback.

Used by permission. Copyright 1994, James A. Fain, RN. In: Fain JA. Assessing nutrition education in clients with weak literacy skills. *Nurse Practitioner Forum.* 1994; 5: 1: 52-55.

Readiness to Learn

Andragogy assumes learners are ready to learn those things that they *need* to learn because of developmental phases they are approaching in their roles as workers, spouses, parents and the like. When the timing is right, the ability to learn a particular task or concept will be possible. This is referred to as the "teachable moment."(7) Before pursuing a counseling relationship, you should determine if the client is prepared to make changes in his health behavior. A candid discussion with the client about his readiness may prevent frustration and misunderstandings down the road.

Stages of Change: Model for Nutrition Counseling

Clients arrive at our doors with varying levels of interest in making lifestyle changes. The Stages of Change Model (See Figure 3.1) has been utilized to describe the processes of health behavior change. Behavioral change can be conceptualized as a shift from a stable behavior to another stable behavior and is influenced by the counseling strategy and interventions selected. Behavioral change has distinctive stages and there can be relapses at any stage, normal for any change process. Prochaska and DiClemente and others (8,9,10) have studied groups of people trying to change risky lifestyle behaviors such as smoking, consuming alcohol, adopting more exercise, and weight loss. They found that participants were more successful making changes if the strategies more closely matched each person's stage of change. For more discussion on this topic and motivational interviewing techniques, see Chapter 19 on counseling people with diabetes.

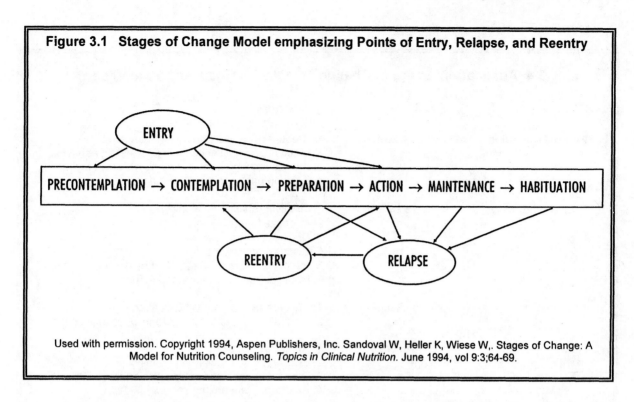

Figure 3.1   Stages of Change Model emphasizing Points of Entry, Relapse, and Reentry

Used with permission. Copyright 1994, Aspen Publishers, Inc. Sandoval W, Heller K, Wiese W,. Stages of Change: A Model for Nutrition Counseling. *Topics in Clinical Nutrition.* June 1994, vol 9:3;64-69.

You can identify which stage a client is in by asking very simple questions like, **"Are you concerned about your cholesterol level being high?"** (A negative answer here would show that the client is in the *Precontemplation Stage* and had not accepted or personalized the risk involved.) Clients in the *Contemplation Stage* believe they have a problem but aren't sure where to begin, and they need lots of help identifying what needs to be done. The *Preparation Stage* is where clients are ready to make a change but haven't yet taken any action, and they need encouragement to make small steps and draw from their past successes. In the *Action Stage,* clients have taken the first steps to change and now need help reinforcing the decision. *The Maintenance Stage* is typified by increasing the coping skills and self-rewards to support sustained change. In the *Relapse Stage,* clients return to old ways and need renewed commitment and motivation. Table 3.4 shows this model adapted to nutrition counseling. (8)

Research has shown that major events (such as illness) stimulate adult learning. However, more research is needed on when is the best time to counsel individuals following an illness. Certainly, we believe in providing the most crucial "survival" information close to the time it is needed in the acute care setting. However, counseling the client more completely when he or she is physiologically and psychologically stable and free from discomfort is much more logical. A number of factors can affect an individual's readiness to learn (see Table 3.5) and some learning needs may be more appropriately addressed in an outpatient setting.

Readiness to learn is greatly influenced by clients' interpretations of their health problems and treatments. It may be necessary for you to talk with the client regarding these concerns before further counseling can take place. Learning readiness can be influenced by many factors such as pain or anything else that affects the client's physical or psychological comfort level. Attempting to proceed with counseling efforts without understanding these circumstances is usually futile.

Acute Care Setting When attempting to counsel the critically ill patient in the acute care setting, there are several counseling issues that should be addressed: (11)
- the nutrition counselor must develop an awareness of what the client is feeling, and
- the counselor must understand her or his own emotional responses to critical illness.

Table 3.4 Application: Stage of Change Model with Goals and Strategies

Stage	Goal	Strategies
Precontemplation	Personalize risk	1. Create supportive climate for change 2. Discuss personal aspects of poor eating behavior 3. Assess nutrition knowledge and beliefs in myths 4. Build on prior nutrition knowledge
Contemplation	Increase self-efficacy	1. Identify problematic behaviors 2. Prioritize behaviors to change 3. Discuss coping strategies 4. Discuss motivations 5. Identify barriers to change and possible solutions 6. Elicit support from family and friends
Preparation	Initiate change	1. Encourage initial small steps to change 2. Discuss attempts to change and ways to succeed
Action	Commitment to change	1. Reinforce decision 2. Encourage self-rewarding behavior 3. Discuss relapse and coping strategies 4. Reinforce self-confidence
Maintenance	Continued commitment	1. Plan follow-up to support changes 2. Reinforce self-rewarding behaviors 3. Increase coping skills 4. Discuss relapse and prevention techniques
Relapse	Reinforce commitment	1. Reassess motivation and barriers 2. Discuss importance of maintaining change 3. Explore new coping strategies

Used with permission. Copyright 1994, Aspen Publishers, Inc. Sandoval W, Heller K, Wiese W.
Stages of Change: A Model for Nutrition Counseling. *Topics in Clinical Nutrition*. June 1994, vol 9:3;64-69.

Table 3.5 Factors Which Can Affect Readiness to Learn

Physical	Pain, fatigue, disability, sensory deprivation
Psychological	Health and illness beliefs, attitude, values, acceptance of illness, motivation to change
Cognitive	Educational level, reading ability, ability to comprehend
Cultural/ Environmental	Ethnic background, religion, health values, social roles, support system, financial standing, home environment

Used by permission. Dietitians in General Clinical Practice, 1992. In: Klawitter B.
The Dietetic Practitioner as Adult Educator: An Overview. *DGCP Newsletter*. 1992; 9; 4: 4-9.

If you are unsure how rigid to make diet limitations for a 78-year-old woman with multiple chronic illnesses, ask her! Say, "How aggressive do you want to be with your food intake now that you understand how it can effect your different medical problems? What are you willing and able to do at home?" You may be surprised! Too often medical practitioners write off people over a certain age and do not expect patients will want to make lifestyle changes that may not increase their life expectancies. But many simple food and lifestyle changes will improve the quality of their lives. It is our responsibility to make patients aware of their nutrition-related options so they can make informed decisions.

It is extremely important that a counselor remain flexible in the acute care setting and return at another time if the patient is vomiting, arguing with a family member, or sleeping during the day when the chart states that the patient has been unable to sleep at night. It is equally important for the intern or dietitian to check the patient's chart and talk to the charge nurse, if possible, about whether the patient knows his or her new diagnosis before entering the room to give a discharge diet instruction.

Many patients and their families are devastated when they find out the patient has diabetes, heart disease, or other life-threatening diseases, and they may not want to talk. The opposite also may be true; they may want and need to talk to someone about what to do. If that is the case, it is a good time to establish rapport by showing concern and empathy, and set their minds at ease by answering their most pressing questions. Of all times, this is a time when the you must avoid overwhelming or confusing the patient with too much information given too fast. If time permits, schedule a second more comprehensive consultation the next day, or if they are leaving that day, let the patient choose which two or three changes he or she will agree to make (from a short prioritized list that you both create) and schedule an outpatient follow-up. See Table 3.6 Communication Techniques for Counseling the Critically Ill.

Orientation to Learning
Maslow's hierarchy of needs describes physiological needs as being the most basic. (12) Safety, belongingness and love, esteem and self-actualization are needs on the progressive steps of the hierarchy. Esteem needs and the motivation to learn are closely related. Consequently, the motivation to learn or change behavior may increase as the client's self-esteem increases. That is why most counselors try to reinforce or build a client's self-esteem during therapy.

Nutrition counseling does not guarantee learning and learning can occur without counseling. The "teachable moment" for the adult occurs when he or she recognizes that a problem needs to be solved. Adult learners want good quality, evidenced-based information so they can actively participate in the decision-making process. However, a client may be motivated to learn by a creative and dynamic counselor. It is important for you to approach adult clients with a positive attitude and believe that they can learn and that learning will have a positive impact on improving their function and well-being. Clients' receptiveness to the counseling experience is influenced by their personalities, attitudes, educational backgrounds, physical characteristics, and even economic situations. (13)

CONSIDERATIONS SPECIFIC TO THE OLDER ADULT

Counseling the older adult presents the potential for ageism. Ageism can be defined as imposing one's own beliefs and values about what an individual can or should be able to do at various ages. A good nutrition counselor must realize there are wide varieties and differences in individual development and that restricting strategies by age may not be valid. Peterson and Eden (14) report that numerous studies have conclusively shown that intelligence does not decline substantially over the lifespan and that healthy older individuals are typically capable of continuing to learn and change behavior into their 60's, 70's, and 80's. Passive learning alone does not engage our higher brain functions or stimulate our senses to integrate new learning. Active learning results in longer-term recall, synthesis, and problem-solving skills than learning by hearing, reading, or watching.

Table 3.6   Communication Techniques for Counseling the Critically Ill

Communication Technique	Suggested Rationale
1. Learn to listen to the patient	Ask patients directly what problems exist. Determine problems then find solutions.
2. Repeat information at least once	The more times a patient hears information, the more it is remembered. When first diagnosed, many people can only remember the most basic information.
3. Provide all pertinent information in writing	Write down pertinent brand names to aid retention. Provide dietitian's phone number for future questions.
4. Urge patients to write down questions	Anxiety of a hospital visit often blocks the memory.
5. Include family members	This emphasizes importance of providers. Provides additional support for patient. Often therapeutic for family to be involved.
6. Always be direct and keep it simple	Avoid medical or nutrition jargon. Do not expect patient to remember names or details. Explain physiology in simple manner to justify changes. Pictures & graphic aids may be appropriate.
7. Compensate for shorter attention span	Medications may make patient unable to concentrate. Make important points first. Reduce length of visit and return more often.
8. Know when enough has been said	Do not pursue counseling when patient is angry or indifferent. Revisit patient on another day.

Used with permission. Copyright 1986 Aspen Publishers, Inc. Adapted from Bell LR.
Nutrition Counseling: the critically and terminally ill patient. *Topics in Clinical Nutrition.* 1986; 1:1: 1-6.

Eldergogy (15) or gerogogy (16) refer to an evolving specialized approach to learning in older adults that utilizes strategies or techniques best suited for the aged. This field of study takes into account the distinct concerns and traits of old age that need to be incorporated into nutrition counseling for the older adult population. Some older adults may appear to have decreased learning abilities because they are physically slower. Research suggests that when adults control the pace of learning, those in their 40's and 50's have the same ability to learn as they had in their 20's and 30's. (17) Speed of perceptions, initiating a response, and of movement are all affected by the neural changes due to aging.(18) In older adults, a brief functional assessment of psychomotor skills (ability to cook food, shop, add more physical activity, and so on) should be carefully done by the nutrition therapist before goals are set and counseling initiated, especially if behavior change necessitates any of these skills.

Deterioration of memory appears to be minor, however, until extreme old age. Research has found inconclusively that the aging adult has increasing difficulty with transfer of information from primary to secondary memory, and particularly in search and retrieval of information from long-term memory. (19) Short-term memory capacity in adults is limited to about 5 to 9 bits of new information at a time. (20) Information in short-term memory is lost with the passing of time and when the memory is overloaded. "Chunking" information often allows the adult learner to increase the short-term memory capacity. (21) Retrieval of information from long-term memory is easier when it has been related to something already known. (20)

Teaching strategies to assist the older adult to adapt to age-associated memory decline are very similar to the guidelines for communicating with a critically ill patient:

- Keep information clear and simple.
- Speak slowly and repeat your major points.
- Support major points with easy-to-understand printed materials.
- Eliminate environmental distractions.
- Correct wrong answers immediately to maintain clarity of your message.

Counseling the older adult includes attention to the sensory changes of aging that have the most significant impact on the teaching-learning process: declines in vision and hearing. These are common physiological deficits in the older age group but may not always correlate with the client's chronological age. Particular strategies to overcome these sensory deficits are listed in Table 3.7.

Research suggests that with increasing age the majority of individuals do become more rigid or set in their ways as one way of coping with stress. (22) Consequently, older adults may be hesitant to learn something new or make changes because they are afraid of failure. Counseling strategies should focus on assessing the client's abilities and pacing the amount and type of information so that success is almost guaranteed. Several studies have identified areas of concern for older adults that can be assessed in the counseling session (23) and may assist the nutrition counselor in the initial assessment process such as age related physiologic changes (i.e., decreased response time, decreased visual acuity) and psychosocial changes (i.e., depression, retirement).

Dietary counseling in long-term care is similar to counseling a resident at home if the person is alert and compliant. (24) When counseling in long-term care, it is important to be warm and cheerful because even if a resident can't hear or see you too well, she or he still can perceive genuineness and respect. Always tell the resident your name and your position and say something like, **"Hello, Mr. Harper, how are you? I'm Jane Jones, the dietitian, and I've come to talk to you about how we can improve your appetite."** Speak slowly and clearly. Unless he is hard of hearing, and that should be in his chart, there is no reason to raise your voice and yell. If it is early in the morning, orient him by saying something like, **"Today is Tuesday and it's snowing outside. The streets are a little icy but it seems to be melting."** Keep your food discussion uncomplicated and practical. Treat the resident as you would a beloved, respected grandparent, not as a child. There are times as a consultant in long-term care when institutionalized residents require creative strategies. This may happen for several reasons: residents may feel angry at restrictions, and they may not want to take responsibility for their health and lives, also, they tend to be frailer with more severe health problems. Since there are many "caregivers" to a resident, there needs to be a collaborative effort to assure adherence to dietary regimes.

CLIENT-CENTERED COUNSELING PROCESS

The focus and purposes of health and wellness counseling are to define the problems, suggest coping behaviors, and facilitate client mastery and control. A counseling process based on a client-centered problem-solving model uses multiple steps: establish rapport with the client, assess the problem(s), determine options and plan strategies, implement opportunities for practice, reassess and adapt strategies, and evaluate the success of the intervention.

Rapport

As mentioned in Chapter 1, possibly the most important single factor that influences the outcome of a consultation is the relationship between the client and the therapist. Careful listening is the most important behavior for building this relationship. You can establish rapport with clients by actively listening to what they have to say, by being genuinely interested in the clients as people not just their health or nutritional problems, by showing an interest and concerted effort in their nutritional well-being, and by being honest, reasonable, and supportive. Adults are more open to learning when they feel they are respected as individuals.

If a client is angry, show concern and respect. Accept responsibility when you are involved and try to make it better. If you are not involved, but could help, offer to communicate on the client's behalf with someone who could help. Don't take abuse and either leave or ask the client to leave if it happens. Document what happened and what was said in case the issue is not over.

Table 3.7 Visual and Auditory Barriers to Learning

Changes of Aging	Teaching Strategies
Decreased visual acuity	Use high-density lighting Use sharp, contrasting colors Use large print and low-vision aids Encourage use of glasses Use taped cassettes as aids
Distorted color perception	Avoid using the colors blue, green and violet
Increased glare	Avoid using shiny surfaces or plastic in teaching aids
Inability to hear high-pitched sounds	Speak slower with greater separation of words Speak in low-pitched tones Use nonverbal communication techniques Use audiovisuals for content communication Avoid background noise

Used by permission. Dietitians in General Clinical Practice, 1992. In: Klawitter B. The Dietetic Practitioner as Adult Educator: An Overview. *DGCP Newsletter.* 1992; 9; 4: 4-9.

Assessment

Assessments serve many functions such as identifying a client's problems or strengths, physical or biochemical abnormalities, abilities or limitations, health risks and so on. As a therapist, you choose how much time and how much value you place on the assessment phase. Some good therapists spend only a few minutes on formally assessing a client at the beginning of the initial consult and instead casually assess the client through one or more sessions. Others using the more medical model, choose to define the situation at that point in time and design future therapy. Whichever style you use is not so important as making sure the results of the assessment actually affect therapy (one diet should not fit all), and that the client is reassessed at each visit to finely tune the therapy to his or her needs.

Assessment is a two-step process: first, information gathering and second, data interpretation by both the therapist and the client. A *learning need* is defined as the difference between the information the client already knows and the information necessary to perform a task or care for oneself. An assessment to determine the client's learning needs is essential so the counseling plan can address the client's deficit in skill or knowledge.

In order to plan and evaluate nutrition counseling, therapists need to assess diet intake with a reasonable degree of accuracy. An evaluation of intake before intervention may help identify problems and target specific areas for modification. Repeating the assessment periodically after intervention will indicate any behavior changes and will provide information to evaluate the effectiveness of counseling.

Assessment should also consider the individual's cognitive function, attitudes, and physical abilities. In certain locales, cultural assessment may also be indicated to elicit detailed cultural factors that may influence intervention strategies. (See Chapter 7 Assessment for more ideas.)

Not all clients may be ready to learn or change behavior and dietetic practitioners do not always have the time to counsel individuals who are not ready either physically or emotionally. With decreasing lengths of stay in the acute care setting, the most that may be accomplished is to assess the level of readiness, document what has been assessed, provide very basic, survival skills/ knowledge, and communicate this to the appropriate referral source after discharge.

Behavioral diagnosis (24) is the systematic identification of health practices that appear to be causally linked to health problems identified in the medical diagnosis. The behavioral diagnosis makes possible the identification of factors that have an influence on health behavior and can aid in selecting

appropriate strategies to aid the client in changing or improving health status. Specific steps in conducting behavioral diagnosis include:
1. Distinguish between behavioral and non-behavioral causes of the problem.
2. Define those behaviors in order of importance.
3. Rank behaviors in order of importance.
4. Assess the changeability of each behavior.
5. Prioritize behaviors in order of importance and changeability.

Behavioral diagnosis may be especially useful for clients with diabetes and weight management concerns in order to achieve specific behavioral changes.

Assessing what information the individual is interested in learning is equally important. Starting with what the client wants to know is recommended even if that information is not what the nutrition counselor feels is most important for the client to know. Client questions may relate to what they believe is of immediate use. If these questions or concerns are not addressed at the onset, an individual may not hear important information being given by the counselor. Providing information that is important to the individual first acknowledges the client's independence in decision making. Meeting the clients' learning needs keeps their interest better and motivates them to stay involved.

The stress of illness can interfere with the ability and motivation to learn. Frustration may result from such factors as lack of experience with the health care system, unfamiliarity with medical terms, and the inability to grasp concepts as rapidly as in the past. Denial of illness is a common defense mechanism, especially in the older adult and in parents of a sick child. Before nutrition counseling can begin, the adult must acknowledge the health problem. The client must believe that learning and changing behavior will have positive results.

Assessment is not complete until data have been interpreted. In making a counseling need diagnosis, the specific illness, physical attributes, and environmental influences must all be considered. Gaining knowledge about a client's strengths, limitations, and coping patterns is fundamental to setting priorities and planning counseling goals, methods, and approaches. Assessment also serves to establish a baseline of data for therapy interaction and conversation, and future evaluations.

Planning

Once a counseling relationship has been established, the nutrition counselor must remain non-judgmental, regardless of the client's feelings, and coordinate a counseling plan of care. The counseling plan is based on the outcome of the assessment and the diagnosis of an individual's learning needs. The plan should contain learning goals/ objectives, information to be covered, and counseling strategies to be utilized. An individual plan, formulated with the client, takes into account any barriers previously identified.

1. Goals and Objectives Danish suggests that the terms "goals" and "objectives" should be reinterpreted to make them more consistent with today's emphasis on smaller steps and permanent changes, especially in weight control. (25) He believes that to "lose 30 pounds" is the *result,* not the goal. Psychologically, clients often become discouraged by goals that are so "far away." He stresses that the goals should be behavioral just like the objectives and within the person's power like "exercise three times per week for 30 minutes" or "eat only when physically hungry and stop when just full" or "set a boundary of 7 hours per week spent on volunteer projects." Goals and objectives would have basically the same meaning, but could be classified as "goals and sub-goals." A sub-goal could be to "make a tub of margarine last two weeks instead of one week," or to "buy new walking-type dress shoes to wear at work" so the client walks more. This new concept helps clients see change as more achievable, and they mentally recognize and acknowledge the importance of small steps in achieving lifestyle changes. Measurable goals help a client gain knowledge and develop skills. See Chapter 8 using this new approach.

Goals state, in very clear and precise terms, what the client will be able to do when the learning is completed. They define content, direct counseling strategies and learning experiences, set up the learning environment, and assist with evaluating program success. They are statements of what is to be achieved and should be clearly stated in terms of expected client outcomes, the result of the counseling process. A goal should describe both the kind of behavior expected and the content/context to which that behavior applies. Performance goals provide direction for clients, helping them understand the specific behaviors they must master to achieve a certain health status. They also allow clients to evaluate their own progress for themselves, which helps them become more independent.

Three Domains of Learning. The objectives of learning are classified into levels of behavior called the three domains of learning. (26) These domains include cognitive, affective and psychomotor skills.

The **cognitive domain** involves intellectual skills and refers to the specific knowledge and understanding an individual has or is given regarding a specific subject. Decision-making skills fall into this area, as decisions are a cognitive process. Beliefs, rational or irrational, can influence how a person chooses to make change.

The **affective domain** relates to attitudes and feelings and is also critical in reaching the desired goals of the client. The individual may have the knowledge and the skills necessary to perform a task but is unwilling or unmotivated to carry it out. The affective domain is sometimes the most difficult to identify but can have a profound effect on the success of nutrition counseling. Responsive listening and other communication skills can assist clients in exploring their own feelings, thoughts, and behaviors to gain insights of themselves and their environment.

Psychomotor skills are the third domain and are a complex interplay of the neurological and musculo-skeletal systems. A client may have the ability to process information necessary to learn a skill but may not actually be able to perform the skill. The focus is on specific, observable behaviors rather than feelings and thoughts. Vision, perception, tactile sensation, coordination, and muscle strength are involved.

Behavior Change Techniques. Practice and the use of behavioral change techniques in counseling imply client involvement. Nutrition counselors can make suggestions to clients and give guidance, but individuals ultimately must decide what they want to do. The nutrition counselor can develop the framework by suggesting achievable goals and approaches to meet those goals, and solicit feedback from the client. Goals should be realistic so they can be achieved within the time frame available for counseling. Short- and long-term strategies need to be designed to achieve the counseling objectives. Accomplishing short-term objectives as a step toward achieving the long-term plan enhances motivation and provides an opportunity for more client interaction.

2. Content The second aspect of the planning phase relates to the content to be discussed with the client. A major component of most nutrition education programs is didactic in nature, focusing on disease characteristics and the relationship of nutrition to treatment and/or prevention. In traditional acute care nutrition counseling, the didactic technique is typically undertaken during a single teaching session. The underlying assumption in presentations of this type is that the more the person knows, the better off they will be and the more willing or able they will be to participate in self-care activities. There is evidence to suggest, however, that the standard presentation of medical facts and treatment regimens is relatively ineffective in fostering the desired behaviors or helping clients cope. (27) It is presumptuous to expect major and lasting lifestyle changes on the basis of such short-term interventions. Long-term intervention with practice of new behaviors, confrontation of old beliefs and adequate time to discuss physiology and disease process when the timing is appropriate, i.e., the blood pressure continues to rise, the person experiences hypoglycemia, or new lab values show improvement, is more effective.

3. Counseling Strategies Counseling strategies like participant modeling and contracting can provide for learning, and when coupled with a strong helping relationship, they can expedite the client's feeling, thought, and behavior changes. Counseling strategies relate to overall approaches to achieving short- and long-term goals. Instructional methods, like viewing a videotape or selecting from a menu, are another consideration of the counseling plan. The method of learning should correspond to the learning style of the client and relate directly to the goals and objectives.

The amount of time available for the counseling relationship is important in the selection of strategies. Some strategies can be implemented in shorter time spans as compared to others; behavioral strategies can be relatively short-term whereas psychoanalytic therapy can last indefinitely. With shortened hospital stays and the resulting limited time for counseling, media can be very useful to the nutrition counselor. Media, including both printed and audiovisual materials, can present repetitive information in an *interesting* manner as well as save staff time. Media, however, should not solely replace individualized one-on-one interaction.

To plan for a positive learning environment, several factors should be considered. When possible, extraneous noise should be minimized, as such distractions can decrease concentration for both the counselor and the client and detract from the counseling session. Other aspects of the environment that should be considered include furniture arrangement, lighting, temperature, a positive atmosphere, and adequate time for counseling. (28)

4. Implementation Once there is agreement on goals and objectives (or sub-goals), opportunities to practice a behavior or skill should be provided. Practice should be integrated throughout daily activities. By having the client practice skills in your office or in the hospital, you provide a clear and precise definition of what the individual is to do at home in terms of diet, exercise or lifestyle changes, and implementation becomes more feasible. Continued practice in diet selection has been accomplished in inpatient and outpatient settings through the use of sample menus and food models. Some health care facilities have access to private dining areas in which clients have a more realistic opportunity to select foods. In this way, learning takes place in incremental steps and clients are not overwhelmed with too much change at one time.

Therapists who treat clients for weight loss admit being particularly concerned about their clients who do not stray from the guidelines and never test their boundaries because they do not develop the coping strategies necessary to handle unexpected events and stresses. It is much better for clients to experiment with eating out and being flexible at social events during counseling so they have support readily available while they learn how to handle the experiences.

5. Evaluation This should be ongoing from the time intervention strategies are implemented. An evaluation aids in determining whether clients have acquired the knowledge or skill to change their behavior. The ultimate evaluation of success is realized when the client has changed his behavior and is complying with the therapeutic regime. This is extremely difficult to evaluate in the hospital inpatient setting since changes in nutrition/diet behavior usually occur after the client is discharged.

Several types of evaluation methodology have been outlined in the literature: (29)

Reaction evaluation: data is collected about how the client is responding to a program or plan of care as the program progresses. This type of evaluation provides information to make program modifications while it is in progress. A summary page with goals/sub-goals, lab values, weight, and other pertinent indicators could be in each chart.

Learning evaluation: data is collected about the cognitive skills the client has acquired. Performance/demonstration activities, recall or problem solving can be used to gauge knowledge.

Behavior evaluation: observations about actual changes in what the client does after learning versus before are evaluated through questionnaires, self-rating scales, and interviews.

Results evaluation: routine records, such as admission data, costs, and lab results are reviewed for changes.

Evaluation has always been difficult because, except for behavioral strategies, there are not always observable criteria. Evaluating whether a skill has been learned may be the easiest to measure, whereas it is more difficult to measure values or attitude changes. Behavioral strategies are more specifically evaluated and easier to limit in a given timeframe whereas those strategies that lean toward the affective domain can take longer to evaluate for effectiveness.

Cognitive learning may be evaluated using such techniques as:

- Application of information (able to use exchanges in planning a meal)
- Verbal rehearsal (rehearse through role-play what to do when offered a dessert)
- Verbal commitment (Client states, "I can walk at least two miles three days a week.")
- Role reversal (Counselor says, "What would you tell a friend who was in this situation and needed sound advice?")

If the right questions are asked, both knowledge and its application can be assessed. Measurements of diet intake as part of an educational evaluation also may indicate diet-related goals that were or were not achieved. Based upon continual evaluations, the counselor and client may decide to utilize another strategy, revise goals, or terminate the counseling relationship.

Documentation of client counseling in the medical record is vital. It is equally important to document client response to the learning. If a brochure is given, a sheet of instructions provided, or a movie shown, the task of nutrition counseling is often checked off as complete. The emphasis was on methodology and content, not the client's response. Knowledge, skills, and behavior changes need to be documented. As Doris Derelian, PhD, RD, JD, says, "You can't write in the chart that you counseled a patient if all you did was hand out written pieces of paper. The patient must know the topic better or be able to do something better than before you began to call it counseling." (See Chapter 6 Measuring Competency regarding documentation of patient care.)

SUMMARY

Nutrition counseling is an important independent function of professional dietetic practice. This overview, based on how adults differ from children in their learning focus, should form a basic philosophy for client counseling. These beliefs and assumptions can serve to help place nutrition counseling into a perspective where the client is the focus. You can facilitate learning and change by incorporating concepts of adult learning into your practice. In years past, the dietitian set the intended outcomes, made independent decisions about what to teach to accomplish the goals, and decided how to present the content. In contrast, the nutrition counselor, using the learning concepts reviewed in this book, would involve the client in setting goals and in deciding how to achieve them.

Nutrition counseling in the acute care setting is a challenge, primarily due to the lack of time available and the acuity of care levels. Using good assessment techniques, sticking to the "need to know" survival content as much as possible, simplifying instructions, streamlining programs, providing opportunities for practice, providing reference and resource materials, and referring clients for further follow up counseling will help get the process done more efficiently and effectively.

Assessment of your counseling strengths should be ongoing. Counseling is both an art and a science. It is an "art" in that the personality, values, and demeanor of the nutrition counselor are important variables that are subjective and difficult to define or to measure. Counseling can be considered a "science" in that much of what we know about human behavior and many of the helping strategies have been developed as structured, measurable, objective concepts. Dietetic practitioners may be skilled in a variety of areas such as group facilitation, individual or family counseling, or the preparation of written materials. Questions nutrition counselors may ask themselves include: (30)
1. Did I help my client achieve their objectives as quickly as possible?
2. Did I use the most efficient strategies?
3. Would a referral source better serve my client?
4. Were my counseling strategies appropriate for this particular client?

Learning Activities

1. Observe a family nutrition counseling session with an older adult patient in an acute care setting. What role does each family member play in the counseling session? What interactions between family members do you observe? What impact does the nutrition problem being addressed play on the family unit as a whole?
2. Counsel (or observe a counseling session) for an adult. What counseling strategies are utilized? How does the client respond to each strategy identified? What changes would you recommend if the session was repeated based on your observations?
3. Participate in a group nutrition education session involving adults over age 55. What age-specific considerations should be made? How would you evaluate whether or not learning or change would take place? How would the same program be altered if the average age of the participants were under age 30?

References
1. Knowles MS. *The Adult Learner: a Neglected Species.* Houston, TX: Gulf Publishing; 1973.
2. Conner ML. *Learning: The Critical Technology,* 2nd ed. St. Louis, MO: Wave Technologies International, Inc.; 1996.
3. Knowles M. Program planning for adults as learners. *Adult Leadership.*1967;16: 267.
4. Johnson DW, Johnson RT. Nutrition education's future. *J Nutr Education.* 1985; 17: 20-24.
5. Napier RW, Gershenfeld MK. *Groups: Theory and Experience.* Atlanta GA: Houghton Mifflin Company; 1973.
6. Kerka S. *Adult learner retention revisited.* ERIC: http://ericacve.org/docs/retain.htm; 1995.
7. Havighurst R. *Human Development and Education.* New York NY: David McKay Company; 1953.
8. Sandoval W, Heller K, Wiese W, Childs D. Stages of Change: A model for nutrition counseling. *Topics in Clinical Nutrition.* 1994; vol. 9 (3): 64-69.
9. Prochaska JO, Norcross JC, DiClemete CC. *Changing for Good.* New York: Wm Morrow; 1994.
10. Prochaska JO. *Systems of Psychotherapy,* 2nd ed. Homewood, IL: Dorsey Press; 1984.
11. Bell LR. Nutrition counseling the critically ill and terminally ill patient. *Topics in Clinical Nutrition.* 1986; 1 (1): 16.
12. Maslow A. *Motivation and Personality.* New York: Harper and Row; 1970.
13. Williams SR. *Nutrition and Diet Therapy.* St. Louis: C.V. Mosby Company; 1989.
14. Peterson DA, Eden DZ. Cognitive style and the older learner. *Ed. Gerontology.* 1981; 7: 51-66.
15. Yeo G. Eldergogy: a specialized approach to education for elders. *Lifelong Learning: The Adult Years.* 1982; 5(5): 47.
16. Billie DA. Educational strategies for teaching the elderly patient. *Nursing and Health Care.* 1980; 256-263.
17. Cross P. *Adults as Learners.* San Francisco CA: Jossey-Bass; 1981.
18. Hicks LH, Birren JE. Aging, brain damage and psychomotor slowing. *Psych. Bulletin.* 1970; 74: 390.
19. Arenberg D, Robertson-Tchabo E. Learning and aging. In: Birren J, Schaie K, eds. *Handbook of the Psychology of Aging.* New York: Van Nostrand; 1977.
20. Cruikshank DR, Bainer DL, Metcalf KK. *The Act of Teaching.* New York: McGraw-Hill Inc.; 1995.
21. Dixon NM. *The Organizational Learning Cycle: How We Can learn Collectively.* London: McGraw-Hill; 1994.
22. Chown SM. Age and rigidities. *J Gerontology.* 1961; 16: 353-362.
23. Kicklighter JR. Characteristics of older adult learners: a guide for dietetic practitioners. *J Amer Diet Assoc.* 1991; 91(11): 1418-1422.
24. Green LW. *Health Education Planning: A Diagnostic Approach.* Palo Alto: Mayfield Publishing Company; 1979.
25. Steve Danish, PhD, speaking on "Advanced Counseling Skills" at Annual ADA Convention, Orlando, FL; 1994.
26. Bloom BS, ed. *Taxonomy of Educational Objectives: The Classification of Educational Goals, Handbook 1: Cognitive Domain.* New York: David McKay Company; 1956.
27. Mazzuca SA. Does patient education in chronic disease have therapeutic value? *J Chron Disease.* 1982; 35(2): 521-529.
28. Hoffman SE. Planning for patient teaching based on learning theory. In: Smith CE, ed. *Patient Education: Nurses in Partnership with other Health Professionals.* Philadelphia: W.B. Saunders Company; 1987.
29. Knowles MS. *The Modern Practice of Adult Education.* Chicago: Follett Publishing Company; 1970.
30. Snetselaar LG. *Nutrition Counseling Skills: Assessment, Treatment and Evaluation,* 3rd ed. Gaithersburg, MD: Aspen Publications; 1997.

HERMAN

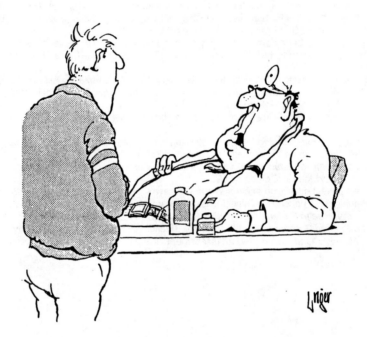

"Are you eating properly and getting plenty of exercise?"

Chapter 4

Personality Styles

Ruth B. Fischer, MS, and Kathy King, RD

After reading this chapter, the reader will be able to:
- ♦ Identify six major factors in personality development.
- ♦ Identify four major types of personal style.
- ♦ Identify dominant personal styles.
- ♦ Determine appropriate counseling approaches for clients based on personal style.

Would you like to increase your credibility and compatibility with others? Would you like to know more about how others think and why they act as they do? Do you wish you were better able to empathize and communicate with others? Can you envision how these skills might be useful for you both personally and professionally? By taking some time to learn more about the concepts of personality development and personal style, you can learn to "read" others better.

PERSONALITY

Just as DNA provides a distinctive genetic framework for each individual, a person's personality provides a unique behavioral framework. A person's personality develops based upon the six major factors described in the Personality Development Model (Figure 4.1). (1)

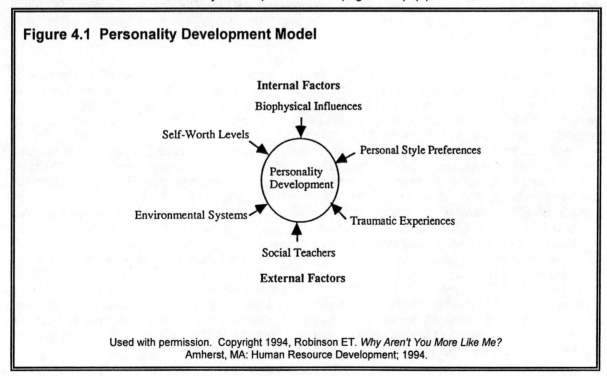

Figure 4.1 Personality Development Model

Internal Factors

Biophysical Influences

Self-Worth Levels

Personal Style Preferences

Personality Development

Environmental Systems

Traumatic Experiences

Social Teachers

External Factors

Used with permission. Copyright 1994, Robinson ET. *Why Aren't You More Like Me?* Amherst, MA: Human Resource Development; 1994.

The Personality Development Model divides factors into internal and external categories.

Internal Factors

Self-worth levels are the part of the personality that governs how a person feels about him or herself. It governs how you evaluate your behavior, appearance, feelings, thoughts, and abilities. It can be influenced by what others say about you, and whether you agree or disagree with what they say. **Those with high self-worth:** (2)

- are less depressed
- evaluate their own performance more positively
- are less prone to addiction
- are more flexible
- think well of others
- are more persistent at difficult tasks
- take more personal responsibility
- are more likely to admit personal faults

Those with low self-worth: (2)

- expect to be rejected
- display little self-respect
- are more resistant to change
- take personal criticism poorly
- are less open with personal information
- suffer more from stress related illness

Biophysical influences are all the biological and physical influences that affect you over your lifetime. Genetics, biochemical occurrences, like puberty, pregnancy and aging, and illnesses all have an impact on your view of yourself.

Personal style preferences are the naturally occurring preferences you have that influence how you perceive, approach, and interact with information and situations. The next section focuses on this factor.

External Factors

Traumatic experiences are any experiences that produce severe stress, whether physical or emotional. It can begin as a positive or negative event; the key is whether or not the experience leaves you feeling victimized. Different individuals will react differently to similar events. Such common events as birth of a child, divorce, promotion, job termination, and even falling off a bicycle, are examples of events that may affect your personality.

Social teachers are the people who directly or indirectly provide positive or negative influence on your personality development. These people, often referred to as role models, have lasting effects on thinking, personality, and behavior, and may include: parents, siblings, school teachers, religious leaders, friends, mentors, supervisors, authors, artists, and so on.

Environmental systems are any other form of experience not specifically covered in the other categories, including your social environment, community, and cultural, ethnic, and religious influences. See Chapter 5 on Cultural influences for more detail.

After becoming more acquainted with what influences and contributes to personality development, it is much easier to appreciate the complexity of your own and your client's personalities. It is apparent why nutrition counselors: work hard to boast clients' feelings of self-worth; probe to discover the client's important behavioral and nutrition-related social teachers; identify traumatic food or body image experiences faced by their clients; and have become more interested in personal styles. Counselors use all of this information and their skills to build on clients' positive experiences and neutralize or retrain the negative ones.

PERSONALITY DISORDER

When counseling, there may be times when a client comes diagnosed with a personality disorder. Usually, however, you don't know much outside of the medical diagnosis. Nor do clients introduce themselves with, "Hi, I'm Mary Smith. I'm passive-aggressive and angry about this diagnosis." Instead, clients will act out who they are: from calm and level headed to suspicious, distant, self-important, and so on. Without advanced training, you should not go beyond your scope of practice into psychological counseling, but you will see these behaviors and they can affect your success.

Table 4.1 Developmental Personality Styles

Style and Positive Aspect	Behavior/Thoughts in Session	Possible Family History	Predicted Current Relationships	Possible Treatment Approach
Antisocial It is sometimes necessary to be impulsive and take care of our own needs.	Acts out; cannot sustain task; involved in crime, drugs, truancy, physical fights; cruel, maltreats family; tries to "con" therapist.	Probable abuse as a child; avoidant family forced child to take matters into own hands; little affection in home.	Abusive; exploitive relationships; fear of abandonment.	Be open, honest; and set clear limits; avoid entanglement; expect client to leave treatment if gets close.
Avoidant It is useful to deny or avoid some things.	Avoids people, shy, unwilling to become involved, distant; exaggerates risk.	Either engulfing family or avoidant family; enacting what the family modeled.	Not many friends; easily becomes dependent on them or therapist.	Use many behavioral and cognitive techniques; assertiveness training and relaxation training useful.
Borderline Intensity in relationship is desirable at times.	Pushes therapist's buttons skillfully; impulsive; intense anger or caring; suicidal gestures.	Enmeshed family during early childhood; lack of support for individuation; probable sexual abuse.	Serial, intense relationships; may have close friends; relationships may move rapidly between extreme closeness and distance.	Confront engulfment and support individuation-- do opposite of family; group/systems approaches are useful.
Dependent We all need to depend on others.	Dependency on therapist even out of session; indecision; little sense of self.	Engulfing, controlling family; not allowed to make decision; rewarded for inaction; told what to do.	Dependent on friends; drives people away with demands.	Reward action; support efforts for self; use paradox, assertiveness techniques.
Narcissistic A strong belief in ourselves is necessary for good mental health.	Grandiose, self-important, sees self as very unique; sense of entitlement; lacks empathy; oriented toward success and perfection.	Received perfect mirroring for accomplishments rather than for self; engulfing family; anxious/ambivalent caregiver.	Focuses on selfish needs, tends to engulf others with needs; is charming to get wishes met, Don Juan type; may pair with borderline.	Interpret behavior; look to past; employ cognitive behavioral, sensitivity training in a group.
Obsessive-Compulsive Maintaining order and a system is necessary for job success.	Perfectionistic and inflexible; focuses on details, making lists; workaholic; indecisive.	Overattached family that wanted achievement; keenly aware of others but limited sense of self.	Controlling; limited affect; demands perfection from others; hard worker.	Reflect and provoke feeling orient to client's personal needs; develop self-concept; orient to body awareness.
Paranoid It is important to watch out for injustice.	Suspicious, takes remarks out of context and interprets them to support own frame of reference.	Probable history of persecution, active family rejection.	Controlling behavior; anticipates exploitation, may mistrust friends and family; quick to anger.	Always be honest, never defensive; structure ahead of time; don't argue, you'll only lose.
Passive-Aggressive All of us are entitled to Procrastinate at times.	Procrastinates; seems to agree with therapist, then undercuts; seems to accept therapist, then challenges authority.	Perhaps obsessive family; moves away from perfectionism and fights back; a more healthy defense needs to be developed.	"Couch potato;" skilled at getting back at and at criticizing others; defends by doing nothing; resents suggestions; not pleasant on the job.	Let client learn the consequences of behavior; do not do things for client, but confront and interpret and pay special attention to client reactions.

Used with permission. Ivey A . *Developmental Strategies for Helpers*. Pacific Grove, CA: Brooks/Cole; 1991.

Developmental counseling and therapy (DCT) reinterprets the word *disorder* as a learned "developmental personality style." (3) They are considered defenses used by the client to cope with environmental stressors. In a session, it is important to note the client's behavior, thoughts, and feelings because they are probably indicative of his other interactive relationships. (3) "Professional helpers are usually "nice" people and find it difficult to work with those who are not nice. *If you react to these clients as others in their history have, you can expect them to continue their behavior.* In short, to help clients you must react to client maltreatment of you with patience, firmness, a clear sense of boundaries, and evidence of caring, but without being manipulated." (3)

EXAMINING PERSONAL STYLE

Becoming more comfortable with personal style will impact on your life, both personal and professional, through building skills to better communicate and lead others. Each person has a style of thinking, behaving, and interacting that is unique. This style acts as his or her anchor or systematic framework for viewing the world. These characteristics are grouped into four behavioral styles or personality dimensions. (3,4,5) Most people have a mixture of all four dimensions in their styles, but usually one and sometimes several styles dominate influencing behavior.

Although this tool is not designed as an in-depth psychological examination of human behavior, it provides a simple way of observing and understanding the differences in people through their behaviors. See Table 4.2 on the Four Types of Personal Style.

Flexibility

Knowing the different styles, their strengths and weaknesses, helps you quickly evaluate your client's style in a counseling setting. You will be able to adapt how you present information—the pace and degree of detail, and how you speak in order to reduce communication barriers. People feel most comfortable in communicating and interacting from their style strengths. People tend to trust and cooperate with people who respond and relate to them in the same style pattern. Being able to interact with others from their strengths shows flexibility or style shifting on your part—changing to what makes the client feel comfortable instead of insisting that the client adapt to your style. Although this sounds easy to accomplish, practice will make you more adept at shifting your style to match your client's. See Table 4.3 on flexibility or style shifting.

Openness

Cathcart and Alessandra describe openness as the readiness and willingness with which a person expresses emotions and enters into relationships. (5) It is the degree to which you reveal *your* feelings and thoughts and the degree you accept other peoples' expression of *their* thoughts and feelings.

Open people are animated and "open up" right away. They are easiest to work with in a counseling setting because you don't have to work as hard to draw out information. Nonverbal behaviors also show a person's openness such as frequent eye contact, hand and body gestures, and changes in posture and facial expressions. (5) These people are more casual and flexible. They are not as specific in terms of numbers or specifics; it is not that important to them. Human relationships count heavily with these people.

Self-contained people are just the opposite of an open person. Cathcart and Alessandra describe these people as taking awhile to show warmth or become involved in relationships. They are task-oriented, well organized, and enjoy the planning process. They like structure and want to know the guidelines and procedures. They are on time and expect you to start your appointments on time. They are rational, logical, detail-oriented. Small talk is not needed with this person and they don't tell a lot of personal stories.

Directness

Another behavior dimension is directness. It shows how a person deals with information or situations. (5) **Direct** people are fast-paced, assertive, competitive, dominant risk-takers who want results NOW! **Indirect** people, on the other end of the scale, are slow-paced, unassertive, quiet, cooperative, and better listeners than direct individuals. They do not want to "rock the boat." They are non-confrontational and will seek roundabout approaches.

Table 4.2 Four Types of Personality Style

(Self- | Contained)

DIRECTOR/ BEHAVIORAL
(Action)

General Orientation: Self-Contained and Direct

To tasks:	Wants results now
To people:	Seeks authority
To problems:	Tactical, strategic
To stress:	Doubles effort, will dictate, "If you can't stand the heat get out of the kitchen."
To time:	Future and present

Typical Strengths
Acts rapidly to get results
Is inventive and productive
Shows endurance under stress
Is driven to achieve goals
Can take authority boldly

Common Difficulties
Can be too forceful or impatient
Can often think their way is best
Can be insensitive to others
Can be manipulative or coercive
Can be lonely or fatigued

THINKER/ COGNITIVE
(Analysis)

General Orientation: Self-Contained and Indirect

To tasks:	Wants quality
To people:	Seeks security
To problems:	Analyzes data
To stress:	Withdraws, "I can't help you any further; do what you want." (5)
To time:	Past and future

Typical Strengths
Acts cautiously to avoid errors
Engages in critical analysis
Seeks to create a low stress climate
Slow, steady, methodical
Complies with authority, "show me" attitude

Common Difficulties
Can bog down in details
Can be too critical and finicky
Can be overly sensitive to feedback
Can seem to be lacking in courage
Can be too self-sufficient, alone

(Direct)

(Indirect)

SOCIALIZER/ AFFECTIVE
(Expressive)

General Orientation: Open and Direct

To tasks:	People come first
To people:	Seeks to influence
To problems:	Intuitive and creative
To stress:	Will confront it, "Listen you turkey I've taken your abuse long enough." (5)
To time:	Future and present

Typical Strengths
Spontaneous, gregarious
Acts creatively on intuition
Is sensitive to others' feelings
Is resilient in times of stress
Develops a network of contacts
Is often willing to help others

Common Difficulties
Can lose track of time
Can "overburn" and over-indulge
Can be too talkative
Can lose objectivity, be emotional
Can be self-oriented, self-assured

RELATER/ INTERPERSONAL
(Harmony)

General Orientation: Open and Indirect

To tasks:	Reliable performance
To people:	Seeks to help others
To problems:	Practical solutions
To stress:	Will submit, "OK, if that's the way you must have it, we'll try it." (5)
To time:	Present

Typical Strengths
Promotes harmony and balance
Is reliable and consistent
Tries to adapt to stress
Sees the obvious that others miss
Is often easy-going and warm
Supports and "actively" listens to others

Common Difficulties
Can be too slow to make decisions
Can Allow others to take advantage of them
Can become bitter if unappreciated
Can feel low in self-worth
Can be too dependent on other

(Open)

Table 4.3 Flexibility or Style-Shifting

If your client is:

DIRECTOR/ BEHAVIORAL	THINKER/ COGNITIVE
Extroverted	Introverted

If your client is:

DIRECTOR/ BEHAVIORAL
Extroverted

Needs	Fears
Achievement	Failure
Autonomy	Restriction
Power	Dependency
Rewards	Poverty
Stimulation	Stagnation

Common Personal Characteristics

Abrupt	Determined
Aggressive	Decisive
Bold	Domineering
Competitive	Productive
Courageous	Restless
Responsible	Self-reliant
Strong-minded	Tough
Unemotional	

Gets Most Upset When Others:
Are too slow
Get in their way
Talk too much
Try to be in control
Waste time

Wants Others to:
Give them summarized facts
Respect their judgment
Support them to reach goals
Cope with unwanted details
Cooperate with them

Responds Best To:
Direct, honest confrontations
Logical, rational arguments
Fair, open competition
An impersonal approach
Getting results quickly

THINKER/ COGNITIVE
Introverted

Needs	Fears
Affirmation	Disapproval
Understanding	Confusion
Order	Chaos
Perfection	Incompetence
Respect	Humiliation

Common Personal Characteristics

Accurate	Indecisive
Analytical	Loyal
Cautious	Organized
Conscientious	Perceptive
Critical	Perfectionist
Strict	Structured
Theoretical	Unsociable
Worrisome	

Gets Most Upset When Others:
Move ahead too quickly
Don't give them enough time
Are vague in their communication
Don't appreciate their efforts
Are too personal or emotional

Wants Others To:
Give them detailed information
Ask for their opinions
Not interrupt their work
Treat them with respect
Do quality work the first time

Responds Best To:
Diplomatic, factual challenges
Arguments based on known facts
Freedom from competitive strain
Friendliness, not personal contact
Doing tasks well and completely

Table 4.3 Flexibility or Style-Shifting

If your client is:

SOCIALIZER/ AFFECTIVE		RELATER/ INTERPERSONAL	
Extroverted		Introverted	

If your client is:

SOCIALIZER/ AFFECTIVE
Extroverted

Needs	Fears
Acceptance	Rejection
Attention	Exclusion
Expression	Repression
Recreation	Boredom
Variety	Routine

Common Personal Characteristics

Appealing	Flexible
Compassionate	Friendly
Convincing	Impulsive
Creative	Intuitive
Enthusiastic	Loud
Open-minded	Restless
Talkative	Undisciplined
Unproductive	

Gets Most Upset When Others:
Are too task oriented
Confine them to one place
Are not interested in them
Compete for and win attention
Seem judgmental of them

Wants Others to:
Give them the opportunity to speak
Admire their achievements
Be influenced in some ways
Take care of details for them
Value their opinions

Responds Best To:
Being challenged in a kind way
An influencing sales approach
Enjoy competitions
Affection and personal contact
Having a good time

If your client is:

RELATER/ INTERPERSONAL
Introverted

Needs	Fears
Appreciation	Ungratefulness
Harmony	Conflict
Stability	Instability
Trust	Deception
Unity	Dissension

Common Personal Characteristics

Careful	Hard working
Calm	Lenient
Dependent	Likable
Faithful	Unassertive
Slow	Stubborn
Understanding	Warm
Shares feelings	Slow to act, relaxed
Relationship-oriented	

Gets Most Upset When Others:
Get angry, blow up or are mean
Demand that they change too quickly
Take advantage of their goodness
Are manipulative or unfair
Are judgmental of others

Wants Others To:
Make them feel like they belong
Appreciate them for their efforts
Be kind, considerate, thoughtful
Trust them with important tasks
Value them as persons

Responds Best To:
A gradual approach to challenging
A factual, practical approach
Comfortable, friendly times
Respecting their boundaries
Conventional, established ways

Used by permission. Copyright 1988, Consulting Resource Group International, Inc.

A person's dominant personal style is his or her natural communication comfort zone. It is important to remember that no style is better than another. Each style has its strengths and weaknesses; however, each style may be preferable in a given situation.

Learning how to be flexible in the use of style or style shifting is an important skill to learn. For example, an entrepreneur may be very outgoing and creative (characterized by the socializer/affective style), but is called upon to act concretely and decisively in a business situation (a director/behavioral quality). A more family-oriented example might be, if you are more of a Director/Behavioral style person who likes quick decisions and direct confrontations, and your spouse has a Relater/ Interpersonal style, communication barriers may develop in the relationship. Referring to Table 4.2, what are some of the approaches that would enhance communication and emotional stability in the relationship?

On Table 4.3, three sections under each style teach you what to avoid doing and what to do more. *You should avoid doing things on this list:* "Get most upset when others." *You should try to do more:* "Wants others to" and "Responds best to."

IN COUNSELING SITUATIONS

Director/Behavioral As a counselor, you support their goals and keep the relationship business-like; if you disagree, argue facts. Be precise, efficient; to influence decisions provide alternatives and probabilities of their success. *To motivate: provide options and clearly describe probabilities of success. (5)*

Direct confrontation with this type client or spouse of a client may win them over to your counseling strategy, rather than turn them away, especially if they have shown some reluctance to the counseling environment. These people respond well to directness, logic and respect for his or her judgment.

Thinker/Cognitive As a counselor, you support their organized, thoughtful approach; give researched facts in some detail; allow plenty of time for the consultation; encourage food records or nutrient analysis of what they are eating as a way to stay on top of their progress. These people are often perfectionists, highly organized and expect the same of you. After an interview, follow-up your personal contact by sending a letter. *To motivate: appeal to their need to be accurate and logical; avoid gimmicks. (5)*

These people thrive on planning and will like detailed handouts. They like to be intellectually stimulated, but not overworked. They can be procrastinators and fear failure.

Socializer/Affective As a counselor, you support their ideas and dreams; don't hurry discussion. You need to show interest in this person not just his nutritional problems. Let these type people tell you about their achievements and allow both of you to have a good time in the session. *To motivate: offer them incentives and testimonials.*

Let them brainstorm some strategies that will meet their need for change. Remember, it is easy for them to get side-tracked.(5)

These people like creative and interactive approaches to learning and problem solving. They become easily bored and like new challenges.

Relater/Interpersonal As a counselor, you support their feelings; show personal interest; accurately explain objectives; when you disagree, discuss personal opinions and feelings; move along in an informal manner; provide assurances that actions or decisions will involve minimum risk. *To motivate: appeal to how it will make them and others feel better.*

These people like personal warmth and friendliness in relationships and enjoy sharing "war" stories.

As a professional, applying the information learned from understanding styles to foster credibility and empathy with others is appropriate and powerful. It should not be used to manipulate others, but for enhancing human relationships.

Learning Activities

1. Using the descriptions for the four personal styles in Table 4-2 to help you, identify your dominant personal style and those of your family members, friends, and a few colleagues or clients. It is helpful to think of the characteristics aligning themselves on two axes: open versus self-contained and direct and indirect. If you can't decide, asking three simple questions will help you place individuals into their dominant style.
    - "Is the person open or self-contained?
    - "Is the person direct (fast-paced, assertive, risk-taker) or indirect (slower-paced, quiet, non-confrontational)?"
    - "Is the person task-oriented (well-organized, detail-oriented, self-contained) or people-oriented (opens up easily, casual, flexible)?"

By plotting your answers, you can easily determine which is the person's strongest style dimension.

References
1. Robinson ET. *Why Aren't You More Like Me?*. Amherst, MA: Human Resource Development Press, Inc; 1994.
2. Robinson ET. *Self Worth Inventory*. Abbotsford, BC, Canada: Consulting Resource Group International, Inc; 1990.
3. Ivey AE, Ivey MB, Simek-Morgan L. Counseling and Psychotherapy: A multicultural approach, 3rd ed. Boston, MA: Allyn and Bacon; 2001.
4. Anderson TD, Robinson ET. *Personal Style Indicator*. Abbotsford, BC, Canada: Consulting Resource Group International, Inc; 1988.
5. Anderson TD. *The Therapeutic Style Indicator*. Amherst, MA: Microtraining Assoc; 1987.
6. Cathcart J, Alessandra T. *Relationship Strategies.* Palo Alto, CA: Cathcart, Alessandra and Assoc; 1984. (Audiocassette program through Nightingale-Conant Corporation)

Ballard Street by Jerry Van Amerongen

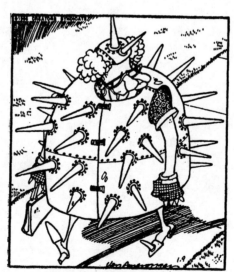

Harmony is no longer a part of Gloria's belief system.

Used by permission of Jerry Van Amerongen and Creators Syndicate

Chapter 5

Cultural Competency in Counseling

Rosie Gonzales, MS, RD, LD and Bridget Klawitter, PhD, RD, FADA

After reading this chapter, the reader will be able to:
- Identify one's own cultural values and beliefs.
- Define cultural competence and determine personal competence.
- Identify the single most important factor in achieving a successful counseling relationship.
- Identify culture-specific characteristics that may impact counseling strategies.
- List communication skills that are of benefit in the multicultural setting.

We live in a society that is growing more culturally diverse at a very rapid rate. According to U. S. Census projections, by the year 2000 more than one-third of the population was racial and ethnic minorities, and by 2010 these population groups will become a numerical majority.(1) It is meaningless to talk of the white majority as multiracial families through interracial marriages, cross-racial adoptions, blended families through divorce and remarriage all bring about families and communities where racial boundaries and cultural differences are blurred. As our society continues to change and become more diverse, it is essential for the counseling professions to develop a multicultural perspective.(1) We must realize that every ethnic and racial group has a unique system of values and beliefs, which influences behavior either directly or indirectly. This means that a "standard" approach to counseling is no longer appropriate. This standard system does not account for the differences and unique needs of diverse populations. In order to meet these needs, we must take responsibility in becoming competent and skilled in working with the culturally different client.

The purpose of this chapter is to help you develop awareness, understanding, acceptance, and the communication skills necessary for becoming a culturally skilled counselor. Although the chapter will discuss several ethnic groups, the goal is not to provide in-depth information about any one group. Rather, it is to make the reader aware of the uniqueness of each culture, and the importance of understanding the barriers to effective multicultural counseling and communication.

Cultural competence is a set of congruent behaviors, attitudes, and policies that come together and enable professionals to work effectively in cross-cultural situations. (2) The word "culture" is used as it implies the integrated pattern of human thoughts, communications, actions, customs, beliefs, values, and institutions of a racial, ethnic, religious, or social group. The word "competence" is used because it implies having a capacity to function effectively. (2) Culture shapes an individual's experiences, perceptions, decisions and how they relate to others. It influences the way patients perceive medicine and healthcare providers.

Cultural knowledge is familiarization with the selected cultural characteristics, history, values, belief systems, and behaviors of another ethnic group. (3) Some use cultural sensitivity and cultural awareness interchangeably, while others believe these are simply steps towards cultural competence. **Cultural sensitivity** is being aware that cultural differences, as well as similarities, exist without assigning values to those differences. (4) **Cultural awareness** is developing a sensitivity and understanding of another ethnic group. (3) This usually involves internal changes in attitudes and values and must be supplemented with cultural knowledge.

The Professional Standards Committee of the Association for Multicultural Counseling and Development produced a basic set of competencies and standards, which define the attributes of a culturally skilled counselor. This chapter will outline these criteria by discussing three essential elements for effective multicultural counseling: a) awareness of your own values and beliefs, b) understanding and knowledge of the clients' world-view, and c) acquiring appropriate communication skills. (1)

AWARENESS OF YOUR CULTURAL VALUES AND BELIEFS

Before you can work successfully with diverse populations, it is essential that you become aware of your own culture. It is not simply your ethnic heritage, but it is everything that influences what you believe, such as your religion, language, social status, level of education, gender, age, family, and ethnic group. (5) Dillard defines culture as the sharing of belief systems, behavioral styles, symbols, and attitudes within a social group. (6)

Depending on each person's background experiences and the culture to which he or she belongs, both the counselor and the client have a variety of characteristics and values that are brought to a counseling session. These influence communication and learning. Understanding your own set of values and beliefs will help you know your limitations and can assist you in becoming more aware of certain biases and prejudices which can affect your abilities as a multicultural counselor. In order to begin thinking about how your background may affect your abilities as a counselor, Ivey, et al (7) suggests that you ask yourself the following questions:

- What is your ethnic heritage?
- Are you monocultural, bicultural, or more?
- What messages do you receive from each racial or ethnic group you have listed?
- How might your cultural messages affect your work as a counselor?

The last question will be most helpful in making you aware of your limitations as a multicultural counselor. For example, let's assume that as a result of your upbringing, you view thinness as a desirable and healthy goal and cannot understand how anyone would want to be overweight. Now, assume that you are counseling a Native American client on diabetes, and part of your diabetic instruction promotes weight loss. However, your client considers thin people to be in poor health and overweight people to be very happy and healthy. If you are unable to accept your client's views about body size without mixing them with your own thoughts and feelings, there will be much conflict in the counseling session, and you can expect very little behavior change. Once you understand your own views, they must remain separate from those of your clients. It is not your job as a counselor to agree with your clients, but to empathetically understand their world-view without placing judgment. (7)

UNDERSTANDING AND KNOWLEDGE OF CLIENTS' WORLD-VIEW

Lack of awareness about cultural differences can make it difficult for both the counselor and client to achieve the most appropriate care. You do not have to be of the same ethnic background as your client in order to provide effective counseling. (6) In the same respect, belonging to a particular ethnic group does not automatically make you a culturally skilled counselor. (1) To be most effective, you must be able to understand the world-view of your client and to communicate this understanding to him or her. (5) American Indians call this "walking in another man's moccasins," and psychotherapists describe this as an empathetic relationship. (7) Research suggests that establishing an empathetic relationship is the single most important and necessary factor to identify successful counseling. (5)

As implied in the previous section, knowledge about your client's culture is a key attribute in the empathetic relationship. You do not need to know everything there is to know about their culture, but it is important to acquire basic knowledge of the cultural groups you will be counseling. Referring back to the example of the Native American woman with diabetes, it would be helpful if you had some knowledge about this client's values, such as the traditional value of harmony with nature. This particular value may provide an incentive for weight loss, since some tribes consider overweight a condition, which conflicts with the laws of nature. (8)

Ivey, et al (7) suggests that a counselor working with diverse groups have knowledge in the following areas: specific knowledge about the client's culture; understanding of the sociological role of minorities in the U.S.; knowledge of the generic counseling literature; and knowledge of barriers that prevent minorities from using mental health services appropriately. The most common way to learn about your clients' culture is through books and audio/visual media. However, you will not fully understand them unless you also make a commitment to listen to and learn from other groups. (7) This may mean becoming actively involved with individuals from other cultural groups through friendships, projects, community events, or social gatherings. (1)

Since it is beyond the scope of this chapter to discuss all ethnic groups in great detail, some of the fastest growing minority groups in the U. S. are outlined in Table 5.1. (1) It should not be assumed, however, that every individual of a group has the same characteristics. Although clients belonging to one of the ethnic groups listed may share common values and experiences, you should keep in mind that acceptance and practice of these values will vary according to a client's acculturation, socialization, and identification with the culture. Thus, the information in Table 5.1 should act only as a guide to enhance your awareness of cultural differences.

MULTICULTURAL COMMUNICATION SKILLS IN COUNSELING

Awareness, understanding, and knowledge of your clients' views as well as your own will be most effective if appropriate skills are also learned. (1,5) When there are cultural and ethnic differences between the counselor and the client, some of the most important skills you can acquire are effective verbal and nonverbal communication skills. Without good communication between you and your client, little, if any, progress toward behavior change can be expected. (6) Understanding what your client says, how he or she says it, and even what he or she doesn't say, are all very important factors that a multicultural counselor must be aware of.

Language

If you have ever been in a foreign country, you know just how frustrating it is for clients for whom English is a second language. The ideal situation is for the counselor to be bilingual, but of course, this is not always possible. In order to overcome the language barrier with clients who have trouble expressing their thoughts in English, counselors need to have extra patience and time for a successful counseling relationship. Counselors must also avoid several language barriers to effective multicultural communication, such as the use of complex vocabulary, technical jargon, and an unnatural communication style. (8,9,10)

It is important to speak slowly and clearly, use simple vocabulary, and avoid the use of slang, or technical jargon. However, you must also be cautious not to treat your clients as if they are uneducated. Just because your client does not speak English well, does not mean he or she is not intelligent. Adults should be treated as adults, just simplify the terminology. It is also important to know that your client may understand English much better than he or she can speak it, and he or she may be able to speak English better than he or she can read the language. (9)

The use of medical jargon and complex ideas can cause much confusion for multicultural clients. For example, there was the case of a doctor who gave a diagnosis of gastroenteritis for a ten-year-old Hispanic girl. However, the little girl's mother understood that her daughter had swallowed an entire cat. The doctor did not realize that "gastro" sounds like gato (cat) and "enteritis" like entero (whole) in Spanish. It is important to explain things in easy-to-understand language, and take time to be sure the client understands. (8)

Do not try to imitate an ethnic group's communication style, which is not natural for you. For example, a Black American client may find it patronizing and disrespectful if an Anglo-American counselor unnaturally tries to use Black slang in order to show that he or she understands the client. As one Black American once put it "anyone who tries too hard to show that he understands Blacks doesn't understand us at all." (11) It is important to be yourself and act natural because clients can see through unnatural behavior.

> **It is important to be yourself and act natural because clients can see through unnatural behavior.**

It may be necessary to have an interpreter if you and the client do not speak the same language. Remember to allow more time for the counseling session and realize it may be difficult to translate certain concepts. Some tips for effective communication with an interpreter include the following:

- Use a bilingual staff member, community volunteer, or adult family member or friend if a qualified interpreter is not available; do not use children as an interpreter for their parents or adult family members.
- Be sure the interpreter understands the goals of the counseling session.

- Maintain visual contact with the client and address him or her instead of the interpreter.
- Use language your interpreter can understand and translate. (9)

Rapport

When you begin a counseling session with a culturally different client, establishing rapport may take a little longer than you are accustomed to in your own culture, but it is very important. The goal is to earn your client's respect and trust by showing him or her that you understand his or her cultural viewpoint. (5) Using "small talk" is a good way to begin communication and to show genuine concern for the client. For example, you might start by saying, **"How may I help you?"** (9) Listen with sympathy and understanding to the client's perception of the problem. Validate your perceptions of the problem from the client's perspective and your strategy for treatment. Another important factor for developing rapport is patience. You must be able to patiently listen and observe your client carefully in order to learn about his or her communication patterns. (5) Always negotiate agreement; it is important to understand the client's perspectives and abilities based on their cultural framework.

Subject

It is important for the counselor to be aware that certain subjects may not be acceptable to discuss with some cultural groups. Some common areas that may be considered inappropriate for discussion include personal matters, family, spouses, and religious beliefs. (9) It is important to know which subjects may be unacceptable for your client. For example, in the Arab culture, family issues are inappropriate to talk about in a counseling session because they should be resolved within the family. Actually, families often meet with elders, not counselors, in the community to resolve problems. Coffee is often served during these meetings, and it is used as a symbol of peace. If the coffee is drunk, then the problems were resolved, but if the coffee is not drunk, then the situation remains unchanged. (12)

Positive Regard

Positive regard means that as a counselor, you are able to find strengths and values in your clients even when their attitudes are opposite from your own. Value diversity. Do not just tolerate differing backgrounds and viewpoints, but consider differences as strengths. For example, let's assume you are counseling a client who has made several attempts to lose weight, but has failed. If you cannot find some positive attributes in this client, it will be very difficult for the client to change his or her behavior. (7) In this case, you might reinforce positive habits by pointing out some changes the client has already made. This should be done before you recommend other suggestions for losing weight. (8)

Body Language

Crossed arms or legs, tightened lips, and a firm handshake, are all forms of body language which may be interpreted differently depending on the culture. The use of the hands varies among the different cultural groups. For example, the Arab culture considers the left hand to be dirty and should not be used during a meal. Anglo-Americans prefer a firm handshake while Native Americans view this as a sign of aggression. (9,12) Hispanics are very affectionate and do not have a problem with touching. A light kiss on one or both cheeks is a very common greeting among most Hispanics. However, being touched by a stranger may be considered very inappropriate for many Asians. (9) It is important for the counselor to be aware of appropriate uses of body language within a cultural group. It may help to carefully observe the client and see how he interacts with you and others. When uncertain about body language, a counselor should be conservative, and remain natural, relaxed, and attentive. (5,9)

Eye Contact

In some cultures, direct eye contact is desired, but in other cultures it is not. For example, Black Americans do not find it necessary to always look at another person while talking. He or she may be actively involved in a conversation with another person while doing other things. A counselor who does not understand this style of communication may interpret this client as being uninterested or fearful. (11) Some groups, such as Asians, believe that staring is impolite. (9) Native Americans and Arabs see the eyes as a powerful tool and they do not make direct eye contact as a sign of respect for the speaker. (8,12) Arabs believe that staring limits the speaker's freedom to talk. (12) It is important to understand that the eyes are used by all cultures to convey meaning and understanding. (5) The key is to know what it means within a particular culture. It may help to observe your client during the counseling session, watching for signs of appropriate eye contact.

Table 5.1 Multicultural Characteristics and Values

Ethnic Groups	Mexican-American	Black Americans	Chinese American
Values	• Identify with family, community, & ethnic group • Status/role in family & community	• Ethnic identity • Kinship bonds • Strong work incentive • Strong religious ties • Adaptable family roles	• Obedience to parents • Respect for authority • Self-control of strong feelings • Praise of others • Individualism discouraged
Family Relationships	• Highly valued • Primary source of emotional, physical, psychological support • Authority with oldest male	• Extended family in rural/ urban communities • Important support system • Authority with mother or father	• Structure varies • Traditional stresses kinship with conformity to family & elders • Authority with mother or father • Obedience to parents
Health Beliefs	• Traditional include folk medicine beliefs, practitioners, & rituals • Hot-cold theory organizes illnesses	• Traditional include folk medicine: supernatural phenomena & herbal • Family responsibility	• Yin-Yang philosophy: a hot-cold classification of foods & diseases with goal to create a balance of Yin and Yang
Dietary Practices	• Staples are rice, beans, tortillas • Others: chicken, lard, eggs, chili peppers, tomatoes, squash, & herb teas • Lactose intolerance common	• Similar to Anglo American • Staples in South are fried chicken, greens & corn bread • Lactose intolerance common	• Traditions are ancient & complex • Diet associated with health & other aspects of society • Common foods: rice, vegetables, eggs, soy, tea • Lactose intolerance common
Religious Attitudes	• Illness is result of punishment from God • Medical care cannot change outcome • Mexican-Catholic ideology	• Important part of culture • Church is central meeting place in the community • Illness viewed as punishment from God	• Traditionally Buddhist and Taoist • Many have adopted Western religions
Language/ Communication	• Spanish speaking • Several dialects among sub-cultural groups	• Varies from standard American English to several Black dialects • Nonverbal behavior important	• Many Chinese dialects

(Sources: 3, 5, 6, 7, 8, 9, 10)

Table 5.1   Multicultural Characteristics and Values (continued)

Ethnic Groups	American Indians	Arabs
Values	• Harmony with nature • Sharing/cooperation • Respect for another's rights • Peacefulness, self-control, wisdom	• Family ties • Family name • Friendship • Hospitality
Family Relationships	• Extended family with strong ties • Respect opinions of members • Important source of support • Respect elders	• Important sources of support • Publicly male is authority, but in private decisions are mutual • Respect family & elders
Health Beliefs	• Tied with religion • Holistic/ herbal remedies • Sacred foods for rituals	• Depends on sub-culture • Tied with religion • Female sees woman doctor
Dietary Practices	• Varies across regions • Wild game, berries, greens prized	• No pork • No animal that eats meat (preditor) • No alcohol in some countries
Religious Beliefs	• Belief in Mother earth • Illness seen as disharmony of nature	• Islam is predominant religion • Follows Holy Koran • Religion & government are the same • Strictness varies with country
Language Communication	• Numerous languages and dialects • Nonverbal communication important	• Numerous Arabic slangs • Basic Arabic spoken in countries close to Mediterranean • Direct eye contact considered disrespectful • Left hand considered "dirty"

Physical Distance

The most comfortable physical distance between the counselor and the client varies among cultures. If the counselor is not aware of the client's preference, he or she may offend the client. (6) Hispanics usually have a smaller personal space than Anglo-Americans, and Asians usually prefer the most distance from another person. (9) In the Arab culture, personal space depends on an individual's gender. Personal space is small when talking to someone of the same gender, but more distance is appropriate with someone of the opposite gender. (12) Asking the client to select where he or she would like to sit may help you determine the preferred distance for your client.

Show of Emotions

Each culture has its own way of showing emotions. Hispanics are very expressive while Asians typically show very little expression. (13) Asian Americans view self-control of feelings as a very important behavior. (6) Even within a culture, you might find much diversity. Some Indian tribes encourage expressing emotions while others discourage it.(13) The counselor must remember that visible signs of happiness, anger, or sorrow are not always an accurate indication of what a person is feeling. Therefore, you must be aware of the form of emotional expression shown by the groups you are counseling. (See Table 5.2.)

Table 5.2

ELICITING CLIENT BELIEFS AND INFORMATION

The following questions may assist clinicians in assessing patients and families from culturally diverse backgrounds.

So that I might be aware of and respect your cultural beliefs...

1. Can you tell me what languages are spoken in your home and the languages that you understand and speak?
2. Please describe your usual diet. Also, are there times during the year when you change your diet in celebration of religious and other ethnic holidays?
3. Can you tell me about beliefs and practices including special events such as birth, marriage and death that you feel I should know?
4. Can you tell me about your experiences with health care providers in your native country? How often each year did you see a health care provider before you arrived in the U.S? Have you noticed any differences between the type of care you received in your native country and the type you receive here? If yes, could you tell me about those differences?
5. Is there anything else you would like to know? Do you have any questions for me? (Encourage two-way communication)
6. Do you use any traditional health remedies to improve your health?
7. Is there someone, in addition to yourself, with whom you want us to discuss your medical condition?
8. Are there certain health care procedures and tests, which your culture prohibits?
9. Are there any other cultural considerations I should know about to serve your health needs?

Adapted from: Carillo J.E., Green A.R., Betancourt J.R. Cross cultural primary care: a patient-based approach. *Ann Intern Med.* 1999; 130: 829-34.

Silence
If your client is silent during the counseling session, it does not necessarily mean he or she is disinterested. For example, many Native Americans consider their personal lives and inner thoughts to be private and do not want to share them with others until those people are known and trusted. If a Native American client appears silent, it may seem as if she lacks interest, but actually she is carefully observing the counselor's behavior. (8) It is not uncommon for Arabs to spend up to 30 minutes together in silence. (9,12) The counselor must be prepared for silent pauses or even interruptions in the communication process with diverse cultures.

CONCLUSION
Culture influences the way clients respond to medical services and preventive interventions. Often in health care, there is a lack of awareness of cultural differences and their impact on client understanding and/or compliance. The LEARN Model can be used to help guide the counselor in designing a culturally sensitive session: (14)
- **Listen** – to the perceptions of the client
- **Explain** – your perceptions of the client's needs
- **Acknowledge** – differences and similarities between perceptions
- **Recommend** – interventions and a plan
- **Negotiate** – culturally appropriate medical nutrition therapy

When counseling other cultural groups, it is important to realize that most people are very proud of their own values, customs, and behaviors. They are unlikely to adopt new ideas or practices if they conflict with their current system of beliefs. Therefore, your goal as a counselor should be to work towards understanding and accepting your clients' cultures. Instead of trying to change their views and beliefs, you must build on them to develop a plan and promote positive change. See Table 5.3. It is also important for you, as a counselor, to determine where you are along the road to cultural

Table 5.3 **Comparing Cultural Norms and Values**

Aspects of Culture	U.S. Health Care Culture	Other Cultures
1. Sense of Self and Space	• Informal • Handshake	• Formal • Hugs, bows, handshakes
2. Communication and Language	• Explicit, direct communication • Emphasis on content – meaning found in words	• Implicit, indirect communication • Emphasis on context – meaning found around words.
3. Dress and Appearance	• "Dress for success" ideal • Wide range in acceptable dress • More casual	• Dress seen as a sign of position, wealth, and prestige • Religious rules • More formal
4. Food and Eating Habits	• Eating as a necessity: fast food	• Dining as a social experience • Religious rules
5. Time and Time Consciousness	• Linear and exact time consciousness • Value on promptness • Time = money	• Elastic and relative time consciousness • Time spent on enjoyment of relationships
6. Relationships, Family and Friends	• Focus on nuclear family • Responsibility for self • Value on youth, age seen as handicap	• Focus on extended family • Loyalty and responsibility to family • Age given status and respect
7. Values and Norms	• Individual orientation • Independence • Preference for direct confrontation of conflict • Emphasis on task	• Group orientation • Conformity • Preference for harmony • Emphasis on relationships
8. Beliefs and Attitudes	• Egalitarian • Challenging of authority • Gender equality • Behavior and action affect and determine the future	• Hierarchical • Respect for authority and social order • Different roles for men and women • Fate controls and predetermines the future
9. Mental Processes and Learning Style	• Linear, logical • Problem-solving focus • Internal locus of control • Individuals control their destiny	• Lateral, holistic, simultaneous • Accepting of life's difficulties • External locus of control • Individuals accept their destiny
10. Work Habits and Practices	• Reward based on individual achievement • Work has intrinsic value	• Rewards based on seniority, relationships • Work is a necessity of life

Source: Gardenswarthz L, Rowe A. *Managing Diversity: A Complete Desk Reference and Planning Guide.*
Burr Ridge, IL: Irwin; 1993: p.57. Reprinted by permission.

competence in order to foster professional development and to heighten your awareness of your own cultural competency. To meet the challenge, counselors must develop a multicultural perspective and make an active commitment to becoming culturally competent and skilled in working with diverse populations.

This chapter outlined three essential elements that should serve as your criteria for working with racial and ethnic minorities:

- You must be aware of your own culture, which will enable you to know your attitudes, values, biases, and limitations as a multicultural counselor.
- You must understand your clients' world-view by gaining knowledge and by taking a proactive role to learn about their culture.
- You must work towards developing culturally appropriate communication skills.

Learning Activities

1. What are areas for professional development you can focus on to gain cultural competence?

2. Spend some time writing down notes about your upbringing. Consider such factors as the socioeconomic environment, important events that occurred, your parents' philosophy about life and their aspirations for you, the importance of social and family traditions as well as the role food played in your growing up. Discuss your notes with a colleague. How does this information impact your food beliefs and practices today?

3. Observe/ participate in meal preparation and the meal presentation in an ethnic setting different than your own. What do you observe? How does this insight change your approach to counseling an individual from this ethnic background? What impact does this insight have on your practice as a nutrition counselor?

4. Choose one ethnic group, and with a colleague, role-play a typical counseling session for a therapeutic diet modification (e.g. weight loss, low cholesterol). What skills and/ or knowledge must you bring to the counseling session? Evaluate your counseling skills after the role-play. What were your strengths? What areas can you improve on?

References
1. Sue DW, Arredondo P, McDavis RJ. Multicultural counseling competencies and standards: a call to the profession. *J Counsel Devl*. 1992; 70:477-486.
2. Cross T, Bazron B, Dennis K, Isaacs M. *Towards a Culturally Competent System of Care, Volume 1*. Washington DC: Georgetown University Child Development Center, CASSP Technical Assistance Center; 1989.
3. Adams DL. *Health Issues for Women of Color: A Cultural Diversity Perspective*. Thousand Oaks: SAGE Publications; 1995.
4. Texas department of Health, National Maternal and Child Health Resource Center on Cultural Competency. *Journal Towards Cultural Competency: Lessons Learned*. Vienna VA: Maternal and Children's Health Bureau Clearinghouse; 1997.
5. Pedersen PB, Ivey A. *Culture-Centered Counseling and Interviewing Skills: A Practical Guide*. Westport, CT: Praeger Publishers; 1993.
6. Dillard JM. *Multicultural Counseling*. Chicago, IL: Nelson Hall Publishers; 1983.
7. Ivey AE, Ivey MB, Simek-Morgan L. *Counseling and Psychotherapy: A Multicultural Perspective*. Boston, MA: Allyn and Bacon; 1993.
8. *Nutrition Education for Native Americans: A Guide for Nutrition Educators*. US Government Printing Office, Washington, DC: US Dept of Agriculture, Food and Nutrition Service; Sept 1984. FNS-249.

9. *Cross-Cultural Counseling: A guide for Nutrition and Health Counselors.* US Government Printing Office, Washington, DC: US Dept of Health and Human Services; May 1990. FNS-250.
10. *Ethnic and Regional Food Practices Series: Mexican American Food Practices, Customs, and Holidays.* Chicago, IL: Diabetes Care and Education Dietetic Practice Group of The American Dietetic Association; 1998.
11. Sue DW. *Counseling the Culturally Different.* New York: John Wiley & Sons, Inc; 1981.
12. In conversation with Tariq Bakri AlAbbassi, BA. November 22, 1994.
13. *Culture-bound and Sensory Barriers to Communication with Patients: Strategies and Resources for Health Education.* Atlanta, GA: US Dept of Health and Human Services, Centers for Disease Control, Center for Health Promotion and Education; 1982. DHHS (PHS) publication 99-1572.
14. *Berlin EA, Fowkes WC.* A teaching framework for cross-cultural health care. *Western J Med.* 1983;139:934-938.
15. Tawara D. Goode, MA, Georgetown University Child Development Center, Center for Child Health and Mental Health Policy, University Affiliated Program, Washington, D.C. (June 1989), revised 1993, 1995 and 2000.

Chapter 6

Assuring and Measuring Professional Competence

Bridget Klawitter, PhD, RD

After reading this chapter, the reader will be able to:
- ♦ Define terminology related to competency.
- ♦ Differentiate between initial and ongoing competency.
- ♦ Identify measurable behavior criteria and methods to determine competency.
- ♦ Discuss importance of competency to the development of nutrition counseling skills.

INTRODUCTION

In recent years, the importance of competency assessment and development has been increasing, especially with the focus on improving patient care outcomes and customer satisfaction. Specifically, the Joint Commission on Accreditation of Healthcare Organizations (JCAHO) competency assessment standards have elevated the interest of many dietetic professionals in how to demonstrate competence in day-to-day practice.

Why be concerned about competence? The focus on whether health professionals in general provided quality care goes back to the 1960's and the rise in consumer involvement in determining their healthcare needs. Today, with the focus on patient-centered care and disease self-management in a world of cost containment, consumers are more selective when choosing health care providers. Word-of-mouth advertising on the quality of services provided and the impact on client outcomes can drive whether a practice or program survives. Dietetic practitioners in any setting should have a vested interest in assuring professional competency in practice, and that competence is assessed, maintained, demonstrated, and continually improved. Healthcare organizations specifically have needed to embrace the competence assessment process more rigorously due to regulatory requirements. However, it is always important to understand the intent of the regulation or standard. The intent may vary depending on whether it is a JCAHO standard, Occupational Safety and Health Administration (OSHA) regulation, federal, state, or licensure board requirement. The most frequent Type 1's (most important standards) in JCAHO surveys are the standards that deal with orientation, training, education, and competency. In the end, understanding the intent will facilitate an effective and meaningful competence assessment program.

Defining Competence
The reason for a formal competence assessment program can vary, but most often are geared towards: (1)
- Evaluating individual performance
- Evaluating group performance
- Meeting regulatory standards
- Addressing problematic issues
- To enhance or replace performance appraisal

It is a tough and time-consuming job to educate staff and maintain their level of competence. A competency program can include several components including: job descriptions, verification of licensure, registration and/or certifications, organization- and department-specific orientation, an initial assessment of competence, annual performance appraisals, ongoing competency validation, age-appropriate competencies, and continuing education. Many definitions have been proposed for competence terminology. JCAHO has provided a general definition of competence (2) stating,"It is the possession of the knowledge, skills, and behaviors to perform assigned tasks." Inman-Felton and Rops (3) have distinguished between "competence" and "competencies:"

Competence is the general state of being competent.

Competencies refer to the specific knowledge, psychomotor skills, critical thinking abilities, and/or interpersonal attributes required for an individual to be considered competent. Therefore, professional competence is multidimensional. This can be visualized as depicted in Figure 6.1.

Figure 6.1 Typical Competency Model

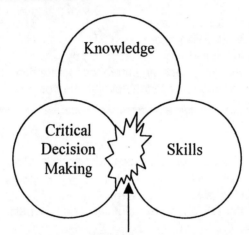

Competent when all three meet to perform a task

Competency assessment is the ongoing process of identifying and validating a practitioner's ability to perform as expected. Competency assessment can provide direction, as well as identify areas for professional growth and development. See side bar on the Commission on Dietetic Registration (CDR) Portfolio System as an example of this for dietetic practice. It is often helpful to develop a broad *competency statement* that defines in a short statement the aspects of performance associated with success in the role. For example, a competency statement for a counseling competency may be, "Provides individualized nutrition counseling for children and adults." Competency statements tend to reflect broad, general behavior, are learner-oriented, measurable, written in action terminology, and free of context, conditions, time limits, and sequencing. (4)

DETERMINING SUBJECTS FOR COMPETENCIES
Ask yourself, what does the practitioner need to know? What critical pieces of essential job functions and expectations must an employee understand and/or demonstrate to perform the job effectively and independently?

The *job description* should be developed to maintain an accurate description of essential and other job functions. A well-written job description can provide the foundation for identifying areas for competency development. Essential functions are a listing of job duties which an individual must be able to perform in this role, such as conduct a comprehensive nutrition assessment, assess educational needs, or provide nutrition counseling. Other job functions are job duties that may not be required for every individual working in that position. Examples may be differences between acute care and outpatient dietitian functions, especially if one "clinical dietitian" job description is used. Sample job descriptions for a variety of dietetic positions are available through ADA (5) and may be helpful in developing or updating job descriptions.

It is often helpful to determine subjects for competency development by looking at *factors*, or reasons that measurement of professional competence may be needed. Such factors may include:

- **High risk**–Refers to a process or skill that if not correctly performed, negatively affects the system's quality, cost, or service.
- **Low volume**–Refers to a process or skill that is not done frequently, and therefore, competency or demonstrated performance is unknown.
- **Problem-prone**–Refers to a process or skill that by virtue of the number of steps or difficulty is susceptible to mistakes.
- **Process improvement**–Refers to a process for which the department or leadership has received unacceptable data, and has recognized the need to develop a competency as part of its process improvement.
- **Performance improvement**–Refers to an individual's inconsistent performance or involvement in a critical incident, and requires additional training and validation of a defined skill or process.

Initial Competence
This reflects the knowledge, skills, and behaviors required in the first 6-12 months in a particular job.
(1) Using the job description and other data, initial competencies are usually based upon:
- Core job functions
- Frequent job accountabilities
- High risk and/or high volume skills

See Table 6.1 for possible core competencies for the dietetic practitioner providing nutrition counseling.

Table 6.1	Core Competencies for Nutrition Counseling
	• Active listening • Age specific care • Assessment • Counseling • Discharge planning • Documentation • Emotional support • Learning facilitation • Quality improvement

Ongoing Competence
This is validated by periodic assessment of selected competencies. These competencies may be determined by quality of patient satisfaction data, new or revised policies and procedures, new technologies, and/or high risk/high volume job functions. Ongoing competencies should also build on established knowledge, skills, and abilities to promote professional growth and development.
Characteristics common to developing all competencies include: (6)
- Specific to role and setting
- Based on real world performance
- Derived from and validated by practitioners
- Practice- and performance-based
- Focused on outcomes
- Structured by competency statements and performance criteria
- May include assessment of knowledge, skills, and critical thinking abilities

Numerous resources are available for the selection of or suggestions on domains for competency development applicable in dietetic practice, as well as additional readings listed at the end of this chapter. (3,5,7-16) See Figure 6.2 Competency Validation Methods.

Figure 6.2 Competency Validation Methods

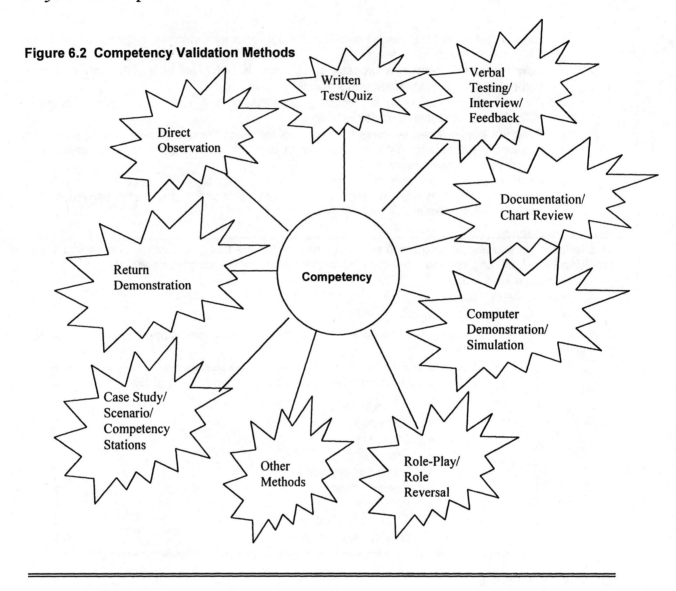

Direct Observation

Observation of technical skills can provide insight into the application of skills necessary for daily job performance. Sometimes simple observation is overlooked as a valid measure of competence. Observation can often be done to validate completion of a process from start to finish.

Return Demonstration

Return demonstration is a good way to measure technical skills. (1) Describing how to do nutrition counseling, for example, and actually doing it are two very different things. Return demonstration can be done in an artificial environment such as a skills lab or class, or in a real-world setting. In return demonstration, the preceptor must maintain control over the situation, especially when real patients are involved. Return demonstrations can be an excellent way to demonstrate proficiency in such clinical skills as blood glucose testing, body fat measurement, or preparing a recipe.

Verbal Testing/Interview/Feedback

Discussion can be used to measure proficiency in cognitive (knowledge), psychomotor (skill), or critical thinking domains. It is often helpful to identify specific questions for the preceptor to ask to determine the individual's understanding of a concept or skill. Peer feedback may also be useful to determine application of competency content to on-the-job situations.

Written Test/Quiz

Written tests work well when measuring cognitive skills; however, they are not as effective measuring behavioral, performance, or psychomotor skills. (1) This method is an excellent way to measure an individual's comprehension of basic knowledge related to a topic or to test cognitive processing using formulas or algorithms. If retention of information is the desired outcome, tests are a good choice.

Documentation/ Chart Review

Documentation review is a quality improvement monitor used to check compliance with policies and protocols, and to collect data on individual performance. Random individual documentation review by peers can also assist in determining consistency of practices. For nutrition counseling, documenting patient education effectively is key to establish consistent practice.

Computer Demonstration/Simulation

This method may be one of the most applicable when assessing competence of nutrition counseling. This is especially useful as individuals practice new counseling skills before using them in practice. Often, videotaping role-play can provide an opportunity for further group/peer discussion and critique.

Role-Play/Role Reversal

This method may be one of the most applicable to assessing competence of nutrition counseling. This is especially useful as

---

COMMISSION ON DIETETIC REGISTRATION (CDR) PORTFOLIO SYSTEM

Over the last few years, increasing attention has been focused on the need for continuing competence of health professionals and on the regulatory board's responsibilities in providing assurances beyond initial certification. Consumer organizations, federal agencies, managed care organizations and legislators are applying increasing pressures for licensure and certifying bodies to require life-long learning of their constituents.

The challenge to CDR was the creation of a professional development system whose value is readily apparent to its various customers: the public, practitioners, employers and regulatory agencies, all of whom have different expectations of the dietetics profession. The *Portfolio* process builds upon the value of CPE. CDR embraces the philosophy of lifelong learning encouraged in ADA's *Standards of Professional Practice*; and believes that CPE activities should be directed towards professional development, personal enhancement, and quality of care improvement. It believes that the *Professional Development Portfolio* process allows the dietetics professional to take responsibility for his or her own professional development. By grounding the process in professional practice, the professional assumes responsibility for selecting learning activities that have a direct relationship to that practice.

Outcomes research shows that effective continuing education is much more complex than information transfer alone, requiring such steps as:

1. Identify what needs to be learned.
2. Use educational methods that optimize learning.
3. Develop strategies to implement and reinforce what has been learned and transfer new learning into practice.

CDR representatives met with JCAHO staff regarding the compatibility of the *Professional Development Portfolio* process with the Management of Human Resources Standards on competence assessment. The JCAHO wants evidence of a system to assess and address competence in the work setting. JCAHO is looking for assessment of performance, identification of learning needs and implementation of a Learning Plan for individuals and the staff of a facility. There are many similarities in the JCAHO and CDR processes. You could use the *Portfolio* as a tool to document competency assessment to meet Joint Commission standards.

The dietetics profession is not alone in evaluating its continuing competency standards. Today, almost all allied health professions and the medical specialty boards have studied, developed, or implemented new continuing competence programs. Some professions (e.g., Physician Assistants and Emergency Medical Technicians) require periodic re-examination to maintain certification. CDR supports putting dietetics professionals in the "drivers seat" of their own professional recertification through the processes of self-assessment, planning and lifelong learning.

For more information on the Portfolio system:
Commission on Dietetic Registration
120 South Riverside Plaza, Suite 2000
Chicago, Illinois 60606-6995
Phone: 312-899-0040 Ext. 5500
Fax: 312-899-4772
www.cdrnet.org

individuals practice new counseling skills before implementing them independently in practice. Often, videotaping a role-play can provide an opportunity for further group/peer discussion and critique.

Case Study/Scenario/Competency Station

Case studies are an excellent way to validate critical thinking skills. (1) A case study provides a situation or scenario and asks individuals their reaction or response to the situation. Often a list of questions is developed to capture the scope of the competency being measured. Case studies can be done independently or in small discussion groups to gain different perspectives.

Documenting Competence

When measuring professional competency, knowledge alone is not sufficient. Just attending a seminar or completing a self-study module, even when continuing professional education (CPE) credit is provided, does not mean one can apply the knowledge effectively and consistently in day-to-day practice. Certification, registration, or licensure, may often be a component of the job description, but does not alone constitute, or ensure, competency.

How often competence should be validated is dependent on various factors. Three general time frames may be considered:

- **Orientation period**–the time allotted for the individual or departments to demonstrate initial competencies.
- **Annual**–assessment of competence required every 12 months due to legal, regulatory, or risk management requirements.
- **Other**–competencies that a department or individual needs to demonstrate on a periodic basis. The supervisor or department should identify a time frame.

Regulatory standards, such as those from JCAHO, require that documentation of initial and ongoing competence is a permanent part of an employee personnel file. It is the intent of the standards that there is evidence of a performance-based assessment of staff proficiency in essential job functions. An excellent overview of competence standards and applications to dietetic practice is available in reference #3.

See Appendix 6-A for Action words for assessment forms. A sample format and examples specific to dietetic practice can also be found in Appendix 6-B. This format was developed by an interdisciplinary Core Competency Team (CCT) at All Saints Healthcare in 2000 and has continued to meet the needs of a large, community-based integrated delivery system.

Focus on Age-Specific Competence

For individual's working routinely and directly with various age groups, age appropriate validation must be conducted to assure age-specific competence. Age-specific competence is the abilities and skills a practitioner must have to provide appropriate care for patients/clients in a given age group. It applies to specific behavioral criteria for a competency in which age specificity is identified. For example, counseling an adult versus a child requires different approaches. (See Chapters 2 and 3 for specifics.)

It is important to know the physical and developmental characteristics of specified age groups for whom you provide care. Without this knowledge base, one may not be able to select the correct size equipment, the correct method of treatment, or the best approach to use with a patient in a particular age group. Some categories of characteristics that may differentiate age groups include:

- General physical characteristics
- Specific safety considerations
- Normal vital signs parameters
- Normal developmental tasks and cognitive skills
- Physiological differences
- Appropriate equipment and techniques
- Incorporation of age specific information into patient counseling, planning, and provision of care

It is critical to assess age-specific aspects of dietetic practice in a variety of settings. However, it is much more advantageous to integrate age-specific criteria into other competencies. As you can see from the examples in Appendix 6-B, age-specific aspects have been integrated into the behavioral criteria where applicable.

Nutrition Counseling Competency Assessment

Nutrition counseling, and the expanding repertoire of skills necessary to build rapport and effectively facilitate behavior and lifestyle change, is a prime area for competence development. The challenges of counseling techniques lend themselves well to the development of competencies.

It is important that practitioners responsible for validating the competence of others are knowledgeable in competency assessment (i.e., purpose, procedures and documentation of professional competency), and they have demonstrated prior competency in the skill area being validated. Experienced, effective nutrition counselors can play an important role in mentoring other dietetic practitioners while they expand their skills in this area.

Competence is a Continuum

Competency assessment should be a fluid, ongoing process reflecting a growth in skills and abilities required to perform a job. Initial job competencies are the validation of actual performance of job duties documented by the end of orientation, and prior to working independently. In the health care setting, an individual's direct supervisor or department manager is responsible for ensuring all staff receives the training and education required to competently perform job responsibilities. Developing an ongoing competency assessment process can often be a challenge for dietetic/clerical managers. Competency assessment and performance appraisal go hand-in-hand. Competency assessment provides the means to expand job skills and address the dynamic nature of ongoing skills to address the changing nature of a job.

Summary

A successful professional competency assessment program will have a strong foundation in adult learning principles. There are four essential components of a competency: competency statement, behavioral criteria, validation methods, and evaluation of performance. (4) Competence assessment is receiving increasing scrutiny from most accrediting bodies. The skills and abilities of dietetic practitioners as nutrition counselors provide a fertile source for competency development and individual practitioner evaluation.

Learning Activities

1. Why is it important to validate competency:
   - At the time of hire?
   - During orientation period?
   - At annual performance reviews?
   - For age-specific care?
   - As technology changes?
   - As new practice guidelines are released?

2. How can developmental tasks and cognitive abilities of a particular age group be used to provide better counseling?

3. How would physiological differences affect your approach to nutrition counseling provided?

4. Review and discuss the sample competencies in Appendix 6-A. Are the validation methods consistent with measurement of the behavioral criteria? Write one case scenario that could be used for each competency.

References
1. Wright D. *The Ultimate Guide to Competency Assessment in Healthcare,* 2nd ed. Eau Claire, WI: PESI Health Care, LLC; 1998.
2. *Joint Commission on Accreditation of Healthcare Organizations. Lexicon,* 2nd ed. Oakbrook Terrace, IL: Joint Commission on Accreditation of Healthcare Organizations; 1998.
3. Inman-Felton A, Rops MS. *Ensuring staff competence: a guide for meeting JCAHO competence standards in all settings.* Chicago: The American Dietetic Association; 1998.
4. Garvis JP, Grey MT. The anatomy of a competency. *J Nurs Staff Dev.* 1995;11(5): 247-252.
5. Hornick BA, ed. *Job Descriptions: Models for the dietetics profession.* Chicago, IL: American Dietetic Association; 2003.
6. Alsbach JG. *Designing Competency Assessment Programs: A handbook for nursing and health-related professions.* Pensacola, FL: National Nursing Staff Development Organization; 1996.
7. American Dietetic Association. Standards of Professional practice for dietetics professionals. *J Amer Diet Assoc.* 1998;1: 83-87.
8. Bruening KS, Mitchell BE, Pfeiffer MM. 2002 Accreditation Standards for dietetics education. *J Amer Diet Assoc.* 2002;4: 566-577.
9. Petrillo T. Lifelong learning goals: individual steps that propel the profession of dietetics. *J Amer Diet Assoc.* 2003;3: 2003: 298-300.
10. Litchfield RE, Oakland MJ, Anderson J. Promoting and evaluating competence in on-line dietetics education. *J Amer Diet Assoc.* 2002; 10: 1455-1458.
11. Brehm BJ, Smith R, Rourke KM. Multiskilling: a course to increase multidisciplinary skills in future dietetics professionals. *J Allied Health.* 2001;30 (4): 239-242.
12. Rops MS. *Helping Dietetics Professionals Learn: A guide to developing learning needs assessment documents.* Chicago: Commission on Dietetic Registration; 2000.
13. The American Dietetic Association standards of professional practice for dietetic professionals. *J Amer Diet Assoc.* 1998; 1: 83-87.
14. Snetsalaar LG. *Nutrition Centered Counseling Skills for Medical Nutrition Therapy.* Gaithersburg, MD: Aspen Publishers Inc; 1997.
15. Arena J, Walters P. Do you know what a dietetic technician can do? A focus on clinical technicians and their expanded roles and responsibilities. *J Amer Diet Assoc.* 1997; (10 Suppl 2): S139-141.
16. Gilmore CJ, Maillet JO, Mitchell BE. Determining educational preparation based on job competencies of entry-level dietetic practitioners. *J Amer Diet Assoc.* 1993; 3: 305-308.

Additional Readings:

Balagun LB, Ward DC, Stivers M. JCAHO update: the nuts and bolts of competency standards including requirements for age-specific competencies. *J Amer Diet Assoc.* 1995; 2: 244-245.

Karp SS, Lawrence ML. Use of the new competencies to access entry-level dietitians. *J Amer Diet Assoc.* 1999;9: 1098-1100.

Harris-Davis E, Haughton B. Model for multicultural nutrition counseling competencies. *J Amer Diet Assoc.* 2000;10: 1178-1185.

Keim KS, Johnson CA, Gates GE. Learning needs and continuing professional activities of Professional Development portfolio participants. *J Amer Diet Assoc.* 2001;6: 697-702.

Jarrett J, Mahaffie JB. Key trends affecting the dietetics profession and the American Dietetic Association. *J Amer Diet Assoc.* 2002;12: 1821-1839.

Section II

Integrating Theory, Skills & Practice

Chapter 7

Physical and Psychosocial Assessment

Michele Fairchild, MS, RD, FADA, Ellen Liskov, MPH, RD, and Bridget Klawitter, PhD, RD, FADA

After reading this chapter, the reader will be able to:
- ◆ Identify at least four types of nutrition therapy assessments.
- ◆ Identify the basic parameters of a clinical nutrition assessment.
- ◆ Identify psychosocial factors that influence food intake.

Assessment is a dynamic, comprehensive, and organized system of gathering information relevant to the nutritional care of your client. It should identify any red flags, which indicate a client is at risk nutritionally. It should identify, along with using good interviewing skills, contributing factors to disordered or inadequate intake, starting points for therapy, and whether goals are met along the way.

The type of assessments you choose to perform will depend upon the tasks at hand. For instance, the information necessary for an outpatient at a cancer treatment center will vary significantly from that of an otherwise healthy, but overweight client. Similarly, the details collected at your initial consultation may not be repeated except at a three-month follow-up, but they may set the course for the goals for the months in between visits.

> **Merely looking over a person's food record at each visit is incomplete and should not be used as the only assessment or counseling strategy.**

During follow-up sessions, you may investigate and assess many of the thoughts, behaviors, and developmental skills that seemed problematic during the first session, or you may expand the first session into a more comprehensive assessment and goal-setting visit.

Assessment should be a part of each and every counseling session. Something so simple as having the client recap his progress, behavior, or cognitive challenges since the last visit more clearly assess whether strategies are working. *Merely looking over a person's food record at each visit is incomplete and should not be used as the only assessment or counseling strategy.* Some examples of nutrition therapy assessments include:

- Evaluation of present nutrition intake patterns (looking at a typical food intake record and computer assessment of present food intake)
- Evaluation of present lifestyle, and health risk status
- Establishing baseline biochemical and anthropometric values, and monitoring them to assess outcomes of diet changes and nutrition intervention
- Understanding psychosocial, cultural, ethnic or literacy factors, use of developmental skills, and physical limitations (e.g. illness, arthritis, poor vision, immobility) which may influence a client's food behaviors
- Identifying economic factors which may limit the client's ability to buy adequate good food
- Evaluation of client's understanding of information discussed
- Identifying the client's personal style
- Assessing motivation and readiness to change eating habits
- Evaluating success with implementing goals set during counseling

The knowledge gained in the assessment process is crucial to developing a plan of action that is consistent with a client's nutrient needs and in helping the client see that problems do exist that need work. The future actions will have a better chance of being realistic given the client's current eating habits, psychosocial milieu, level of understanding and motivation. Good interviewing skills are essential in order to elicit the details required in a fashion that does not bias the client's responses.

THE ASSESSMENT PROCESS

Nutrition assessment is a comprehensive approach, completed by a registered dietitian, to define nutritional status that uses medical, nutrition, and medication histories; physical examination; anthropometric measurements; and laboratory tests. (1) Details of assessment calculations are beyond the scope of this chapter and are very adequately covered in other books on the subject. (2 - 6) This chapter will cover an overview of the process and potential tools and resources for counselors to use. The process may be broken down into sections including:

- Medical history, biochemical parameters, clinical examination
- Anthropometrics and fitness evaluation
- Food intake, preferences, allergies, and needs
- Psychosocial factors, family influences, developmental skills, motivation, and readiness
- Lifestyle and health risk appraisal
- Personal and preferred learning style

As dietetic practice expands into new areas and nutrition therapy skills mature, assessments will change and the usage of the assessments will become even more foundational to the course of the therapy. Many sources are available to assist the practitioner in developing data collection forms or that offer charts, equations, and assessment tools.

Screening

Nutrition screening is the process of identifying characteristics known to be associated with nutrition problems. (1) The screening process has the following characteristics:

- May be completed in any setting
- Facilitates completion of early intervention goals
- Includes the collection of relevant data on risk factors and the interpretation of data for intervention/treatment
- Determines the need for a nutrition assessment
- Is cost-effective

Nutrition screening is appropriately used in pre-admission surgical interviews, upon admission to the hospital, in private practice nutrition therapists' and physicians' offices, corporations, clinics, HMOs, senior centers, at health fairs and schools, and wherever else target populations meet. See Appendix 7-A for sample screening and assessment forms.

Screening tools can be developed for any population group. Nancy Clark, MS, RD, sports nutritionist at Sports Medicine Brookline, developed a "Nutrition Checklist" for athletes to use as they sit in the lobby waiting for an appointment with a physician or physical therapist. The self-graded tool creates awareness of possible nutrition-related problems, as well as serves as a marketing tool for Nancy's services. Other references for evaluation of exercise readiness are also available. (9)

In acute care settings where dietitians and dietetic technicians must prioritize care of patients, screening for nutritional risk is appropriate to identify those in need of a more comprehensive nutritional assessment. This process should assist in the implementation of timely, outcome-based, cost-effective interventions. Screening can be done by dietetic practitioners or, especially in the acute care setting, as a multidisciplinary process. The key components of an acute care screening process are chart review and the patient/family interview.

New computer and software technology can make basic screening of the client commonplace. In some settings, clients can sit in front of a screen and answer questions (or a helper will sit at the screen, ask the questions, and input the information). Hand-held technology enables dietetic practitioners to input basic information and perform calculations or do screening and assessments and download the information. Many such programs are available free or at a nominal cost on the Internet. (10)

As more hospitals go to paperless, computer-based systems, nutrition screening is not

> **The dietitian must practice at a higher level where he or she interprets the data, makes critical assessments and calculations, works collaboratively with the medical staff, counsels patients to improve outcomes, and with appropriate training, makes nutritional diagnoses.**

performed manually by dietetic practitioners unless on a laptop or handheld computer. Eventually, all hospitals will use computers to facilitate collaboration on patient care and manage information better. It is important that dietitians recognize that tasks that do not require interpretation will be put on software and delegated to a lesser-paid person.

MEDICAL—BIOCHEMICAL—CLINICAL

Medical History

In the inpatient setting, the medical history is readily available in the patient's chart. In the outpatient setting, when you do not have access to the client's medical record, it is recommended that the practitioner contact the client's primary care or referring physician's office prior to the initial consultation for nutritionally relevant medical history information. This is essential in order to identify all the factors that are influencing nutritional status or nutritional requirements. While there are many clients who can provide accurate information about their medical background, prescribing inappropriate nutritional therapy to a client can threaten your practice if he or she is a poor historian or chooses not to reveal pertinent information. After the visit, send a summary of the visit and nutritional plan of care to the client's physician.

Health Status. Identify any chronic or acute conditions that are affecting nutritional status, nutrient needs, food intake, digestion, absorption, or metabolism of nutrients. In the outpatient setting, diabetes, hyperlipidemia, obesity, eating disorders, food intolerances, hypertension, and gastrointestinal disorders are commonly seen. Burns, infections or prolonged fever, liver or kidney disease, AIDS, complications from chemotherapy, congestive heart failure, chronic obstructive pulmonary disease, failure to thrive, cystic fibrosis, or multiple trauma are powerful risk factors for poor nutritional status in hospitalized patients. A thorough medical history should also investigate appetite as well as dentition or other mechanical problems that may preclude adequate food intake.

Medication Usage. Many clients will be taking medications routinely, either prescription or over-the-counter, which creates the possibility for a food-drug interaction. When a food-drug interaction is suspected or likely, be sure to incorporate information into your counseling sessions on timing of meals, food selections, or supplementation. (11-13)

Be sure to ask the client about any vitamin, mineral, and herbal supplements currently being used, as this is commonly overlooked in a medication history. (14) Many health conscious clients self-prescribe potentially harmful doses of fat-soluble vitamins, niacin, minerals, or herbs. In addition, some supplements may have adverse bleeding or anesthesia effects if taken prior to or after any surgical procedures.

Biochemical Parameters

Laboratory measurements of visceral protein, immune function, or vitamin and mineral stores may be used to evaluate nutritional status in the assessment process. (6) Serum albumin is a commonly ordered test for measuring visceral protein status but it cannot detect short-term changes in nutritional status due to its relatively long half-life of about 21 days. Acute or short-term changes in nutritional status may be detected with the use of prealbumin or transferrin due to their shorter half-lives of 2-3 days and 8-10 days, respectively. Since malnutrition can depress immune function, the total lymphocyte count (TLC) can be used as a marker of nutritional status. Extreme caution must be taken with the interpretation of these parameters, as they are all highly influenced by non-nutritional factors such as age, fluid status, stress, drugs, infection, AIDS, and liver or kidney disease.

Lastly, any biochemical parameters associated with a particular health condition (i.e., glucose, glycosylated hemoglobin, serum lipids, etc.) should be noted at the time of the initial consultation and then monitored during follow-up to assess the efficacy of nutritional therapies.

Clinical Examination

Physical signs of poor nutritional status may be identified by visual examination, particularly loss of somatic fat and protein stores. A very skilled practitioner may be able to detect clinical signs of protein or micronutrient deficiencies in a client's hair, skin, eyes, and mouth areas. Such physical findings, however, are often due to non-nutritional causes or are indicative of more than one deficiency state. Any suspicions about nutritional deficiencies, as detected by physical examination, should be confirmed with biochemical testing. Sources are available for further reading regarding clinical examination for detecting malnutrition (see references 1,2,15).

ANTHROPOMETRICS

Anthropometric variables such as weight, circumference measurements, and skinfold thickness are commonly used to assess nutritional status and body composition. All of these measurements are relatively simple and inexpensive to obtain but are not without error. Standardized techniques for obtaining anthropometric indices should be documented in the practitioner's standards of care so baseline values and changes in serial measurements can be accurately evaluated.

Weight

The most commonly performed type of anthropometric evaluation is weight relative to height. Many tables are available to determine ideal body weight (IBW) based upon height (15-17), where a percentage of ideal weight can be calculated (% IBW = Actual Weight/ IBW). Accurate use of the Metropolitan Life Insurance weight tables (15) necessitates calculation of body frame size using elbow breadth, which makes this process more complicated and prone to error. Thus, many practitioners are using body mass index (BMI), which is derived by dividing weight in kilograms (kg) by height in square meters (m^2). Bray (17) has defined BMI as:

Underweight	< 18.5
Normal/healthy	20.0 – 24.9
Overweight	25.0 – 29.9
Obesity Class I	30.0 – 34.9
Obesity Class II	35.0 – 39.9
Obesity Class III	≥ 40

For hospitalized patients, evaluation of weight and weight change are simple methods of screening for nutritional risk. Rapid weight loss is associated with protein catabolism. Loss of more than 5% of usual body weight in the previous month or more than 10% loss in the previous six months indicates protein malnutrition and dictates that a more comprehensive nutritional assessment is in order.

In children, growth charts are commonly used to identify the child's height and weight as compared to the norm. Weight-for-stature index and BMI for age is used to identify infants and children with obesity or acute protein-energy malnutrition (PEM). Weight-for-stature index is calculated by dividing the child's actual weight by the 50% weight for length. Children with an index equal to or greater than 1.1 (110% of standard) require further evaluation for overweight/obesity; those falling below 0.9 (90% of standard) require assessment for acute PEM. (19) The growth charts consist of a series of percentile curves that illustrate the distribution of selected body measurements in U.S. children. (20) The 2000 Center for Disease Control (CDC) growth charts represent a revised version of the 1977 NCHS growth charts. The addition of the BMI charts is probably the single most significant new feature of the revised growth charts. *Growth charts should not be used as diagnostic instruments.* Instead, they are tools that can determine a trend in growth and an overall impression of the child being measured.

The detriment of using weight alone as a measurement of nutritional status is that it does not provide any information on body composition such as muscle mass reserves or subcutaneous fat stores. It is also affected by the person's fluid status.

Circumference Measurements and Skinfold Thickness

Caliper skinfold measurements can be taken by a trained individual to estimate subcutaneous fat stores or total body fat. Somatic protein reserves can be determined by calculating Mid Arm Muscle

Circumference (MAMC) that is derived from the upper arm circumference and triceps skinfold measurements.

Standardized techniques to perform and evaluate skinfold measurements are widely published in sports nutrition, fitness and sports medicine books, in physical assessment books, and by pharmaceutical companies.(1,4,21) These measurements provide the most useful information when monitored over time. Skinfolds are not recommended for routine screening in children, but they may be beneficial in assessing a child's status when it is above the 90th or below the 10th percentile of weight-for-stature. (4)

Currently, waist-to-hip ratio (WHR) is one of the most common circumference measurements performed as an assessment of body fat distribution. (13) A simplified technique of calculating WHR involves measuring the individual's waist at the smallest circumference and hips at the largest circumference below the waist. The waist measurement is divided by the hip measurement where a WHR of >1.0 in men and > 0.8 in women is indicative of android obesity. Upper body, or android obesity, is associated with greater risk of diabetes, gout, and heart disease. (22)

Fitness Evaluation

Using information from screening and guidelines established by the American College of Sports Medicine (ACSM), the dietetic practitioner can stratify clients according to health and/or risk status prior to beginning an exercise program. Although the details of a fitness evaluation are beyond the scope of this chapter, several references can assist in expanding your knowledge in this area. (23,24)

DIETARY INTAKE AND NUTRITIONAL NEEDS

Determining Current Intake

One of the more time consuming aspects of nutritional assessment is determining what a client is eating. The details about food selections, preparation methods, and portion sizes can be obtained in a variety of ways. However, it is always a challenge as factors such as poor memory, limited knowledge of preparation methods, poor estimation of portion sizes, and client bias in reporting intake

---

SCREENING IN THE ONCOLOGY SETTING

Maintaining quality of life is important for patients with cancer. It is also known that maintenance of nutritional status can play an important role in treatment outcomes. Physically, nutrient depletion can adversely affect morbidity and mortality, length of hospital stay, wound healing, immune function, and response to chemotherapy and radiation treatments.

A questionnaire, called the Functional Assessment of Anorexia Cachexia Therapy (FAACT) Subscale, has been developed by Cella and associates to measure the nutritional quality of life. The tool is comprised of 27 general questions and 12 questions specific to anorexia/cachexia.

To view the FAACT tool, visit the web site at www.accc-cancer.org/publications/faact.pdf.

The Patient Generated Subjective Global Assessment (PG-SGA) is another validated nutrition screening tool appropriate for use in all oncology outpatient settings. This tool provides a global assessment of the patient's nutritional status based on nutrition-related history and physical symptoms and has been used to evaluate nutrition quality of life. The first part of the tool is completed by the patient and includes questions related to weight, food intake, nutritional impact symptoms, and activity patterns. These answers can be used to identify patients at risk for malnutrition or a decreased quality of nutritional life. The rest of the tool is completed by the health professional, including a physical exam and lab work. An overall global assessment and a patient score are derived. The score then determines intervention pathways.

To view these pathways and the tool, visit www.accc-cancer.org/publications.pgsga.pdf.

---

can negatively affect the reliability of the information. Food models are helpful when assessing portion sizes, especially when a client has not measured or weighed foods eaten. Underestimation of amounts is a common phenomenon. (25) As always, the practitioner should try to make clients feel at ease, do not act judgmental and clients will feel more like writing their actual intake on the food record.

It may be helpful to explain your purpose in gathering a diet history. It helps you provide assistance in identifying potential areas for change (i.e., food selections, preparation methods, or portion sizes). However, remember it takes multiple counseling sessions to fully understand what a client is eating and all relevant information need not be gathered in the initial consultation.

Twenty-four Hour Recall. One of the quickest ways to get a general idea about a client's eating habits is to ask the individual to recall everything he or she ate and drank within the past 24 hours. However, in addition to the inaccuracies described above with food records, the previous 24 hours may not be representative of the client's normal diet. In such cases, substitute a "typical day's" intake.

Food Records. Food records kept by a client prior to the consultation, provides more information than the 24-hour recall, and allows more time for intervention than a recall assessment in the counseling session. In this method, have the client complete food records, inclusive of food selections, name brands, preparation methods, and portion sizes, for at least five typical weekdays and one weekend. Bias in reporting food intake often occurs with food records when a client preferentially completes them on "optimal" eating days or based upon what he or she believes constitutes a healthy diet. Food records are also invaluable in subsequent follow-up sessions for helping both counselor and client understand the eating behavior at hand. Additional details such as location of meal or snack, hunger, mood and related thoughts can be instrumental in identifying behaviors or attitudes in need of modification during the counseling process.

Food Frequency. This type of questioning is used to identify how often specific foods or food groups are consumed by the client. Food frequency questionnaire forms can be general to all the foods commonly eaten or specially developed to quantify intake of a nutrient of particular concern, such as sodium. A food frequency can be used as a crosscheck method of validating the accuracy of a 24-hour recall.

Additional information such as food preferences, food intolerances or allergies, and dining out habits can be elicited during the interview either through closed or open-ended questioning. Combined with details regarding psychosocial factors influencing food intake, the practitioner will have a reasonable understanding of what the client is eating and why.

Evaluation of Current Intake

Once you have gathered information regarding a client's intake, the next step is evaluating it in accordance with his or her prescribed diet or nutritional needs. Thus,

---

Nutrition Screening Initiative

The Nutrition Screening Initiative (NSI) was founded in 1989 and is a broad, multidisciplinary effort coordinated by the American Academy of Family Physicians and The American Dietetic Association with more than 25 national health, aging and medical organizations. The goal of NSI is to promote the integration of nutrition screening and intervention into the provision of health care for older adults. Through these collaborative efforts, screening tools, and resources to help prevent malnutrition were developed. The screening tools are:

1) DETERMINE Your Nutritional Health Checklist
(available in English and Spanish)
This checklist is a public awareness tool for patients to assess their risk for poor nutritional status. It can be self-administered or administered by someone who interacts with older family members, friends, or clients. Actually, the screening tool questions can be appropriate for all ages. This tool is one page long and can be left in lobbies or handed to clients in physicians' offices, senior citizen centers, health fairs, home health agencies, health screening events, other community or group settings, and one-on-one with a family member.

2) Strong and Healthy
This tool is a companion pamphlet to the DETERMINE checklist that gives simple steps individuals can take to improve nutritional health.

3) Level I Screen
This screening tool can be administered as a follow-up to the *Checklist* or it can be utilized as the initial screen in the home health or other setting. It can identify people who should be more carefully evaluated for referral to other medical or community services.

4) Level II Screen
For someone whose *Checklist* or *Level I Screen* indicates a potentially serious nutritional or medical problem, the *Level II Screen* includes more specific diagnostic information. This screen must be administered by a qualified health professional to collect and interpret the information and then implement the most appropriate intervention.

These forms, instruction manuals, and additional resources are available on line or through the Nutrition Screening Initiative:

The Nutrition Screening Initiative
1010 Wisconsin Avenue NW, Suite 800
Washington DC 20007
www.nutritionscreening.org
www.aafp.org/nsi.xml

---

estimating nutritional needs is a prerequisite to this step in the assessment process. The purpose of this evaluation is to assist the practitioner in identifying areas of focus in the counseling process.

Quantitative assessment of food intake for macronutrients can be accomplished using computerized nutrient analysis software, the American Diabetes/Dietetic Associations' Exchanges for Meal Planning (26) or a food composition handbook (27), when sufficient details are obtained from the diet history. Semi-quantitative methods for diet evaluation have been developed for several nutrients such as fat intake. (28) The most time efficient manner of quantifying micronutrient intake is by using computerized nutrient analysis software, although food composition handbooks will also be accurate. Intakes of vitamins and minerals which are often less than two-thirds of the Dietary Reference Intakes (DRI) (29) is a nutritional risk but does not necessarily constitute a deficiency state. The DRIs are actually a set of four reference values: Estimated Average Requirements (EAR), Recommended Dietary Allowances (RDA), Adequate Intakes (AI), and Tolerable Upper Intake Levels (UL) that have replaced the 1989 Recommended Dietary Allowances.

A qualitative assessment of food intake can be performed by comparing overall intake from each food group in accordance with the Food Guide Pyramid (31) or Dietary Guidelines for Americans. (32) This type of evaluation can be rapidly performed to judge the overall balance and adequacy of an individual's diet. In May 2003, the Department of Health and Human Services (HHS) and the Department of Agriculture announced they have begun the process of developing the 6th edition of the Dietary Guidelines for Americans, scheduled for release in 2005. Although counseling efforts may focus on only one or two nutrients, such as saturated fat or sodium, it is important not to overlook other aspects of a healthy diet.

Estimating Nutritional Needs

Energy. Many formulas, such as the Harris-Benedict equation (33) and calories per kilogram (cal/kg) (34) are available for estimating energy requirements in hospitalized patients. Some simplified formulas are available to provide a reasonable estimate of calorie needs based upon level of stress for hospitalized patients and activity level and age in outpatient settings. While indirect calorimetry is likely to be the most accurate way of calculating calorie needs, it is not cost effective nor is it practical under most circumstances. (35)

Protein. For healthy adults, the Recommended Dietary Allowance for protein is 0.8 grams per kilogram ideal weight. (29) Protein intake for hospitalized or acute care outpatients should be estimated based upon disease state, degree of stress, unusual losses, and visceral protein status as assessed by the biochemical parameters previously reviewed. (35)

Vitamins and Minerals. The Dietary Reference Intakes (29) for vitamins and minerals are appropriate for use by healthy individuals. Recommendations for dosages can be adjusted upward for deficiency states, conditions which increase demands, or when absorption or utilization is impaired. As research identifies preventive benefits to taking additional nutrients, recommendations will change.

Fluid. This is especially crucial for pediatric and geriatric clients, for workers or athletes in warm environments, and when a person has a fever, vomiting, or diarrhea. For a child the recommendations are: (4)

1-10 kg	100 ml/kg
> 10 kg	1500-1800 ml/m2/d
> 20 kg	1500 ml plus 20 ml/kg for each kg > 20 kg

The general recommendations for fluids are 1 cc/kcalorie or the more common 6-8 glasses of fluid per day. Workers and athletes should drink at least the 2 quarts of fluid plus replace each pound of weight lost each day through dehydration with one pint of water. (36) Thirst is not a good indicator of dehydration in geriatric clients. When calculating fluid needs for the older adult, the amount should be based on body size and medical status. (37)

PSYCHOSOCIAL FACTORS AFFECTING FOOD INTAKE

One of the greatest determinants of food behaviors is an individual's psychosocial domain. (38,39) Counselors who have long-term relationships with their clients and are assisting them with changing their lifestyles should devote a considerable amount of attention to this area of assessment. One of the most challenging aspects of counseling is helping a client identify and overcome barriers to change. When these barriers are not identified in the assessment process and addressed during counseling, many clients will continue to make poor food choices, in spite of their knowledge of nutrition. These very personal details about a client's eating habits are best gathered through open-ended questioning, after rapport is established with a client.

Social Influence. Family and friends may have positive or negative effects on the client's eating behaviors based upon their own practices or the level of support offered to the client. (39) Also, social obligations and activities may influence dining out patterns and the food selections available. It is often valuable to gather information about other members at home, the person that does the shopping and cooking, and social activities that necessitate a deviation from the normal diet.

Food Availability Issues. Poor economic resources, sub-optimal preparation, poor storage facilities in the home, an inability to shop and prepare food due to illness, and lack of transportation to the grocery store will all impact upon the consumer food choices. After identification of these issues, referral to outside agencies may help remove such barriers. The Nutrition Screening Initiative for the elderly pointed out that 40 percent of people over 60 years in the United States live on less than $6,000 per year. (7)

Cultural and Religious Background. The environment in which we are raised will be a strong determinant of food preferences, consumption, preparation, and storage behaviors. (40) Be sensitive to a client's cultural food behaviors in all counseling interventions. See Chapter 5, "Cultural Competence in Counseling," for more information on this subject.

Stress and Emotions. How does the patient cope with feelings of stress, anger, depression, frustration, boredom and happiness? Often, eating is not from hunger but instead it is in response to these external cues. The antecedent to overcoming emotional eating in behavioral counseling is identification of these triggers in the assessment process.

When people are depressed, they may admit to sleeping too much, especially through the morning, or not resting well at night. The person may seem to lack enthusiasm for life in general, including interest in making or staying with behavior changes. The person may have difficulty identifying goals and strategies that he or she feels can be accomplished. Depression can interfere with a person's ability to work and maintain good relationships with family and friends. During a counseling session, a client may disclose many of these signs and symptoms to a nutrition therapist. If the person is dangerous to him or herself or to others, a referral to a mental health professional or referring physician is in order. If the person just needs small, achievable goals, enthusiastic guidance, and encouragement, the nutrition therapist is qualified to fill those functions.

SCREENING in the LONG-TERM CARE SETTING

The Resident Assessment Instrument (RAI) is a standardized approach for assessing, planning, and providing individualized care for residents of extended care facilities. Components of the RAI include:

- Minimum Data Set (MDS)
- Triggers
- Resident Assessment Protocols (RAP's)
- Interdisciplinary Care Plan (ICP)

The MDS is a basic multidisciplinary screening tool to identify factors associated with possible functional decline. Factors included that may impact nutrition status include cognitive and communication patterns, mood and behavior, psychosocial well being, physical functioning, oral/dental status, skin condition, activity level and special treatments and procedures.

Triggers are specific resident responses for the MDS elements and identify individuals who have, or are at risk of developing, specific functional deficits.

The RAP's are problem-oriented frameworks for additional assessment of triggered conditions. The triggers most applicable to the dietetic practitioner include nutritional status, nutrition support, dehydration/fluid balance, dental status, and pressure ulcers.

The ICP is a comprehensive nutrition care plan based on the results of the MDS assessment and the RAP's. It has three major components: problem identification; measurable time-limited goals designed to rehabilitate and prevent deterioration; and a plan of action, including follow-up. The ICP is reviewed regularly to ensure planned interventions remain appropriate to improve or maintain the resident's functional status.

Reference: Department of Health and Human Services, Health Care Financing Administration, Section 4145, specifications of RAI for use in LTC facilities, Appendix R. In State Operations Manual, Transmittal No. 272. Baltimore MD: DHHS, HCFA;1995.

Developmental Skills. When clients don't learn how to set boundaries or be assertive as an adolescent, they often have problems with these lifeskills for the rest of their lives. By not knowing how to control their time and by allowing other peoples' priorities to become their own, clients can remain confused about their own goals and direction. Danish (41) teaches high school students how to teach junior high students how to develop developmental or lifeskills. These skills can be the missing link between nutrition-related problems and developing the behaviors to eat healthy. For example, the reason a client may overeat each evening is because work is too hectic to leave for lunch. The more assertive person will bring this to the management's attention and request that changes are made in the schedule to allow time to eat a noon meal. For more discussion on this topic, see Chapter 13, Teaching Developmental Skills.

Motivation and Readiness. Different factors motivate individuals to change their eating behaviors. Fear of illness, feelings of improved well being due to the changes made, and the belief in one's ability to carry out the recommended actions are signs of motivation. (42) Conversely, when the client believes there are too few benefits in making changes, there are too many barriers, or he lacks feelings of competence, it is unlikely he will be able to modify his diet. Motivational factors should be assessed such as the client's perception of self-competency, his perceived threat from not taking action, and the benefits of change as opposed to the burdens. This will assist the practitioner in identifying attitudes in need of change in the counseling process. Some practitioners recommend using "Diet Readiness" tests as predictors of compliance and success in a weight loss program. (43,44) (See Appendix 7-B for sample "Weight loss Readiness" test.)

LIFESTYLE AND HEALTH RISK APPRAISAL

In the outpatient setting at corporations, wellness programs, fitness centers, health fairs, and private practice offices, lifestyle and health risk appraisals are becoming commonplace. Through a series of questions about family and personal medical histories, food habits, stress management, exercise, smoking, alcohol intake, safety habits, and so on, a client's lifestyle decisions and health risks can be determined as compared to a norm. The forms are often handed out to private clients at the first visit or they are mailed ahead of time so they can be filled out and turned in at the first visit. You can merely review the answers, or the answers can be scored by hand or by computer. Some companies that specialize in developing these tools also sell software for private offices, customized software (for large accounts), or they will run the program and mail back the results. (See Appendix 7-C for sample questionnaire.)

CONCLUSION

Assisting the client in making dietary changes requires a counselor to not only understand nutritional requirements related to both health and disease, but also the complex determinants of food behaviors. The comprehensive assessment process reviewed will enable the practitioner to better identify areas in need of modification in the client's diet and develop action plans, which are considerate of the client's domain.

Learning Activities

1. Select a particular type of client for nutrition counseling. Based on your assessment:
   - What are the specific medical nutrition problems for this client?
   - What are the nutrition goals for this client?
   - What psychosocial, cultural, ethnic or literacy factors must you consider?
   - How will you evaluate the client's motivation to learn or meet established goals?

2. Visit a medical clinic or ambulatory care setting. How are clients screened for nutrition risk? Who does the nutrition screening? What methods of assessment are used? Evaluate the effectiveness of the screening process and develop recommendations for the process if you were to make changes.

3. Interview a dietetic practitioner in private practice. How are clients screened and assessed for nutritional risk? What tools are used? How is baseline nutritional information utilized in designing the counseling sessions?

4. Research and then compare and contrast 3 computer systems available for nutrition screening and/or assessment. What are the strengths and weaknesses of each? In what settings would each be appropriate for nutrition counseling? What software considerations would a dietetic practitioner need to consider based on various practice environments?

References
1. American Dietetic Association. Definitions for nutrition screening and nutrition assessment. *J Am Diet Assoc.* 1994; 94:838-839.
2. Escott-Stump E. Dietary and Clinical Assessment. In: Mahan LK, Escott-Stump E, eds. *Krause's Food, Nutrition & Diet Therapy.* 10th ed. Philadelphia, PA: W.B. Saunders Co.; 2000.
3. Nieman D, Nieman DC, Lee RD *Nutritional Assessment.* 3rd ed. New York: McGraw-Hill Science/Engineering/Math; 2003.
4. Queen PM, Helm KK, Lang CE, eds. *Handbook of Pediatric Nutrition.* 2nd ed. Gaithersburg, MD: Aspen Pub.; 1999.
5. Niedert KC, ed. *Nutrition Care of the Older Adult: A Handbook for Dietetics Professionals Working Throughout the Continuum of Care.* Chicago: Consultant Dietitians in Healthcare Facilities and The American Dietetic Association; 1998.
6. Grant A, DeHoog S. *Nutrition Assessment Support and Management,* 5th ed. Seattle WA; 1999.
7. White JV, Dwyer JT, Posner BM, Ham RJ, Lipschitz DA, Wellman NS. Nutrition Screening Initiative: Development and implementation of the public awareness checklist and screening tools. *J Am Diet Assoc.* 1992; 92: 163-167.
8. Sanders P, Albarado M, Baldwin D, Newyear P. *The Handbook of Medical Nutrition Therapy.* Lake Dallas, TX: Helm Publishing; 1996.
9. McArdle WD, Katch FI, Katch VL. *Sports and Exercise Nutrition.* Philadelphia PA: Lippincott, Williams and Wilkins; 1999.
10. Aronson D. Personal Digital Assistants: Toys or Necessities? *Today's Dietitian.* 2003; 15 (5): 34-37.
11. Pronsky ZM, Redfern CM, Crowe J, Epstein S, Young V. *Food Medication Interactions.* 12th ed. Pottstown, PA: Food-Medication Interactions; 2001.
12. McCabe BJ, Wolfe JJ, Frankel EH, eds. *Handbook of Food-Drug Interactions.* Boca Raton FL: CRC Press; 2003.
13. Burke P, Roche-Dudek M, Roche-Klemma K. *Clinical Indications of Drug Nutrient Interactions and Herbal Use.* Riverside IL: Roche Dietitians, LLC; 2001.
14. Lyons TR. Herbal medicines and possible anesthesia interactions. *AANA J.* 2002 Feb; 70(1):47-51.
15. The American Dietetic Association and Dietitians of Canada. Nutritional Assessment. In: *Manual of Clinical Dietetics.* 6th ed. Chicago: American Dietetic Association; 2000.
16. Metropolitan Life Insurance Co., data adapted from the 1979 Build Study, Society of Actuaries and Association of Life Insurance Medical Directors of America. Phil., PA: Recording and Statistical Corp.; 1980.
17. Bray GA. *Contemporary diagnosis and management of obesity.* Newton PA: Handbooks in Healthcare Company; 1998.
18. Master A, Lasser R. Tables of average weight and height of Americans. *J Am Med Assco.* 1960; 172:658.
19. Waterlow JC. Classification and definition of protein-calorie malnutrition. *Br Med J.* 1972; 3: 566-569.
20. Centers for Disease Control (CDC), www.cdc.gov/growthcharts/
21. Heyward VH, Stolarczyk LM. *Applied Body Composition Assessment.* Champaign IL: Human Kinetics Publishers; 1996.
22. Despres JP. Lipoprotein metabolism in visceral obesity. *Int J Obes.* 1991; 15:45-52.
23. American College of Sports Medicine. *Guidelines for exercise testing and prescription.* 5th ed. Media PA: Williams and Wilkins, 1995.
24. Roitman JL, ed. *Resource manual for guidelines for exercise testing and prescription.* 3rd ed. Baltimore MD: Williams and Wilkins, 1988.

25. Litchman SW, Pisarska K, Berman ER, Pestone M, Dowling H, Offenbacher E, Weisel H, Heshka S, Matthews DE, Heymsfield SB. Discrepancy between self-reported and actual calorie intake and exercise in obese subjects. *New Eng J Med.* 1992; 327: 1893-1898.
26. The American Diabetes Association and The American Dietetic Association. *Exchange Lists for Meal Planning,* 2003.
27. Pennington JAT, Bowes AD, Church HN. *Bowes and Church's Food Values of Portions Commonly Used.,* 17th ed. Philadelphia PA: Lippincott, Williams and Wilkins; 1998.
28. Remmell PS, Benfari RC. Assessing dietary adherence in the Multiple Risk Factor Intervention Trial (MRFIT). *J Amer Diet Assoc.* 1980; 76: 357-360.
29. Food and Nutrition Board, Institute of Medicine, National Academy of Sciences. *Dietary Reference Intakes.* Washington, DC. 2002.
30. Kristal AR, Andrilla CH, Koepsell TD, Diehr PH, Cheadle A. Dietary assessment instruments are susceptible to intervention-associated response set bias. *J Amer Diet Assoc.* 1998; 98(1): 40-43.
31. *Food Guide Pyramid.* Washington, DC: US Dept of Agriculture, Center for Nutrition Policy and Information; Home and Garden Bulletin No. 252; 1996. www.usda.gov/fcs/cnpp.htm
32. *Nutrition and Your Health: Dietary Guidelines for Americans,* 5th ed. Washington, DC: US Dept of Health and Human Services; Home and Garden Bulletin No. 232; 2000. www.usda.gov/fcs/cnpp.htm
33. Harris JA, Benedict FG. *A biometric study of basal metabolism in man.* Publications No. 279, Carnegie Institute of Washington. Philadelphia PA: JB Lippincott; 1919.
34. National Research Council. Recommended Dietary Allowances. Washington DC: National Academy Press; 1989.
35. Gottschlich MM, ed. *The science and practice of nutrition support: a case based core curriculum.* Dubuque IA: Kendall/Hunt Publishing Company. 2000.
36. Rosenbloom CA, ed. *Sports nutrition: a guide for the professional working with active people.* Chicago IL: Sports, Cardiovascular and Wellness Nutritionists DPG and The American Dietetic Association, 2000.
37. Chidester JC, Spangler AA. Fluid intake in the institutionalized elderly. *J Amer Diet Assoc.* 1997; 97: 23-28.
38. Blum LS, Horbiak J. *Take the Lead. Person-Centered Counseling Skills.* Chicago, IL: National Center for Nutrition and Dietetics, 1990.
39. Stuart MR, Simko MD. A technique for incorporating psychological principles into the nutrition counseling of clients. *Top Clin Nutr.* 1991; 6: 32-39.
40. Dwyer JT. Steps to take in primary care for achieving lasting dietary change. *Top Clin Nutr.* 1991; 6: 22-31.
41. Terry DR. Needed: A new appreciation of culture and food behavior. *J Amer Diet Assoc.* 1994; 94: 501-503.
42. Danish S. *Advanced Counseling Skills.* Presentations at ADA Annual Convention, Orlando, FL, October 1994.
43. Rosenstock IM, Strecher VJ, Becker MH. Social learning theory and the health belief model. *Health Education Quarterly.* 1986; 13: 73-92.
44. Brownell KD, Wadden TA. *The LEARN Program for Weight Control.* Dallas, TX: American Health Pub. Co.; 1999.
45. Carlson S, Sonnenberg LM, Cumming S. Diet readiness test predicts completion in a short-term weight loss program. *J Amer Diet Assoc.* 1994; 94: 552-554.

Chapter 8

Counseling Skills for Behavior Change

Idamarie Laquatra, PhD, RD and Steven J. Danish, PhD

After reading this chapter, the reader will be able to:
♦ Identify four reasons for using counseling skills in their practice.
♦ Discuss appropriate counseling situations for the use of confrontation.
♦ Identify influencing skills used in a counseling session.
♦ List potential barriers to client goal achievement and methods to overcome these barriers.

What does nutrition counseling really mean? What are you trying to achieve through your counseling? More importantly, what are the client's goals for the nutrition counseling process?

As mentioned earlier, dietitians have not received adequate training and supervision in counseling skills, yet they are expected to be powerful forces in the lives of the clients they see. Some succeed and others do not.

Armed with loads of nutrition facts and figures, too many dietitians flood clients with information in the hopes their behaviors will change. How effective is giving information on behavior change? Not very. (1) Patients forget most of what they hear during informational sessions; the more information that's given, the more that's forgotten. (1,2) *You may lull yourself into thinking that if you can just figure out the right piece of information or point out their problems, you will motivate clients to change their behaviors. Nothing could be further from the truth.* This is not to say that giving information is without merit.

The real issue is learning to understand clients and their problems so well that you know the obstacles they face when trying to reach their goals. A lack of information is likely to be just one of the roadblocks present.

Incorporating specific skills into your nutrition counseling demands a commitment, and it often requires some significant behavior changes on your part. Just like the clients you see, making behavior changes often turns out to be quite difficult. Yet, dietitians expect clients to make incredible changes in their lives. Should you expect anything less of yourself? The authors don't think so.

Rationale for Learning and Using Counseling Skills

To change the way you counsel requires acceptance of a rationale for doing so. Specific reasons for making the effort to learn and use counseling skills are to:
• Facilitate change
• Empower clients to make their own decisions
• Empower dietitians
• Produce results

> **Perfection is not necessary to be successful in life, learning to cope and manage are.**

Facilitating change. In order to help clients change, you must first understand the problem from *their* perspective. The counseling skills help you zero in on the problem so you can work with clients to develop appropriate behavior change strategies.

Empowering clients. The skills enable clients to make their own decisions and control their behaviors. A major hurdle you must face is letting clients be less than perfect. New for some practitioners is the idea of encouraging "coping" or "managing" instead of "perfection." For example, dietitians learn specific dietary measures for specific diseases, and unfortunately, they often teach the diet in absolutes. They go over lists that contain foods that are allowed and those that should be avoided. Clients then tend to think in absolutes and feel as though they are failures if they cannot follow the program to the letter. Everything is black or white, right or wrong. Steps aren't small; they are the whole problem at once.

It's almost as if counseling is backwards: the diet is given in absolutes, the client follows the diet perfectly for a week or so (or until the first obstacle derails adherence efforts). Then the client backslides, berates his or her efforts and continues to fail to measure up to perfection. The dietitian, in an attempt to salvage the effort, suggests taking smaller steps and finally asks the client what he or she feels is possible. If a client is on a low saturated fat diet, instead of eating his usual four tablespoons of butter per day, he can start with eating only two. This is progress. *Wouldn't it be better to start off with a small step and then build on each success?* In the long run, the client is further ahead. In addition, the client and not the dietitian would be setting the goals, increasing client participation in the process of change.

Empowering dietitians. Counseling skills help you use your time more effectively because they help focus the direction of the counseling session. They position dietitians as more than information-givers, and allow you to use your training in nutrition and food in new and creative ways.

Increasing effectiveness. Using counseling skills will help clarify the problem. However, we must understand that the problem does not exist in isolation. Counseling skills help us understand how the problem fits into the client's life. They also help clients talk about themselves and increase self-awareness.

A GUIDE TO CORE COUNSELING SKILLS

Counseling is a two-part process. (3) During the first phase, the goal is the development of a strong, trusting relationship. The second phase involves the generation of behavior change strategies. You can't bypass the first phase for two reasons. First, you can't help clients develop strategies to address a problem until you understand what the problem is from the client's perspective. Second, a good relationship is an integral part of the second phase. You don't stop listening and start changing behavior. Listening attentively while you develop behavior change strategies will keep you from putting words into the client's mouth or making erroneous assumptions. Also, as mentioned earlier, the relationship with the counselor is often as therapeutic for the client as the counseling process.

Success in counseling is based on the counselor's level of skill in both phases of counseling. To build a good relationship, counselors must hone the skills that develop the core counseling conditions of empathy, genuineness, and unconditional positive regard (respect). To generate behavior change strategies, counselors must acquire the skills, which promote the process of change.

PHASE 1.   DEVELOPING A HELPING RELATIONSHIP

Nonverbal Attending Skills
You have heard and read about the importance of "good" nonverbal skills, but how recently have you evaluated yours in a counseling session? The message you communicate involves so much more than the words you say: 55% is communicated through body language, 38% through the tone of voice you use, and only 7% through words. (4) You must ensure consistency between your verbal and nonverbal messages. The following list should refresh your memory.

> *Eye contact:* In most cultures good eye contact without staring demonstrates that you are attending to the client and what the client says is important. It also communicates confidence.
> *Tone of voice:* Tone of voice means inflection and loudness. You can communicate your sense of caring, and your enthusiasm, friendliness, and warmth.
> *Body language:* Leaning forward with arms at your sides and hands relaxed or gesturing shows interest, openness, and a calm demeanor. Head nods communicate understanding.

> *Practice Activity. Working with a colleague, have him or her discuss a problem with you while you communicate your understanding with nonverbal gestures only. Do this for two minutes, afterward, discuss how you felt and how your colleague felt. Switch roles.*

Verbal Relationship-Building Skills: Active Listening
One of the keys to developing rapport and empathy entails "active listening." Active listening creates an accepting environment. You can capture the client's thoughts and feelings and communicate your understanding. Active listening requires you to reflect the thoughts and feelings of the speaker without adding your interpretations, solutions or information until you fully understand what is going on. Do not confuse active listening with parroting (repeating back what the person says). It is not a "technique" to manipulate the client. There is no game in counseling. As the nutrition counselor, you must work to clearly comprehend what the problem is, let the client know you understand, and then work together to solve the problem. (See Table 8.1 The Basic Listening Skills.)

Reflective Responses are basic to developing rapport, empathy and a trusting relationship. They summarize what the client said or target the feelings expressed. They serve three purposes: they help the client to continue to talk, they clarify, and they communicate a willingness to help. You must listen carefully to make an appropriate response. Following is an example of a client who is undergoing hemodialysis. He has experienced nausea and vomiting and has had problems with his appetite.

  Client Concern: "I find it difficult to eat all the calories I need to. I'm finding it bothersome to keep track of my salt and fluid intake, it takes so much energy. Sometimes I feel like it's all so useless. I'm not getting any better."
  Reflective response that summarizes the <u>content</u>: "Sounds like you think your diet is more work than it's worth."
  Reflective Response that targets the <u>feeling</u> being expressed: "You're feeling hopeless about your health right now."

  Practice Activity. Tape your next counseling session (if your client agrees). Try to use at least three reflective responses during your counseling. Listen to the tape and rate your success. After you succeed in using three, try increasing the number of reflective responses you give.

Leading Skills
Some clients can grow if you use only active listening skills. Many clients can work through their problems and concerns very effectively and need clarification and understanding rather than advice, direction, or suggestions. (1) However, when clients are seeking direction, leading skills can be used when nutrition therapists understand the nature of the problem, have specific suggestions to help deal with the problem, and feel comfortable assuming significant responsibility helping the client work with the problem. For example, a client may not have all of the information necessary to handle a new renal or hiatal hernia regime. Or, a client is at a loss for ideas for incorporating some exercise into his daily routine. Nutrition therapists may therefore need to advise, question, influence or educate, as well as coach and facilitate.
There are four different types of leading skills: **questions, influencing responses, advice, and giving information.**

Questions are used to gather <u>new</u> information. Verbal responses are like tools, and there are specific tools for specific tasks. There are different types of questions: open questions, closed questions, and ones that begin with "why." Unfortunately, dietitians overuse questions in counseling sessions. Rather than gathering significant information, dietitians often rely on questions to add more minutia to the assessment, to satisfy some curiosity, or to replace silence.

Table 8.1

The Basic Listening Skills

Skill	Description	Function in Interview
Active Listening Skills		
Silence or minimal response	Nod of head; "um-um"	Provides neutral feedback that the message was heard but does not indicate judgment.
Reflective responses	Statements which summarize the content or feelings of the client	Encourages elaboration and discussion, shows understanding and a willingness to help, checks clarity of counselor understanding, elucidates emotions underlying client's words and actions.
Leading Skills		
Open questions	"What?": facts "How?": process or feelings "Tell me more" "Could you be more specific?"	Used to bring out major data and facilitate the helping interaction. Elicits client response in open-ended yet focused manner. Can be in form of questions or open statements.
Closed questions	Usually begin with "Do," "Is," "Are" and can be answered with a "yes," or "no" or 1 or 2 words.	Used to quickly obtain specific data. Use with caution.
Why questions	Questions that seek the reason, cause, or purpose.	Can result in learning more about how the client reasons. Caution: May put the client on the defensive. Use sparingly.
Influencing responses	"That's a good idea."(encourages), "Maybe that's not the real issue." (interprets), "It's self-defeating to think that." (discourages)	Encourages or discourages the client's ideas, thoughts, or course of action to change or reinforce their behavior.
Advice	Provides suggestions, instructional ideas, homework, advice on how to act, think or behave.	Used sparingly, may provide client with new and useful ideas to try.
Information	A statement made to instruct the client on appropriate nutritional practices.	Provides clients with more data to enable them to design their own solutions. Note that too much information is overwhelming. Counselors must determine the amount that is really necessary.
Self-Referent Skills		
Self-involving responses	The counselor shares a present reaction to the client through a personal response to what the client said or did.	Can be used to provide feedback, praise, or to gently confront. Gives counselors a way to use their own feelings and reactions to the client during counseling.
Self-disclosure	Counselor shares personal experience from the past or present information about him or herself with the client.	Can build a mutual relationship with the client through similar, shared experiences.

To help break this habit, think, "If I already know the answer, don't ask the question!" By using a reflective response instead, you will show that you are perceptive of the client's point-of-view. This will save precious counseling time by getting to the underlying issues, and it shows a higher level of counseling skill. To help you learn how to do this effectively, when you wish to ask a question of your client, **First** ask the question to yourself. **Second,** answer the question, as you would expect the client to answer it. **Third,** make a reflective response that captures how the client would respond.

> Client: "I had been doing so well, and then the holidays hit. First, I started eating sweets as soon as I arrived at work. It's really hard...they're only available at this time of year, and I hate to see the holidays go by and not even get a taste. But then, at night when I get home, I look in the mirror and ask myself what I'm doing. Then, the next day comes and it's back to the sweets. Oh, I don't know...."
>
> Dietitian wants to ask: "Do you think you can break out of this cycle?"
>
> How the dietitian expects the client to respond: "I don't know, even though I resolve to stop doing it at night, the next day, all the resolve melts away."
>
> Reflective response the dietitian can use: "Sounds like you're frustrated about the cycle you're in right now."

Open questions put few parameters on clients, leaving plenty of room for them to respond. They allow the client to explore an issue instead of simply answering "yes" or "no." Open questions usually start with "what" or "how." Statements such as "Tell me more" and "Can you be more specific?" can be classified as open because their use elicits open-ended responses from clients.

> "How do you think your new behaviors will affect your family?"
> "What obstacles will you face when you try to implement these ideas?"
> "Tell me more about what you felt when you knew you wanted to binge?"
> "Can you be more specific about your exercise?"

Closed questions can usually be answered with "yes," "no," or in one or two words. They do not encourage exploration and they can lead to a dead-end in counseling. Closed questions pose the risk of providing little information beyond the short answer to the question. There may be times when closed questions are appropriate, like to obtain specific data or close a lengthy answer; however, as a general rule, choose open questions if at all possible.

> "Do you understand why eating is so important when you're taking insulin?"
> "Were you able to choose low saturated fat foods at the reception?"
> "Do you have any questions?"
> "Have you tried to decrease your sodium in the past?"

"Why" questions can put clients on the defensive because they seem to require an excuse. Also, sometimes clients respond to "why" questions with "I don't know." This type of answer provides little information for counselors. Questions that begin with "why" are common among friends, and we usually do not think about the unintended consequences that may result when used in counseling. Exercise caution when using "why" questions; opt for open ones if you can rephrase the question. If you feel that you must use a "why" question, watch your tone of voice to remove any judgmental tone or threat the client may feel. (See discussion on Confrontation and when it is appropriate.)

> *Practice Activity. Listen to a tape of one of your counseling sessions. When you hear a closed question, stop the tape and try to change the closed question to an open one.*

Confrontation

Confrontation is used as an invitation and challenge to examine, modify, or control some aspect of a client's behavior. It helps individuals see more clearly what is happening, what the consequences are, and how they can assume responsibility. It is hoped that clients will learn how to confront themselves and take corrective action in the future. Failure to confront when you see and hear self-defeating or unreasonable behavior implies support for the behavior.

Clients are frequently unaware of the games they play and do not realize the confusion they produce in their lives through conflicting messages. Most clients do not recognize the consequences of their maladaptive behavior. Confrontations help clients admit ownership of how they truly feel (without distortions or denial) and that they rule their own destinies. Common discrepancies include:

1. *A discrepancy between the way the client sees himself and the way others see him.* For example, a man with a strong family history of heart disease sees himself as a victim and it doesn't matter if he takes care of himself or not. The dietitian views him as someone who should be motivated because of his family history.
2. *A contradiction between what the client says and the way she behaves.* An obese woman says she wants to lose weight and yet she still binges on food.
3. *A discrepancy between two statements by the client.* The same client talks about not being sedentary in the same interview that he states he has never liked exercise.
4. *A discrepancy between what the client says he is feeling and the way most people would react in a similar situation.* A client tells the counselor that he feels good about not achieving a short-term goal because it makes him try harder.
5. *A contradiction between what the client is presently saying she believes and the way she has acted in the past.* A client describes her present nutrition philosophies, which vary greatly from how she has described her past food intake.

The guidelines to keep in mind when formulating a confrontation response are:
- Mutual trust and empathy must already be established in the counseling relationship.
- It should come across as a positive, caring act, not as an attacking, judgmental one.
- It addresses specific, concrete attributes of the client's behavior that the client can change.
- It points out discrepancies in how clients view their assets (strengths). Responses can constructively focus on these strengths that clients may overlook.

How to Confront

A self-involving response can be used successfully in confrontation. For example, suppose the client sets a goal each week and then reports time and again that he could not follow through with achieving the goal:

Client: I just couldn't follow through on eating one portion at dinner again this week. I just had so much on my mind.

Counselor: I'm confused. You seemed enthusiastic about working on your goals when you set them, yet you haven't been able to achieve this one for the last two weeks. Help me understand what's going on. (self-involving response)

You might also try the following to gently confront clients:

"Have you ever noticed that you...."

"Did you hear what you just said...."

"What you are telling me now is different than what you said awhile ago about ...."

"You say you want to eat fewer high fat foods, but what I see you doing is...."

"One of the reasons that people may respond to you that way is because ...."

Always remember that confrontation is an act of caring and a desire on your part to become more intimately involved with the client.

Used with permission. © 1983 American Dietetic Association. Adapted from Engen HB, Iasiello-Vailas L, Smith KL: Confrontation: A new dimension in nutrition counseling. *J Am Diet Assoc;* 83 :34, 1983. (5)

Influencing Responses are used to reinforce or discourage the client's ideas or statements. They can also offer an interpretation of what the client says or does. Influencing responses can be used to indirectly change client behavior. Following are examples of influencing responses.

Client: "I'm thinking of taking a herb cooking class to get away from using salt when I prepare meals."
Counselor (reinforces): "That's a terrific idea!"

Client: "I want to try out that new weight loss herbal treatment---a friend of mine said it was quick and easy."
Counselor (discourages): "You already know that weight loss requires some lifestyle changes. Have you read the ingredients to figure out how it works? It could be dangerous."

Client: "I know I should be eating more, but I don't like the food. I don't know anybody; they all seem so old, so I sit alone. I don't think they like me."
Counselor (interprets): "Maybe the food isn't the whole problem here."

Advice provides clients with thoughts or behaviors they haven't tried (or at least you think they haven't tried) to help solve the problem. Think about your past week. Did you receive advice from anyone, even when you didn't ask for it? Did you follow the advice (even if you DID ask for it)? Good advice is specific and realistic, and it's given in a tentative manner to allow the client an "out" if needed. "Perhaps you might try..." or "You might consider..." are good tentative openers for advice.

You have to listen well to know what the client has tried, what has and hasn't worked in the past, and why the solution did or did not work. Unfortunately, counselors often give advice before they fully understand the situation or before they know what was already tried. In these instances, you hear words like "Yes, but..." from the client:

Client: "I'm going on vacation, and I just don't think I can follow this program while I'm away."
Counselor: "What makes you feel that way?" (Open Question)
Client: "Well, we'll be eating out, and I'll be staying with friends and relatives for parts of the trip."
Counselor: "Perhaps you could do the grocery shopping while staying with friends and relatives, and buy the foods you would normally eat." (Advice)
Client: "Yes, but we'll only be with friends on one weekend, and I really don't feel comfortable enough with my relatives to ask that."
Counselor: "Maybe you could tell them in advance what your needs are." (Advice)
Client: "Yes, but I hate to be a bother."

This counseling session is going nowhere fast. The dietitian needs to spend more time exploring the problem before offering solutions. For example, the dietitian could ask, "What do you eat on a typical day when you are on vacation?" and then they could identify simple ways to alter the food choice or cut the volume. Or, the dietitian might say, "Imagine that you are on vacation and you are also in control of your eating habits, how would you eat?"

Not only can giving advice be a waste of precious time, but poor advice can also undermine your effectiveness. With a dependent client, giving advice can encourage dependence on the counselor because the counselor is making the decisions.

Practice Activity. For one week, record any advice that people give you. Keep track of whether you asked for it and whether or not you implemented the advice. See how often advice is given and how seldom it is implemented.

Information about nutrition or the diet seems to be the mainstay of dietary counseling. (7) As discussed earlier, dietitians too often overwhelm clients by trying to teach them everything they will ever need to know about their diet for the rest of their lives. *Clients can't remember THAT much information.* Break it up into more manageable pieces and let the client have time to review it before the next visit. Evaluate every piece of information you give. Will it really help? Does it classify as a "so what" piece of information? For example, some interesting tidbit to you may not be so interesting to a client who happens to be a novice at assessing his or her eating behavior. To solve problems and overcome barriers, use attending skills and cognitive-behavioral, psychoeducational, or other approaches.

Self-Referent Skills
Using self-referent skills provides nutrition counselors vehicles for talking about themselves and their feelings during a counseling session. Self-referent skills can increase openness, give feedback to clients, provide a model for how to talk about oneself, and make the counseling session less impersonal. The focus shifts from the client to the counselor. Although these skills can be extremely effective, using them too often or too early during counseling can have some negative effects: 1) counselors may spend more time talking about themselves than listening to the client; 2) counselors may unintentionally offend the client; and 3) counselors may turn the counseling into "chatting" visits rather than helping sessions.

Before you use self-referent skill, you should be able to answer the following questions: What personal needs am I fulfilling by using this response? How will the client respond? What effect will my response have on the relationship? Counselors can use two types of self-referent skills: self-involving responses and self-disclosure.

Self-Involving Responses actively put the counselor into the session. This response follows the format: I (the counselor) feel (this way) about what you (the client) said or did. You can use a self-involving response to gently confront or to provide feedback to the client about how you feel.

Client: "I'm sorry I couldn't stick to that program to lower my cholesterol. I know you were counting on me and I let you down."
Counselor: "I'm concerned that you're following the program for me and not yourself."

Client: "My blood sugar has been great, and I really feel like I'm starting to understand the diet."
Counselor: "I'm thrilled with your progress."

Self-Disclosure is often used without thinking about the consequences. With a self-disclosing response, a dietitian talks about himself or herself. On the positive side, self-disclosure provides a model to the client of how to talk about personal subjects, and it changes the relationship from an impersonal to a personal one. On the negative side, the dietitian can end up taking up most of the time talking about his or her experiences and learning nothing about the client. For example, imagine you are working with someone who has diabetes, and you have diabetes too. Dealing with restaurant eating poses a major problem for your client and it used to be a problem for you. Suppose the counseling session went like this:

Client: "I worry about eating out, now. I'm not sure how to count some things, and I always seem to eat more when I'm with a group."
Counselor: "Well, I have diabetes, too, and I remember how difficult I thought it was to eat out."
Client: "Really? What did you do?"
Counselor: "I asked what ingredients were in some entrees, and I just asked the waiter to serve sauces and dressings on the side. I always tried to order first, so I wouldn't be influenced by someone else."
Client: "How did your friends feel?"
Counselor: "They're dietitians, too, so it didn't bother them."
Client: "Oh."

From this short interchange, you can see that the focus changed from being on the client to the dietitian, and the shared information gave little help or direction. The dietitian could have used reflective and leading skills only or the dietitian might have said the following:

Client: "I worry about eating out, now. I'm not sure how to count some things, and I always seem to eat more when I'm with a group."

Counselor: "Well, I have diabetes too, and I remember how difficult I thought it was to eat out."

Client: "Really? What did you do?"

Counselor: "I soon learned to control my portions by eating the same amount as I would at home. We're talking a lot about me. (reflective) Tell me more about your situation so we can design a strategy to deal with it." (open-ended question)

> ***Practice Activity.*** *Listen to a tape of one of your counseling sessions. How often do you discuss your personal life? How often do you bring in your feelings? What effect does each have on the counseling session?*

> ***Practice Activity.*** *Tape a counseling session and as you listen to the tape, record the responses you made, identify them, and rate them. If you were not happy with some responses, think of a more appropriate one. Part I and Part II of the Counselor Evaluation System in Appendix 8-A can be a helpful tool in this process.*

PHASE 2. DEVELOPING BEHAVIOR CHANGE STRATEGIES

To empower clients is to enable them to achieve and to take control of their lives. If you want to enable clients to do something, you have to help them develop the necessary skills to do so. Ultimately, you want your clients to have the skills they need not for a short-term diet but to change their eating styles permanently. Telling clients what to do and simply giving information are short-term fixes; empowering offers a long-term solution.

One of the best ways to help clients gain control over their situation is to teach them how to set goals. Now this sounds simple, but it is truly amazing how few people are skilled at setting reachable goals. Setting goals involves three steps:

Step 1 You help clients identify the goal.

Step 2 Assess its importance.

Step 3 Analyze the roadblocks which hinder goal attainment.

Let's look at each step in more detail.

Step 1 Goal Identification

In order to identify a goal, you must have a very clear picture of the problem. A goal is simply the flipside of the problem (if the problem is skipping breakfast and overeating in the evening, the goal is to do the opposite). *Achievable goals are positive, specific, and under the goal setter's control.*

As discussed earlier, the newer thinking on goals is that they should be *much smaller steps and even more achievable so that clients feel empowered.* Therefore, "losing 35 pounds" should be seen as a *result* that goals were met and achieved. In weight loss counseling when you create a potentially overwhelming end goal, it can seem extremely distant to some clients. *It often fails to motivate the client after a few weeks, and there are several generations of dieters who prove the approach doesn't work.* **It also diminishes the recognition paid to the true contributors to change like new cognitions, more mature developmental skills, healthier eating or lifestyle choices. These are the changes that must be recognized and maintained for the result to be maintained.**

Goals that have the words "not" and "avoid" are negative and difficult, if not impossible, to achieve. Focusing on the negative expends energy on what the client doesn't want to do. Because it's not a constructive exercise, clients start to feel frustrated or deprived, increasing the likelihood that they will give up and feel like failures. Helping clients set positive goals reveals the control and power they have in a situation.

For example, a client with diabetes may have a problem eating on a regular schedule: "I just can't seem to eat my meals and snacks regularly because my schedule is so hectic." A positive goal would be: "I want to eat my meals and snacks on a better schedule." While the goal is positive, it is vague and hard to reach. How does the client define "a better schedule"? How will the client know when the schedule improved?

Reachable goals are specific, and expressed in behavioral terms. A positive, specific goal would be: "On Monday and Tuesday of this week, I plan to eat breakfast at 8:00, a snack at 10:00, lunch at 12:30, afternoon snack at 3:00, dinner at 7:00 and an evening snack at 10:00." The goal is small, clear, and practical. The client will know when it's achieved.

Making sure the goal is under the client's control involves two aspects:

- **First, the goal must involve the <u>client's</u> behavior and not the actions of someone else.** For example, a goal such as, "I want my wife to use low fat cooking methods like baking or broiling instead of frying" is an admirable goal, but it is dependent on the wife's behavior not the client's. The dietitian must help the client refocus and concentrate on <u>his </u>behaviors. In this instance, the client may decide to set a goal of asking his wife to cook using lower fat methods: "Tonight, I'll ask Joan to bake the chicken instead of frying it." Notice that the client can achieve the goal of asking regardless of whether or not Joan cooperates.
- **The second aspect of control pertains to distinguishing <u>goals</u> from <u>results</u>,** as mentioned above. Lowering blood cholesterol is a result; eating low saturated fat foods is a goal. Losing weight is a result; eating fewer calories and exercising three times per week for 30 minutes are goals. Goals that are achieved often lead to positive results.

Step 2 Goal Importance Assessment

Critical to the entire goal-setting process, *goal importance assessment defines the motivation.* The goal must be most important to the client. Goals that physicians, spouses, or nutritionists find important may or may not be meaningful for the client. Always check to see if clients feel they <u>should</u> reach the goal or if they <u>want</u> to reach it. *"Want" goals are more often achieved than "should" goals.* Clients say "should" to themselves so often when it comes to diet and lifestyle change it may take time to uncover the "want" goals.

Step 3 Goal Roadblock Analysis

Four obstacles impede goal achievement:

- Lack of knowledge
- Lack of skills
- Inability to take a risk
- Lack of support

A client may have one, two, three,or all four of these roadblocks.

Lack of knowledge **means the client doesn't know the "what."** For example, he or she may be unaware of the calorie content of different food choices; a person just diagnosed with diabetes may not know what the consequences are of skipping meals; or an individual with kidney disease may not know what the lower potassium fruits are. If clients lack knowledge, it is appropriate to provide information or show them how to access that information.

Lack of skills **means the client lacks the "how to."** Ms. Jones may not know how to control her intake at a social function; Mr. Smith may not know any other way to relax besides eating; Jennifer may be unaware of rewards beyond the refrigerator; Sam may not believe he can change the way he eats. Clients often focus on their weaknesses, failing to identify strengths they already have. Teaching them to focus on their strengths will eventually help them see how they can transfer different abilities to more than one life situation. When clients lack developmental skills, dietitians can help teach the client new skills in a systematic way. Skill learning requires demonstration and practice.

Inability to take risks **refers to the fear associated with goal achievement.** Clients may have certain costs associated with reaching their goal, and their perception is that the costs outweigh the benefits. For example, Mr. Brown, who has a concern about his cholesterol level, may be afraid that he will never succeed in changing his level so he chooses not to try. Ms. Jones may be afraid her dates will feel she has a serious illness and won't want to pursue a relationship if she tries to adopt a diabetes diet. As their dietitian, the focus needs to be a realistic weighing of both the real and perceived costs and benefits of changing behavior. What do they have to gain by reaching the goal? What do they have to lose?

Lack of social support **may require clients to look beyond their traditional support structure to help sustain behavior changes.** Sometimes, spouses or family members sabotage life change efforts. Often, the dietitian becomes the support during the initial part of counseling. The dietitian must help the client identify what support is needed, who can best or most likely will provide that support, and what is the best way for the client to ask for the support.

Using good listening skills will help you determine if the obstacles interfere with goal achievement and what they are. Once you have a clear understanding, you and the client can develop a program to achieve the goal. Make sure the program consists of small steps so that the client will not fail during the early stages. As the client gains self-confidence, more difficult steps can be undertaken. Clients feel a sense of accomplishment when they can evaluate their progress.

Goal Setting Guide
Included in Appendix 8-A is a sample Goal Setting Guide (Part 3) of the Counselor Evaluation System. Feel free to use the guide, think of it as a blueprint for counseling. You do not have to ask all or any of the questions on the guide; use active listening skills to determine the answers.

APPLYING THE SKILLS IN YOUR COUNSELING
While the process of counseling described above sounds simple, the authors have found that helping dietitians change their behaviors can be just as challenging as helping clients! They've conducted numerous workshops with dietitians, and the response is usually the same: there is excitement about the skills and a sincere desire to incorporate them into nutritional counseling. When the participants return to their work environments, many fall back into old habits and fail to use the skills. Why are the skills hard to implement once they return to work? Why is it so hard to change? (1)

There are basically four roadblocks that they face when trying to implement a change. (Sound familiar?) They are lack of knowledge, lack of skills, inability to take risks, lack of support, or a combination of these. Note that these obstacles have nothing to do with the merits of using the skills. If you believe in the importance of the skills and have a desire to use them, the roadblocks just mentioned will be all that stand in your way.

Lack of Knowledge. If the obstacle is a lack of knowledge, you're not alone. Lack of training in this area is the primary reason for the dilemma. (1) Traditionally, dietitians are taught about the importance of developing rapport and tailoring dietary interventions to fit the client's lifestyle without being taught the actual skills. Dietitians are also taught how essential it is for clients to accept the responsibility for change, but not taught the methods for helping clients become involved in the process. Unfortunately, most learning is through a lecture format. Your practice may occur during an internship when you observe dietitians (who may or may not know specific counseling skills) as they work with clients. You then imitate what you see. In this chapter, the authors explained the nonverbal and verbal skills needed to build an effective helping relationship and to encourage behavior change. Learning what the skills are should help you hurdle the obstacle of the lack of knowledge. Use this chapter as a reference for the counseling skills. Recognize that reading this book still may not be enough to cause a change in your behavior because other obstacles may stand in your way.

Lack of Skills. This is the most difficult obstacle to deal with through the written word. You may need to go through the process of skill development to increase proficiency in using the skills. There are specific steps for this and they include:

- Evaluating your motivation
- Assessing your current skill level
- Setting a goal
- Practicing
- Evaluating progress

Note that the first step is evaluating your motivation. If adopting the skills is not a priority, it just won't happen. To be actively involved in the process of learning a skill, you have to be convinced that the skill is worth pursuing. Some questions you might ask yourself include: Why bother with these skills? Why are the skills important for me? What makes me believe that I can learn these skills? Are the skills worth the trouble?

Next, assess your current skill level. Audiotape or videotape a counseling session, it is an incredible learning process. Review the tapes with someone more knowledgeable than you (a supervisor or therapist colleague), or use the system in Appendix 8-A. Assessing where you are will help you determine the exact skills you need to develop. If you can, have a skilled therapist model the skills so that you can observe the skills in action and then discuss their uses.

The third step in skill development involves setting a goal. Refer to Part 3. A sample of a goal might be: "I will ask an open question at least once during my counseling session with Ms. Dean."

Once you set the goal, practice under supervision by having someone observe you or by making an audiotape. And don't forget to evaluate your progress on a regular basis. Compare your skills on a week-to-week basis through audiotapes to assess progress.

Dealing with Problems
Kathy King, RD, LD

When you see patients in the hospital or clients walk into your office, they bring along their emotions, anxieties, moods, and personalities. You are not expected as a nutrition therapist to deal with everything and make it all better. To be effective as a counselor, however, you cannot act clueless and go ahead with a diet instruction when the client is clearly very upset, too ill, or reacting to another agenda. There may be times when clients are in denial about their diagnoses. They may be too upset about something to listen. They may listen, but abuse at home or some other barrier makes behavior change improbable. You cannot fix them all. These are times when you need to listen and determine what's best for the client or patient. It may be to act as a conduit to getting them help in other ways. You may need to listen and offer a supportive environment for their venting. It may be a time to postpone or reschedule the appointment. At times logic and a few kind words will change the mood and help move the client to reassess his temperament or resistance to change.

For example, a client came for a weight loss follow-up appointment to a private practitioner's office. The client was agitated with darting glances and furrowed forehead. When the dietitian asked how he was doing, he answered angrily that the diet was worthless. He didn't know why he had come because nothing was working. This was the client's third visit and he had never been negative or so abrupt. The dietitian started out by saying, "I'm so sorry that you are frustrated. Please tell me what has happened." She showed empathy instead of taking his comments personally and becoming defensive. He answered with a description of his eating during the week, which was not bad. He then started talking about his job, an incident at work that upset him, and how his boss had "laid into me just as I was leaving today." The dietitian responded, "You are feeling a lot of stress at work?" He responded, "Yeah, a lot of unfair stress." The dietitian queried, "What can you do to handle the stress?" He said, "I'm going to write down what happened from my point of view and talk to my boss tomorrow." "Good," responded the dietitian, "Tell me, how you feel about your food choices this past week?" The client said, "I really didn't do that bad. I just ate smaller portions and didn't skip meals." The initial anger was gone and they both knew its source had nothing to do with the client's food intake. By quietly listening and asking a few open-ended questions, the dietitian was able to show positive regard, help the client identify his source of anger, and get the nutrition therapy back on track.

As a counselor, you are not responsible for entertaining or mothering the client. You should keep professional boundaries in place by showing concern and empathy without delving into highly private affairs or allowing the client to use you as a buddy, girlfriend, or social outlet. When a client exhibits mood swings and emotional outbursts, try to keep a level head, don't take comments personally, and don't take on the client's problem and feel you have to "make it all better." If the problem is within the nutrition therapist's scope of practice (nutrition-related or lifestyle choices), the therapist can help the client determine his goals and strategies, help him overcome barriers, and practice new choices until they become automatic. This does not include abuse counseling, suicide prevention, or deep-seated emotional counseling. These needs require intervention by other therapists with more advanced training. As mentioned earlier, do not allow yourself to be verbally or emotionally abused by a client. See the discussion on page 39.

Inability to Take Risks. If this is your roadblock, you might feel afraid to use the skills because you don't know what the effects on your clients will be; you might be worried that you won't appear expert enough to your clients or you may be worried that your superiors won't accept your new approach. Whatever the problem, weigh the advantages and disadvantages of using the skills. Because the actual consequences of using the new skills in your situation are uncertain, there is a tendency to guess about the potential outcomes. In guessing, people often confuse what is likely to happen with what is probably *not* going to happen. You might want to ask yourself the following questions: What can be gained by using the skills? What can be lost? What positive outcomes will likely occur? Are there any negative consequences to consider? What is the best possible outcome and how realistic is this? What is the worst possible outcome and how realistic is this?

Lack of Support. To change the way we counsel requires a supportive environment. If we don't create an atmosphere that encourages skill use, the chances of maintaining the skills will be slim. Don't just hope that your supervisor or co-workers will see how great the skills are and support their use. If you need to, be prepared to sell them on the counseling skills. Take a win-win approach. Find out what their needs are, figure out how using the skills will fill their needs, and then tell them about it. Don't be put off by objections. Try to think of objections as a desire on their part for more information. Listen actively to the objections until you understand them so that you can provide whatever is necessary to sell your point.

CONCLUSION

As a final note, dietitians just learning this approach believe it will work well with individuals struggling with obesity. They hesitate to use the approach with clients suffering from other diseases such as diabetes, renal disease, or cardiovascular disease. Why? Dietitians may think that these diseases are more serious, or that when clients have such problems, they need to be told what to do or suffer dire consequences. Despite what you may think, dietary adherence, no matter what the problem, is notoriously poor over the long-term. Also, today's recommendations for just about every disorder focus on individualizing the program to meet the client's needs and requirements. If the old approach doesn't work, why not try something new? Start with small steps and you'll see the self-esteem of clients grow as they make progress in reaching their attainable goals.

Learning Activities

1. Observe a one-on-one nutrition counseling session. Identify the basic listening skills utilized by the counselor. Were they effective in moving the session along?

2. With a colleague, role-play a counseling session in which the "counselor" utilizes confrontation to deal with client behaviors. What skills are needed to use confrontation effectively?

3. Observe a counseling session where the counselor is providing nutrition education information. What influencing skills did the counselor use to increase the client's knowledge level? Critique the session; what would you have done differently based on your knowledge of effective nutrition counseling techniques?

4. For one of the counseling sessions observed above, how were goals set with the client? Were the goals client-centered? What obstacles did you observe that may interfere with client goal achievement?

References
1. Laquatra I, Danish SJ. A challenge to change the way we help. *J Am Diet Assoc.* 2001; 11:1318.
2. Green LW. Educational strategies to improve compliance with therapeutic and preventive regimes: The recent evidence. In: Haynes RB, Taylor RB, Sackett DW, eds. *Compliance in Health Care.* Baltimore, MD: The Johns Hopkins University Press; 1979.
3. Danish SJ, Ginsberg MR, Terrell A, Hammond MI, Adams SO. The anatomy of a dietetic counseling interview. *J Am Diet Assoc.* 1979; 75: 626-630.
4. Mehrabain A. Communication without words. *Psych Today.* 1968:9.
5. Tamminen AW, Smaby MH. Helping counselors learn to confront. *Personnel Guid J.* 1981; 60:1.
6. Danish SJ, D'Augelli AR, Hauer AL. *Helping Skills: A basic training program.* New York: Human Science Press; 1980.
7. Laquatra I, Danish SJ. Effect of a helping skills transfer program on dietitians' helping behavior. *J Am Diet Assoc.* 1981; 78: 22, 181.
8. Laquatra I. Helping Skills for WIC Nutrition Education Counselors. University Park, PA: The Pennsylvania State University; 1983. Dissertation.

Chapter 9

Cognitive-Behavioral Therapy
Alison Murray, EdD, NCC, CCMHC, LMHC, RD

After reading this chapter, the reader will be able to:
♦ Distinguish between behavioral, cognitive, and psychoeducational theories.
♦ List three categories of disordered eating and potential counseling strategies.
♦ Recognize behavioral, cognitive, and psychoeducational treatment strategies in given scenarios.

One of the most important functions served by nutrition therapists is as a facilitator of change. Changes in eating behavior may improve your health, sports performance, or medical condition. Dietitians, therefore, are behaviorists. You may also be a cognitivist because you might first focus on changing clients' thoughts, beliefs, or attitudes with respect to food, eating, or some other dietary related behavior.

This chapter will focus on techniques used within the cognitive-behavioral category of counseling theory, including behavioral theory, cognitive theory, and psychoeducational theory, which involve both a cognitive component and a behavioral component, such as hunger and fullness training. Basic premises of each approach will be explored, as well as techniques that are representative of that discipline. Following the explanation of each technique will be a discussion of clinical utility and an example of its use. (See Table 9.1 Cognitive-Behavioral Techniques.)

Table 9.1 Cognitive-Behavioral Techniques

Behavioral Techniques	Cognitive Restructing Techniques	Psychoeducational
Classical conditioning	Decatastrophizing	Distraction
Operant conditioning	Challenging Shoulds, Oughts, Musts	Delay
Self-monitoring	Reattribution	Parroting
Stimulus control	Decentering	
Imagery		
Role-playing		
Real-life performance-based		
Self-reinforcement		
Modeling		
Systematic desensitization		

Ethical Considerations
As a practitioner, you are cautioned with regard to using techniques without first developing a caring relationship with the client. Techniques should be used in a spontaneous way, as they are needed to help the client. In their book on *Family Therapy Techniques,* Minuchin and Fishman describe this situation more fully. (1)

... technique alone does not ensure effectiveness. If the therapist (dietitian), becomes wedded to technique, remaining a craftsman, his contact with patients will be objective, detached, and clean, but also superficial, manipulative for the sake of personal power, and ultimately not highly effective. (1)

Corey outlines numerous questions a counselor might consider in monitoring your use of techniques. (2) Some of these questions, adapted to the work of a dietitian, are summarized below.

- Do you first give advice, or do you allow clients to explore their eating problems fully?
- Do you give your clients guidance and reassurance? Do you allow clients to express how they feel about their diet, circumstance, and dilemmas? Or, do you immediately tell them how to solve their dilemma?
- Do you clarify and checkout what you think clients are telling you with regards to their story, how they feel about their story, and what their concerns are?
- In what ways do you use techniques? To get clients moving? Or, do you wait until you have more information about what a client might need, discuss what might help, and direct communication to a more personal level?
- Do you use techniques that you feel comfortable with? That you have studied, practiced, and received supervision on (a mentor has discussed your use of techniques with you)? Are your techniques mechanical or unforced? (2)

In using techniques then, nutrition therapists must consider spontaneity as well as ethical issues. Involved in spontaneity and ethics are outcome considerations. Techniques should not be *applied* indiscriminately, but rather, with concern for the client's well being, capacity for change, and expectations of treatment. (2,3,4) In this regard, the client should be as much a part of the selection of techniques as the dietitian. The dietitian might ask the client such questions as illustrated in the example below.

Dietitian: What do you think will help you change your eating behavior?
Client: I don't know. That's why I'm coming here. (This client might also be experiencing anger, which will make the *application* of techniques that much more difficult.)
Dietitian: Well let us review some of what brought you here and some of your expectations for nutrition counseling. First, your doctor referred you so that you might lose weight. Your doctor thought this might help lower both your blood pressure and cholesterol level. You describe your eating as spontaneous—you just don't think about it much. We might begin by helping you understand more of your eating habits, and specifically, the triggers in your environment that may stimulate your eating. To accomplish this, you might record everything you eat and drink, and the conditions under which this takes place, for about one week. How does this sound to you?
Client: Well, I hate to keep records. I'm not good at doing it, but I do want to lose weight.
Dietitian: Let's discuss what will keep you from recording what you eat (barriers) and what will make it easier (positive reinforcements). Why don't we start with what will make it easier? Can you imagine for a moment (imagery) it is Monday morning, you are eating breakfast, and you remember you should record what you eat and drink? What might help you here?
Client: Well, let's see. I might keep a reminder, say; on my refrigerator so that when I grab the milk for my cereal I see a note that will remind me to record my intake.

This example illustrates a discussion between a dietitian and client that brings into consciousness, for both the dietitian and client, specific difficulties encountered by the client in the process of keeping food records (self-monitoring). It also illustrates that the dietitian does not demand that a client participate in treatment in a predetermined way. Rather, the dietitian helps the client explore the utility of a particular technique in his/her life. In doing so, the dietitian does not merely *apply* a technique. The dietitian empowers the client by providing a forum to participate in planning treatment. The client may feel encouraged because of the following:
- Obstacles to reaching goals are illuminated.
- There may be greater self-understanding (that the client can make a decision; has a sense of what she or he needs and wants; and has a sense of what will make achieving the goal difficult).
- The client is given a measure of control over his or her problem. (2-5)

Other ethical considerations that may be useful in making the decisions of which techniques to use are described below: (2,3,4)

- Clients should be fully informed of the dietitian's education, training, experience, and qualifications.
- Clients should be provided clear explanations, goals, expected outcomes, and risks (i.e., emotional, behaviorally, socially) of techniques, before techniques are used in a counseling session.
- Clients should be at liberty to choose when to participate in certain activities.

Dietitians should be aware of their own values and expectations relative to eating, weight, behavior change, and other life values, so the dietitian is careful to not impose these values on a client.

DISORDERED EATING CATEGORIES AND SELECTION OF TECHNIQUES

Does the usage of a technique vary with the degree of change required? For example, might a dietitian use a different technique for a client with an *older* eating problem, established in childhood, versus a *new* eating problem, recently acquired due to a change in the client's environment? This question will be explored and answered throughout the chapter; however, a brief description of each category is explored below.

New Eating Problems

Some clients complain of *new* problems. They struggle with dietary problems that occurred with the advent of some change in their environment or daily routine. Perhaps the client is eating in a restaurant more often, socializing more because of work, or has had a change in family status (i.e., recently married or divorced and meals are different). Further, something or someone likely reinforces these changes in the client's environment or value system (i.e., it saved time, the food tastes good, or another's validation or approval).

A variety of techniques might be used to change *new* behaviors that are problematic. A dietitian and client may establish treatment goals that:

- Change the environment.
- Change the client's behavior in an environment.
- Change the client's thoughts or cognitions regarding the environment.
- Identify methods to reinforce the learning of new behaviors and thoughts (called operant conditioning).

A combined approach is likely more effective to produce the behavior change required to sustain an improved health status.

Old Eating Problems

Old eating problems may be different however from *new* eating problems. One with an *old* eating problem likely developed this problem many years earlier, perhaps in childhood. In this case, *old* eating behaviors have been well learned and well reinforced, and may be more difficult to change. Strategies, which produce the change of old behaviors, may include both operant conditioning and classical conditioning (to be discussed). For example, when the client eats some food it may reinforce a memory of a person, which yields a positive, warm feeling. The food may precipitate a feeling of affection (classical conditioning).

Loss of Control Eating Problems

A third category of eating behaviors, different from the *new* and *old* eating behaviors described above, may be experienced by a client who suffers with a sense of *loss of control* with regard to eating or weight. This is a client whose degree of suffering is very intense, much beyond that of one who suffers with a change in environment. A client who suffers to this degree may be diagnosed with a mental disorder, according to the *Diagnostic and Statistical Manual of Mental Disorders* (6), in one of three diagnostic states: Anorexia Nervosa, Bulimia Nervosa, or an Eating Disorder Not Otherwise Specified. Cognitive-behavioral therapy is also effective with this group; however, it is used somewhat differently from the two categories of eating behavior described above. Excellent summaries of cognitive-behavioral techniques for eating disorders are available in the literature. (4,7,8,9,10)

It appears that some techniques may prove more effective than others relative to the problem treated. In addition to ethical considerations and the client's expectations of treatment, the nutrition therapist might use two other considerations to select techniques. First, you might consider if the problematic eating behavior is well learned. Second, you might consider whether the client has any degree of control over the problem eating behavior. Three categories of eating problems (old problem, new problem, out of control problem) are used throughout this chapter to help dietitians conceptualize and select appropriate treatment strategies.

Fit The Technique To The Client

> Dietitians must not forget to explore the individuality of the client's dilemma, how the client feels about the dilemma, what has worked, and what has not worked in trying to solve the client's problem.

One last factor, and definitely most important, is selecting a technique to fit the client. The dietitian must not forget the person. Despite the intensity of the struggle with food or weight, inside there is a person who possesses an *individual* history, *individually* prioritized needs, expectations, values, and an *individual* set of circumstances. Dietitians must not forget to explore the individuality of the client's dilemma, how the client feels about the dilemma, what has worked and what has not worked in trying to solve the client's problem. The client should be invited to explore his or her problem, and should be invited to both plan and implement a treatment strategy in a personal way.

BEHAVIORAL TREATMENT STRATEGIES

This discussion starts with behavioral strategies because dietitians tend to be more familiar with these strategies; cognitive and psychoeducational strategies will follow. Behavioral strategies employed for the purpose of changing eating behavior and maintaining dietary change is not only increasingly more popular, strategies included under this umbrella are effective. Efficacy is well established in hypertension programs (4), smoking cessation

> Behavioral programs offer hope, new coping mechanisms, and perhaps most importantly, an opportunity for autonomy.

programs (4), cholesterol lowering programs (4,11-15), diabetes mellitus (16,17), weight reduction programs (18-29), and in eating disorders programs. (30-33) The utility and value of a behavioral program extends far beyond that of producing change, however. *Behavioral programs offer hope, new coping mechanisms, and perhaps most importantly, an opportunity for autonomy.* The provision of hope is perhaps best illustrated with clients who suffer with a sense of *lack of control* of eating behavior, as in those suffering with compulsive eating, anorexia, or bulimia. (33)

Behavioral programs offer clients new strategies for coping with difficult situations. Moreover, those in all behavior categories can use the strategies (old, new, and out of control). *Eating serves some function for a client.* Some clients use food to cope with anxiety and disappointment. Food provides a source of nurturance. In some ways food itself becomes a reinforcer (stimulus--as a reward or the removal of discomfort). *It is important for dietitians to be aware of the reinforcing nature of food, the function of food in the client's life, and to imagine how a client might feel if this reinforcer is suddenly removed from his or her repertoire of coping strategies.* You may, in some cases, actively explore with the client the purposes and functions of food in his or her life. After accomplishing this, you may proceed to a second level of counseling which entails behavior change. (34)

Finally, behavior programs offer clients self-efficacy. (35) Clients learn they can indeed manage their own behavior without the assistance of a counselor. It should also be made clear to a client that it will not be frowned upon, nor is it a sign of failure when he or she seeks continued assistance. Instead, it is seen as a high level of self-understanding. A client may merely require a "refresher course." Indeed, one study in the area of obesity management revealed that clients might actually wait too long before seeking additional help. (21) Behavioral strategies are useful and appealing to nutrition therapists. It is likely that most dietitians already employ many of these techniques, although they may not call them by their name. The basic assumptions of behavioral theory are listed in Table 9.2; however, the following quote summarizes this approach nicely. (36)

Most behaviorally oriented therapists believe the current environment is most important in affecting the person's present behavior. Early life experiences, long time intrapsychic conflicts, or the individual's personality structure are considered to be of less importance than what is happening in the person's life at the present time. The procedures used in behavior therapy are generally intended to improve the individual's self-control by expanding the person's skills, abilities, and independence.(36)

Table 9.2 Basic Assumptions of Behavioral Theory

1. All behavior is learned, and is directly related to the events, stimuli, and reinforcers in one's environment. Therefore, all behavior can be unlearned through corrective learning experiences.
2. A personal relationship between the dietitian and client is not required for recovery to occur.
3. Symptomatic behaviors are considered nothing more than the result of learning maladaptive solutions to common problems.
4. Behavior theory relies on the principles of the scientific method; data is quantifiable and based on empirical research.
5. A client's problem can be better conceptualized by gathering precise, concrete data on the client's behavior and action.
6. Assessment focuses on current determinants of behavior; rather than historical determinants. Indeed, one need not *understand* historical factors to experience changes in behavior.
7. Treatment focuses on changing target behaviors; goals are explicit and well defined.

Adapted from Corey, 1984 (3); Eysenck, 1987 (37); Ivey, 1987 (5); Wilson, 1984 (41)

You may find that as a counselor, you don't agree with all of the above premises. That is why most counselors today use many of the behavioral techniques along with other counseling theories and closer interpersonal relationships. As discussed earlier, techniques may vary with the degree and manner in which behaviors are learned (new, old, out of control behaviors). The actual differences between such problems may be better conceptualized with a discussion of classical and operant conditioning.

Classical Conditioning

Give me a dozen healthy infants, well-formed, and my own specified world to bring them up in and I'll guarantee to take any one at random and train him to become any type of specialist I might select-- doctor, lawyer, merchant, chief, and yes, even beggerman and thief, regardless of his talents, penchants, abilities, vocations and the race of his ancestors. (Watson, 1930)

Watson's quote above summarizes the ideology of classical conditioning. (38) That is, in spite of knowledge, one can be conditioned to behave in a specified way. While the assumption has been "humanized" today, classical conditioning continues to consider environmental factors as more important than other factors (i.e., intrapsychic, contextual, maturational) in the shaping and influencing of behavior. The validity of this assumption may be observed in the context of eating. That is, eating may indeed be conditioned. Many dietitians are acquainted with clients who, intellectually, are quite astute and yet behaviorally, practice behaviors, which are not consistent with their goals. This includes those with diabetes mellitus who eat too much fat and sugar, those trying to lose weight who eat excessive calories, and those with heart disease who smoke. Their problem is not one of insufficient knowledge, but rather, the learning or conditioning of unhealthy and problematic behaviors.

Classical conditioning may provide one framework to understand this phenomenon. *It refers to involuntary processes (i.e., blinking, security, fear, or preferences).* Pavlov first described these processes of conditioning in the early part of the twentieth century. With this technique Pavlov taught his dogs to salivate at the sound of a bell instead of the presence of meat. To accomplish this, Pavlov first presented a dog with an *unconditioned stimulus* (US)—the meat. This US produced the *Unconditioned Response* (UR)—salivation. Pavlov then paired the US with a *Conditioned Stimulus* (CS)—the sound of a bell. The result of this pairing, when the pairing occurred at the same moment in time, was a *Conditioned Response* (CR—salivating at the sound of a bell and the presence of meat. In time, Pavlov's dogs learned to salivate only with the sound of a bell, without the presence of meat.

Classical conditioning has been used by others to condition fear, as with little Albert and his fear of white mice, rabbits, and men with white beards. (38) Watson's research demonstrated that *the object of such conditioning could generalize conditioned responses*. That is, you can *auto condition* yourself. (39,40) The process of generalization occurs when the object of conditioning responds to similar stimuli in a predetermined way. That is, many stimuli may yield a certain conditioned response. For example, one may learn to eat other foods, in addition to chocolate, and drink alcohol, and smoke cigarettes when experiencing anxiety, with the goal of producing a conditioned response of security, nurturance, and peace. Two other examples of classical conditioning are listed below in Table 9.3.

Table 9.3 Examples of Classical Conditioning

Unconditioned stimulus (US)	produces	Unconditioned response (UR)
flash on a camera	produces	blinking
mother's affection	produces	security, nurturance
US + Conditioned stimulus (CS)	produces	Conditioned response (CR)
flash on camera + camera	produces	blinking
mother's affection + eating	produces	security, nurturance
Conditioned stimulus (CS)	produces	Conditioned response (CR)
camera	produces	blinking
eating	produces	security, nurturance

Extinction. In light of the examples above, classical conditioning may be used successfully in changing a client's dietary behavior. The therapeutic process is known as *extinction*. Through extinction a person that is conditioned unlearns the conditioned response. That is, with time and the intentional omission of pairing the UCS with the CS, one can unlearn that the CS produces a CR (merely seeing the camera doesn't cause blinking). After a client learns this, a new, more adaptive behavior can be learned. For example, if a client learns to eat when anxious to feel security, the first step in unlearning would be to avoid eating when anxious. Then you can help the client learn new ways of handling anxiety that don't involve eating. For example, a client may begin learning relaxation techniques to the extent that relaxation is paired with anxiety to produce a new response, security.

Operant Conditioning
Operant conditioning refers to voluntary processes, and is based on the premise that behavior is controlled mainly by consequences in the environment. (4,17,42) Thomdike demonstrated this principle with mazes. Thomdike placed cats in a puzzle box and rewarded only those cats that learned to solve the puzzle. Thus, he used food as a *positive reinforcer.*

Positive Reinforcers. *Positive reinforcers* increase a desired behavior—the more frequently the cats solved the puzzle the more they were rewarded with food. Dietitians likely hear many examples of how clients reward their "good behavior" with food. A client might reward himself with chocolate cake because he met an important business deadline, or reward herself with pretzels for enduring a tedious afternoon at the office. A man might reward himself with a cigarette for having endured a fight with his wife. When a client engages in such behaviors, operant conditioning is at work.

Negative Reinforcers. Negative reinforcers work on a different principle. A certain behavior is increased to *avoid* a negative outcome. For example, one may learn to eat chocolate to avoid the unpleasant situation of low blood sugar in the afternoon. Or, one might take aspirin to avoid a headache. The degree to which you participate in an activity (eating, taking aspirin) increases because you learn that low blood sugar and headaches can be successfully avoided when a particular behavior is increased. Conditioning through negative reinforcers implies that a client may be aware of how a particular behavior is reinforced. For example, one is aware aspirin stops or decreases headaches.

Diets work off the principle of negative reinforcement. One might diet, that is, consume fewer calories, to avoid gaining weight. Thus, the incidence of dieting behavior increases to avoid the negative outcome. One might vomit to avoid gaining weight. Thus, the incidence of vomiting, in a client who suffers with bulimia, may increase in frequency. There is danger in such thinking however, while effective, one is at risk of thinking irrationally. For example, a dieter might starve to avoid the negative outcome, weight gain. Moreover, this behavior may become cyclic, frequent, and result in significant health problems. While at times they are adaptive and useful, negative reinforcers may go too far and prove harmful.

Punishments. A final consequence that influences behavior is punishment. *Punishment* yields a different behavioral outcome from both positive and negative reinforcers. Punishment serves to *decrease* the frequency of a particular behavior. Many parents are familiar with this phenomenon. Time out may be sufficiently negative to correct the inappropriate behavior of a child, as it removes a child from an enjoyable activity. Thus, a child may learn, through punishment, to avoid the undesired behavior (i.e., hitting, yelling). This principle is also applicable to dietary behavior. For example, a client might eat smaller portions to avoid requiring the use of diets. One might smoke fewer cigarettes to avoid the dizzy sensation that accompanies them.

In review then, eating behavior may be influenced by both classical conditioning (involuntary behavior) and operant conditioning (voluntary behavior). The difference is teased out through the process of assessment. During assessment, a nutrition therapist will determine how food is used, and the outcome of using food. Other assessment procedures may include an interview with the client and/or significant others, client self-monitoring, observation of a client's behavior *in vivo*, role playing, self-report measures, and through testing (i.e., self-esteem scales, etc.). (4)

Assessment Procedures

During the initial interview, the dietitian should first question the general nature of the client's problem and then itemize specifics of the client's problem. It is important to proceed slowly to allow trust and rapport to develop. When you sense trust from the client, you may move to deeper material. Trust is enhanced when the dietitian engages in four activities: (4)

1. Attends closely to a client's message, focuses on the client's verbal and nonverbal messages, encourages the client's discussion of the problem, and withholds bias, judgment, and purposeless conversation.
2. Avoids allowing one's own values and biases from influencing the client's discussion of the problem, listens objectively.
3. Listens and responds empathically. It is important for the client to know that his/her feeling will be validated and acknowledged. For example, when hearing about the client's struggle with losing weight, a dietitian might respond, "I can really hear how you have suffered with your weight and in your attempts to lose weight."
4. Ensures client confidentiality. Clients must know that their stories are safe and will not be repeated carelessly to other staff, other clients, and/or the client's family, without prior approval.

Simple questions, regarding the nature of the client's work, place of residence, and educational experience, may be used during the first interview to ease a client's anxiety. (4) You might then proceed to questions that relate to reasons for the appointment. O'Leary and Wilson outlined several questions (4), listed below, to interpret the exact nature of the problem.

When did the problem begin?
How frequently does it occur?
When and in what situations does it occur?
What occurs before and after it?
What has been done to change the problem?

Once the nature of the problem is conceptualized, the dietitian may then inventory both the strengths and vulnerabilities of the client. Concluding this first visit with strengths may encourage the clients to feel good about themselves, to the extent that they may leave the counseling session with a positive feeling. It may be this positive feeling that keeps a client in treatment.

During the second assessment appointment, you may again inventory the client's dietary problem. A functional analysis is often used to further clarify the client's problem. With this assessment technique, you identify how the client behaves in his or her *natural environment.* (4, 5, 34) A functional analysis reveals the ABCs of one's behavior, that is, more information is revealed about the target problem. The *antecedents* (A) of behavior (triggers, what leads to eating, i.e., seeing cookies on the counter), the *resultant behaviors* (B) (what occurs after eating, i.e., exercise, vomiting, more eating), and the *consequent behaviors* (C) (system of positive reinforcers, negative reinforcers, and punishments, i.e., losing weight, avoiding discomfort, gaining weight, feeling full). An example is outlined below.

Dietitian: Can you help me understand your problem more fully? It may help us both to know what happens before or after you eat, and what reinforces your eating. It may help to recall a specific example when you experienced trouble controlling your eating. Tell me about the last time this happened to you.

Client: Well, let's see. Today is Monday. Friday I got home from work. I was really tired and anxious. It was a Friday, and I had a difficult week. First, I hung up my coat then I went into the kitchen for a drink. As I opened the refrigerator I saw the cookies. Then I felt the craving. So I ate some. Then I ate some more. Then I ate some more. Before I knew it, I ate half the package. I couldn't stop!

Dietitian: Let me see if I understand you correctly. You arrived home from work feeling tired and anxious (antecedent). You hung up your coat, walked to the kitchen, opened up the refrigerator, and ate some cookies (resultant behavior). Then you ate some more, but you did not really describe what happens after eating. Do I understand you so far?

Client: Yes, you got it. Then I feel just terrible. I feel depressed. Then I don't eat dinner because I'm too full and feel really bad. Sometimes I just go and read.

Dietitian: So the consequence of eating for you is really severe. You feel depressed, overfull, and really "bad." Sometimes you just go and read (consequent behavior).

In this example, the dietitian effectively engages with the client, inviting the client to tell her story. Without significant prompting, the client sufficiently delineates the details of her experience, to the extent that antecedents, resultant behaviors, and consequent behaviors are identified. Not depicted in the example, however, is information regarding how the target behavior is reinforced in the client's natural environment.

A final part and critical aspect of the assessment interview is to ascertain what maintains the problematic behavior in question. (4, 5) If a client is aware that an eating problem exists, understands, but is not happy with the ramifications of this problem, how is it that the problem continues to exist?

From a behavioral perspective, life problems take on a life of their own. The reinforcers in the client's environment maintain problems. Relative to the example above, you might presume that eating is maintained through the taste of the food. A second hypothesis might be that the client receives more attention through eating poorly. Perhaps the client calls a friend and commiserates about how terribly her diet is going. A third hypothesis relates to the experience of the client. Perhaps the positive feeling this client experiences after eating is related to committing to begin a diet "tomorrow," and buy new dresses after losing weight. Indeed, reinforcers may not be rational.

Through assessment, the dietitian experiences and conceptualizes the depths of a client's problem. With this information, the client and you may proceed to treatment planning. Appendix 9-A represents a sample format that might be used by you and the client to achieve this end.

First, the client and you should describe the desired goals of treatment. Some behavioral goals might include: 1) learn relaxation techniques that can be used in the car on the way home from work, 2) decrease fat consumption to no more than thirty percent of total calories, 3) walk at least five times per week for twenty minutes.

Second, both the client and dietitian should agree on treatment modalities. (4,5) Treatment techniques are described in the next section.

The treatment plan should be signed by both parties and stored in the client's medical record. It provides a forum for the client and you to continually rework the course and context of treatment.

Outcomes should be measured or reevaluated to determine the extent to which goals for change have been met.

Treatment Strategies

Self-Monitoring. A technique used both during assessment and treatment, self-monitoring refers to the monitoring, overseeing, observing, or regulating of an aspect of one's behavior. During assessment, it provides the client a forum to identify aspects of eating that are troublesome. For example, a client may not be aware that the time of day is a trigger for eating until all foods and beverages consumed are recorded on paper for a specified period of time. The information revealed with self-monitoring, therefore, establishes the context and course of treatment.

A client might monitor a variety of eating behavior factors, as appropriate to the client's needs and problem. Factors that may be monitored with this technique include time of day, type of food, amount of food, place of eating, activity while eating, with whom eating, rate of eating, degree of hunger or fullness, mood (i.e., angry, sad, happy, afraid, lonely), and physical state (i.e., tired, fatigued) (see Appendix 9-B). An adjective list of moods and physical states may assist a client in identifying states of being (see Appendix 9-C,9-D).

In treatment self-monitoring serves two purposes. First, and perhaps most important, it provides the client a forum to make decisions about the behavior that is monitored and, therefore, allows the client to maintain a level of awareness.

A second function of self-monitoring in treatment is to monitor progress. Indeed, it is the basis by which you might judge efficacy. A variety of self-monitoring tools might be used in this endeavor including diaries of food consumed, cigarettes smoked, exercise completed, or records of blood sugar, blood pressure, or pounds lost.

Stimulus Control. Once identified, problematic stimuli can be better managed so that the desired outcome can be achieved. These stimuli are managed through the technique of stimulus control. Stimulus control is used in the phase of treatment where solutions to problems are identified and implemented. *The focus should be on managing or coping, rather than controlling perfectly.* Controlling implies that a stimulus may be extinguished, where in reality the best that may be hoped for is management. Management implies coping differently with a given stimulus.

Before stimuli can be managed in an orderly and coherent way, however, goals for treatment should be identified. (3-5,18,34) What stimuli are problematic? In what way is it problematic? Under what specific conditions? What outcome do the client and dietitian agree is desirable and achievable? Finally, in what way will the stimuli best be managed? It is upon these, and other questions, the client and dietitian might reflect so that a strategy or strategies for change can be identified, and implemented in a sequential manner. The technique of stimulus control has clinical utility with old problems, new problems, and out of control problems. While there are three methods by which this technique may be used, primarily stimulus control modifies food exposure and/or availability, and alters food associations. (18) For example, some clients are at risk of eating simply because they saw cookies on the counter top. A stimulus control strategy strives to decrease exposure. Thus, cookies might be stored in the cabinet.

Second, stimulus control may be aimed at changing and/or limiting eating times and eating places. Thus, one might be encouraged to only snack on fruit between four and six in the evening, and only in the kitchen. Such a technique will break food associations between time of day and eating, as well as location and eating.

Finally, stimulus control is aimed at breaking the automaticity of eating. Thus, food associations between home from work and cookies, or television and popcorn, might be broken with stimulus control. An example of a stimulus control form is found in Appendix 9-E .

The case of Roger clearly explains the technique of stimulus control. Roger, a forty-seven year-old man who sought treatment in a weight loss clinic, complained of excessive eating, usually during the day at fast food restaurants. Roger traveled a great deal during his workday, and he often stopped at fast food restaurants where he ordered two or three large burgers, fries, and sugared sodas. He was over stimulated with the sight and smell of a fast food restaurant and was unable to change his response. This problematic eating situation was corrected, in part, by changing Roger's driving route. Further, he carried healthy snacks with him and ate these, rather than stopping for a "quick" snack. Finally, Roger broke the automaticity of his response near fast food restaurants by finding other ways to cope with triggers that prompted eating, such as stopping on the side of the road and practicing relaxation techniques. Upon doing so, he often found he no longer desired to eat. Over time, Roger lost his desire for fried burgers and fries.

Imagery. This technique is where a counselor assists the client in recalling or creating a hypothetical problematic situation, and then solving it. (41) This technique provides the client a forum to envision healthy coping. Further, problematic situations are categorized on a hierarchy from least difficult to most difficult.

Imagery has clinical utility with all three eating categories; however, it may require one who has an ability to think abstractly. The case of Tom best depicts the utility of this technique.

Tom is a forty-three year old man who sought treatment in a weight management clinic. He was sufficiently able to describe his struggles with eating; however, he was not able to control his eating. The dialogue below further describes Tom's eating difficulties and the use of imagery.

Dietitian: It seems your eating struggles are pretty well defined. You are able to identify both situations and specific foods which give you trouble. Let's review once more what your struggle is.

Tom: Well, I just cannot control my eating at buffets, social events where there is a lot of food, and restaurants. I also cannot control my intake of donuts, cookies, and ice cream. If I have them in the house, I eat them within a relatively short period of time, within a few hours. Also, a most dangerous time for me is when I am home on a cold winter day. I have nothing to do; so, I eat.

Dietitian: You really understand your struggle with food. Let's take a moment now and create a hierarchy of situations and food from least troublesome to most troublesome. 10 will represent the least troublesome food or situation and 100 will represent the most troublesome food or situation. Does this sound okay to you, Tom?

Tom: Yes, it sounds okay. Let's see, I think 10 is restaurants, 40 is social buffets, 60 is cookies, 70 is ice cream, 80 is an all-you-can-eat buffet, 100 is a donut. I just can't stop with one.

Dietitian: Very good, Tom. You completed this without much difficulty. I imagine you have reflected on this quite a bit. You seem to understand your struggle well. Let me see if I understand you correctly. Let's construct your hierarchy together.

100	donuts
90	
80	all you can eat buffet
70	ice cream
60	cookies
50	
40	social buffets (work)
30	
20	
10	restaurants

I see, however, that you did not list "in the house on a winter day." Where would it go, Tom?

Tom: Let's see, I would put that at 50. Come to think of it, at 30 I would put the teacher's lounge. At 20 I would put the lunch cafeteria at work. Let's see, 90, what is as difficult as donuts for me? I would have to say steak. I guess that's it.

Dietitian: The next step in our imagery is to begin with the situation that provokes the least amount of worry and anxiety. You described this as restaurants. I imagine then, Tom, you could walk into a restaurant and order your chicken meal without too much anxiety or struggle. Is this true for you, Tom?

Tom: It sure is. It's the easiest one on my list.

Dietitian: Okay, Tom. Try to relax in your chair. Close your eyes. When you are completely relaxed, I'd like you to imagine yourself at your favorite restaurant (note: the dietitian would likely spend time training Tom on relaxation techniques before actually trying out the imagery exercise). You walk in the door. The host seats you and your wife at your table. You feel slightly anxious, hungry, and happy to see your wife after a long workday. You sit at your table, review the menu. You feel this is a special time and you want to eat something special. Then you see baked chicken with black-eyed peas, a meal you think would be healthier, yet still tasty. I want you to imagine yourself ordering the chicken meal, completely relaxed and without struggle. Imagine yourself able to stop eating when full. You experience no struggle over whether you should finish all of the food on your plate. You simply stop eating when comfortably full, and focus your attention on your conversation with your wife. The waiter comes, removes your plate with some food left on the side, you smile and ask for the check instead of dessert......STOP

Okay, Tom, let's talk about your experience. (Ask one question at a time.) What did it feel like? What were your thoughts about the situation? How do you think you might actually feel in that restaurant experience? Suppose you were to eat in a restaurant this evening with your wife, could you act out this imagery experience with her?

As Tom completed imagery experiences at the lower level, he would slowly move up the hierarchy until achieving success at the level of 100. The focus on treatment would likely be comprehensive in that as Tom successfully imagined eating at each level, he might try out new behaviors with real-life performance-based techniques.

Imagery techniques, combined with other cognitive-behavioral approaches, may be very successful in helping a client move in an ordered fashion through treatment. Imagery, as described here, provides a context and framework for treatment.

Role-Playing. Like imagery, this is a treatment technique used in the presence of the counselor. It differs from imagery, however, in that the counselor takes an active role in the imagery (hypothetical or actual) situation. (17,18,35,41)

Role-playing provides the client a forum to practice new behaviors in a safe environment. The case of Edith nicely describes this technique.

Edith is a sixty-year-old woman who cannot say "no" to others when they offer her food. Edith role-played this dilemma with her dietitian. This was an important opportunity for Edith, as she was both able to imagine, in an emotive (emotional) and cognitive (mentally clear) manner, her dilemma. At the same time, Edith was able to practice a new ending to her story, in a safe and protected environment. While the dietitian offered some challenge, she did not overly confront Edith, and did not require that Edith behave in a specified manner. With practice, over three role playing exercises, Edith was able to say "no" to the extra, undesired chocolate cake calories that her hostess prepared for dessert, and without feeling guilty. Instead, Edith described feeling that when she did say "no," she felt empowered, as if she was nurturing herself.

Real-Life Performance-Based Techniques. These techniques are similar to role-playing, however in addition, they allow the client to practice new behaviors *in vivo*. That is, clients are given an opportunity to practice newly learned behaviors in their natural environment. With time and practice, new behaviors come more easily, and the likelihood that old, less adaptive behaviors may surface decreases. (41,42)

This is an important clinical technique for all groups of eating behavior, and especially those who feel a sense of control over eating. A simpler term to describe this technique is that of "practical homework." It is an important technique, as it teaches clients they can indeed cope in a new way with problematic eating situations. Real-life performance-based techniques are illustrated with George.

George complained that he just could not enjoy a holiday meal without the "normal" fixings. The dietitian disagreed with him and contracted with George to begin practicing new eating behaviors as early as June. Both George and his dietitian agreed that if he practiced lower calorie and fat habits sufficiently, he would develop coping strategies, which allowed him to eat smaller amounts and less fat during the upcoming Thanksgiving Day meal. George practiced moderate eating on three occasions. During each experience he consumed a "typical" holiday meal at a restaurant, while noting both his feelings and the content of his thoughts during each event. Of particular interest was his attitude that "it's just not a holiday meal unless I'm totally full."

With time, both George and his dietitian noticed a transformation in his thinking. After three months of practicing new eating behaviors, exploring triggers to eating, and "trying on" new thoughts and behaviors, George experienced a change in basic attitudes about holiday eating. He no longer felt the need to eat until overfull; instead, George consumed smaller portions of food, feeling both physically and emotionally satisfied.

Self-Reinforcement. Positive reinforcements (operant conditioning) are the methods by which new behaviors are rewarded; therefore, they are the means by which new and more appropriate behaviors increase in frequency. (35,18,42) Perhaps the most basic of self-reinforcers is the positive mood state that occurs with a sense of achievement. Other, more tangible, reinforcers may include smaller sized clothing, a vacation, or a day at the spa.

Self-reinforcement is an important component of behavior change programs. Indeed, self-reinforcement is a predictor of weight loss success. (24,43) A dietitian's task, therefore, is perhaps to continually focus discussions on *what worked* for the client rather than *what went wrong*. This is empowering for clients. Clients want to feel good about what they are achieving and a dietitian can be instrumental in helping clients achieve this mood state.

While dietitians are important sources of reinforcement, they must not be the only provider of positive reinforcement. It is equally important that clients self-reinforce, and also receive reinforcement from those in their social network. First, clients should learn to reinforce their own behavior. (3) This is important to increase one's sense of control over the problematic situation and to decrease dependence upon others as continual sources of support. A relationship characterized by merely positives is not necessarily ideal or mutual. Mutual relationships are characterized by those where both members feel a sense of increased zest, empowerment, self- and other knowledge, self-worth, and a desire for more connection. (44)

Not only must a client begin to self-reinforce, others in the client's life may behave in a similar fashion. During a treatment session, therefore, the dietitian and client may determine who most often provides the type of support or reinforcement so desired by the client. With such an exploration, clients may learn how others reinforce them (through attention, affection, praise, approval, support), and how clients themselves may provide support and reinforcement to another. *In effect, what a client may be learning is how to relate mutually, and how to develop a level of emotional intimacy with another.*

The efficacy of reinforcement is well documented in research. A weight loss program compared treatment modalities: (20)

1. Behavior therapy alone
2. Behavior therapy plus post-treatment counseling
3. Behavior therapy plus post-treatment counseling plus aerobic exercise
4. Behavior therapy plus post-treatment counseling plus social support
5. Behavior therapy plus post-treatment counseling plus aerobic exercise plus social support

The only group to continue losing weight at 18 month follow-up was the treatment group characterized by all four treatment modalities: behavior therapy, post-treatment counseling (26 weeks), aerobic exercise, and social support. Clearly, more comprehensive programs appear more effective than programs that offer fewer components.

Modeling. Derived from social learning theory, modeling was first described by Bandura. (45) It is a form of imitation and occurs in a four-step process. A client should first <u>observe</u> the model's behavior (i.e., eating, speech, thought processes) to a sufficient degree so that some of *how* the model performs is <u>remembered.</u> Next, the protégé or client may <u>reproduce</u> the behavior and/or state of being previously observed. Finally, clients should receive reinforcement and <u>feedback</u> for their newly learned behaviors. **It is through this process of observation—remembering—reproduction—feedback, that new behaviors are formed and imprinted.** Once achieved, new behaviors may become a part of the client's coping repertoire. (Incidentally, this is also how dietitians and students learn new counseling skills best.)

Clients do not easily model the behavior of strangers. Clients actively discriminate between persons and select, unconsciously, the most desirable model available. (45) Models share certain similar attributes with their protégés. They are of similar age, sex, race, and attitudes. Further, models are prestigious, competent, and often work in distinguished and important positions. Such research has important implications for dietetic practice.

First, a dietitian may be a model for some and not others. This is normal. The key to a dietitian's experience is to know with *whom* she or he may be an effective model. Perhaps this explains why some dietitians feel completely ineffective with certain clients, and yet so successful with others.

Second, dietitians can explain the principles of modeling to clients and assist clients in their journey to find prospective models in their *natural* environment. Once identified, and a trusting relationship is developed between model and protégé, the client may seek advice, reinforcement, praise, or coaching from his or her model. (46) Indeed, there is a certain order to the modeling relationship.

The principle of modeling applies to mentoring relationships, and to self-help groups where one selects a sponsor. Models are invaluable sources of methodology, reinforcement, praise, trust, and other positive experiences, and perhaps provide some of the social support many behavioral therapies declare is so important in behavioral change.

Systematic desensitization. A technique used to relieve a person of the pains associated with phobias (extreme anxiety in relation to objects, animals, or people), systematic desensitization may not be appropriate for use by a dietitian. (3-5,39-41) Still, it may be useful information for the dietitian, when making a referral.

The process of systematic desensitization is achieved with three steps. (5) First, a client is taught methods of deep muscle relaxation. Second, a client is instructed on how to construct an anxiety hierarchy (similar to the hierarchy constructed during imagery). Finally, anxiety producing phobias, objects, or animals from the hierarchy are matched with relaxation training.

The goal of systematic desensitization is to teach a particular client a new way of coping. Instead of coping by using anxiety, one learns to substitute the relaxed state for the anxiety state, to the degree that the relaxed state becomes automatic. It may be clear to some that the assumptions of this technique are rooted in classical conditioning; thus, it is a technique particularly suitable for one who feels a sense of *loss of control.* Those who suffer with compulsive eating, bulimia, and/or anorexia may benefit from systematic desensitization.

This technique is included, not with the intention that a dietitian may use this technique upon reading, but rather, for the purpose of information. Indeed, many clients dietitians counsel may benefit from such a technique. It is important for dietitians to know, therefore, when to refer a client to a behaviorally oriented counselor.

Those who may benefit from systematic desensitization may suffer with a variant of anxiety disorders (6), as well as those who feel *out of control* with eating or eating-related behavior. (35) Symptoms of generalized anxiety disorder include persistent anxiety as manifested by excessive worry concerning many life events, an inability to control the worry, and worry that is associated with motor tension, restlessness, apprehension, or vigilance. (6,47)

COGNITIVE RESTRUCTURING TREATMENT STRATEGIES

Men are disturbed not by events, but by the views they take of them. Epictetus (4)

The actual assumptions of cognitive therapies are perhaps as old as Epictetus, described as a stoic Roman philosopher who lived around the time of 55 AD. He professed that a person's problem is rooted in how he perceives his problem, rather than what the problem may actually be. Indeed, your problem is a function of your values, beliefs, ideologies, and philosophies of living. When these beliefs and values are absolute in nature, as opposed to relative, you will likely experience emotional responses (anxiety, guilt, shame, depression), as well as behavioral responses (eating problems, punching a wall, drinking alcohol, smoking). Moreover, these responses or sequelae are viewed as maladaptive answers to a mismanaged problem. Basic assumptions of cognitive therapies are further outlined in Table 9.4.

Table 9.4 Basic Assumptions of Cognitive Therapy

1. People are born with powerful aptitudes to think both rationally and irrationally.
2. People have vast resources for growth, and therefore, can indeed change their destiny in personally significant ways.
3. Family and culture exacerbate people's tendency for irrational thinking.
4. To understand disturbed behavior, the therapist must understand how people perceive, think, emote, and act.
5. When people experience life disturbances, it is because they care too much about what others may think.
6. Cognitive-behavioral techniques effectively change behavior and cognitions in a brief period of time.
7. The technique is designed to help people examine and change their most basic values.

In the quest to correct a maladaptive problem, a client might first explore his or her basic ideologies. These ideologies are often a reflection of early learning in the family and in society. For example, his family may have taught, *"You must always eat all of the food on your plate; you must never cry; you must never show others when you are vulnerable."*

The problem of adopting irrational ideologies is further exacerbated when you attend school during middle childhood, and thereafter, as your exposure to irrational ideologies is expanded. Indeed, irrational ideologies (racist, sexist, or other bigoted ideas, use of violence to solve problems, the idea that material goods will lead to happiness and popularity, and so on) are ubiquitous---they emanate from teachers, television, music, media, most any place people are. The problem, therefore, becomes one of exposing, eluding, and circumventing irrational ideology. Once exposed, irrational ideologies can be replaced with ideologies that are more consistent with one's goals for healthy living. The process by which this occurs is perhaps best described by Albert Ellis in his Rational-Emotive Therapy (RET). (3,5,48)

Albert Ellis developed a cognitive-behavioral counseling technique called Rational-Emotive Therapy(RET) in 1950.(3,5,48) Ellis believed undesired emotional consequences (anxiety, depression, shame, etc.) are created by an individual's faulty belief system. These beliefs can be challenged, however, and replaced with more adaptive beliefs. Doing so may help the client avoid not only the undesired emotional consequence, but the undesired behavior, as well (eating, weighing, exercising, smoking, etc.). You may help clients with RET by disputing their irrationally held beliefs and helping them to think more rationally.

Any faulty belief that predisposes the client to aberrant eating, weighing, or exercising behavior is an area upon which the dietitian might focus. Clients may abandon treatment because they may think they *cannot* change these undesired behaviors until they understand the origins of their problem. *It is a premise of this theory, however, that clients need not understand why they eat as they do to change behaviors. Clients need only to understand the ABCs of their behavior and cognition. Relaying such a message may be freeing for a client.* Some do not care to explore to a level deeper than the immediate problem of weight.

Assessment
The cognitive-behavioral theorists will ultimately be interested in knowing how the individual developed ideas or cognitions about reality, how the individual chooses and decides from the many possibilities, and how the individual acts and behaves in relationship to reality. (5)

Like behavioral therapy, a functional analysis is used during cognitive assessment to identify faulty and absolutist attitudes and beliefs. However, the functional analysis used with cognitive techniques differs somewhat from that of behavioral therapy, as thoughts, attitudes, and beliefs are considered a part of the formula (see Appendix 9-F). (3,5,48)

During assessment you might first identify the event that precedes eating. Subsequent to this you assist your client in identifying his or her attitudes, values, or beliefs about the event. It is often their attitudes that result in both excessive eating and a dysfunctional mood, as these attitudes are often irrational. Irrational attitudes are clearly evident when clients think they *should, must, ought, always, never do something.* Irrational beliefs are absolutist. Thus, clients may never feel satisfied because they cannot achieve their goals, and may be left feeling badly (shamed, depressed, anxious). Clients may act out this "bad" feeling by eating. The case of Marie illustrates assessment using RET.

> *Marie complained of overeating and lack of physical activity, especially when anxious. She often ate when feeling as if she could not control a problem in her life. This out of control feeling resulted in significant anxiety. Marie blocked or coped with the anxiety by eating handfuls of jellybeans or chocolates. Eating further exacerbated her dilemma because as she ate she gained more weight and her mobility was further limited. Thus, her goals of weighing less and increasing mobility were yet more distant.*

Further discussion between the dietitian and Marie reveals the following information (Figure 9.1).

Figure 9.1 Therapy Discussion Flow Chart

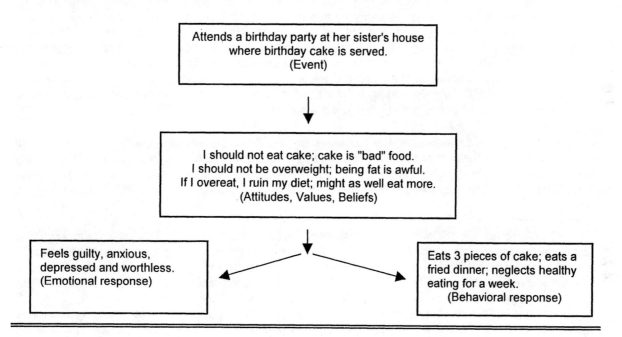

Treatment

Decatastrophizing. This technique was used by Ellis to abate anxiety, which was often an exaggerated negative response to a specific situation. (3,5,48) The technique involves evaluating the client's fear of an identified situation and the *horrible* negative outcome, and helping the client to acknowledge the ridiculousness of the belief and resulting emotion, fear. The case of Adrian illustrates this technique.

> Dietitian: Adrian, you described never eating chocolate because you see it as a *horrible* food. You further said, if you did eat chocolate you would not be able to stop. Can you help me understand more of your experience here? (The dietitian suspects that chocolate is not the real issue here.)
>
> Adrian: Well, if I ate chocolate it would be horrible. I would get fat. That's why I can't eat it.
>
> Dietitian: What is the worst possible outcome you can imagine might occur if you got fat?
>
> Adrian: Well, my friends wouldn't like me. I wouldn't fit into my clothes. I just wouldn't fit in with the group. You know, they are all popular, pretty. They have the boyfriends. If I got fat, I wouldn't have that.
>
> Dietitian: Why would that be horrible?

Adrian: Well, then I would be alone.

Dietitian: It sounds like being alone carries with it a greater fear than being fat carries. Would you say that's true? What seems most scary to you, being alone or being fat?

Adrian: I don't know, being alone I guess. But I still can't get fat.

Dietitian: So your friends might not want to be with you because fat people are horrible. Why would that make you horrible?

Adrian: Well, I shouldn't be fat.

Dietitian: It might be nicer if you were not fat. You might be able to walk easier. But being fat does not mean that you are *horrible*. Who told you that you should never be fat? Who told you that you would be horrible if you were fat?

Adrian: Well, I guess when I was seven, my Mom did. She put me on these diet pills. I was a chubby little kid. So I lost some weight and it was like everything changed. I got new clothes. My Mom took me places with her. My friends liked me more. I had more friends. I just became a better person. Before that I only got the chubette clothes. My friends made fun of me. I stayed home a lot.

Dietitian: So being thin means you will not be horrible because you will have more friends, your Mom will give you more attention, and you can buy different clothes. Being fat means you are horrible because you have fewer friends, and your Mom won't take you places. It might be *nicer* to have more and different clothes and friends and your Mom's attention. But being fat does not mean you are horrible. Why is it that you feel it necessary to berate yourself? Do you see where your logic goes astray? You believe and family and friends told you that being thin somehow means being more worthy. You might replace this logic with, *it would be better to weigh less. But being fat does not mean that I am a bad person.* Do you see the difference in what I said and what you are saying?

Using the client's response, the dietitian can help the client become aware of other ways of thinking. Further, the dietitian can help the client see the outcome she may imagine as *horrible* is really quite manageable. Thus, the dietitian might use this questioning to move the client to imagining alternative emotional and behavioral reactions, and finally to problem solving and empowering the client.

Challenging the Shoulds, Oughts, and Musts. According to Ellis (48), "shoulds" and "musts" are the foundation of irrational beliefs. Without the dichotomous thinking inherent in these self-imposed rules, irrational thinking would not occur. Perfectionist beliefs upheld by clients always lead to failure because they cannot be achieved; therefore, clients are left feeling even more inadequate than before the rule was imposed. (See Appendix 9-G Irrational Beliefs Daily Log.)

The goal of the dietitian is to help the client dispute irrational beliefs, and develop awareness that such beliefs are absurd or unachievable. By comparing facts with fantasies, observing real life phenomenon, trying out behaviors and waiting for the *horrible* event to occur, clients find they can indeed cope with the *horrible* event.

Reattribution. This technique challenges faulty self-perceptions, and is described by Garner and Bemis. It is used in cognitive therapy with those suffering with anorexia when one experiences distortions in body image. (32)

This technique helps clients perceive an attribute of themselves differently. The nutrition therapist helps the client question the validity of self-perceptions, and therefore, creates an atmosphere of ambiguity where other cognitions may be considered. Questioning and exploring the evidence of one's beliefs are the primary methods by which this ambiguity is achieved.

Because this technique is confrontational, to be effective it requires a good relationship. That is, there must be a high level of trust, to the degree that the client will not feel criticized or abandoned when irrational thoughts are challenged. Dietitians must, therefore, attend to the client's affect (emotions), verbal responses, and gestures, searching for gestures of hurt and insult. Should you notice such behavior or feelings, this should be openly discussed.

Decentering. Piaget first described decentering in his theory of cognitive development. (49,50) Piaget asserted that developmentally, a person is not able to decenter until middle childhood, between the ages of six to twelve years. In the context of Piaget's theory, decentering means taking into account more than one perspective or explanation, perhaps many, of a particular situation or problem.

A person who can decenter is able to hold, to understand, to explain that there may indeed be various and very different explanations for one particular problem.

The principle of decentering may be applied to your self-understanding and to relationships. Relative to your self-understanding, decentering implies that you may understand an aspect of self from many perspectives. For example, a person who decenters sufficiently understands that an overweight condition occurs because he has consumed quantitatively and qualitatively too many calories, and has exercised too little. One who does not decenter sufficiently might understand weight gain only and completely in terms of eating a "bad" food.

Decentering might also be understood in the context of a relationship. With regard to your relationships, decentering implies a social situation where both persons in the relationship understand, *I understand you, you understand me, and we both understand a third, more objective perspective.* These are the principles of Selman's social perspective, and are very applicable to the dynamic that should exist between a client and a dietitian. (51) For example, a client who does not sufficiently decenter may not understand that you can know his or her experience. Your task, therefore, is to help the client understand that you can indeed feel the experience of the client. It is the experience of the author that clients like and want to know this. It helps them feel understood, significant, and cared for. In fact, conveying to a client that you understand (cognitively) and can feel (emotionally) a client's experience, is being empathic and is a core requirement of a therapeutic relationship. (34)

While decentering is an ability acquired and used in cognitive processing during middle childhood, researchers who studied this phenomenon in years after Piaget have demonstrated that even during adolescence, some individuals maintain a level of egocentricity. In his work with adolescence, Elkind demonstrated that adolescent egocentricity is apparent in behaviors such as fault finding, argumentativeness, self-consciousness, self-centeredness, indecisiveness, and identifying hypocrisy. (52) Many adults behave in a similar fashion. Thus, this issue of decentering, and helping clients to decenter, is seemingly important to many of the clients dietitians treat.

Garner and Bemis (32) used this technique with those suffering with anorexia. The outcome of this technique is your ability to acknowledge a perspective different from your own perspective. For example, a person with anorexia might imagine that others might detect when she or he gains three pounds, and everyone notices. Through decentering, this person can begin to understand that others may not notice something so overly important to the client.

Decentering is a technique applicable to clients other than those suffering with anorexia. Actually, it is a very personal technique because it has to do with what you imagine others know about you. It is applicable to a person of any weight, and perhaps most applicable with persons who are overly concerned with how others regard them. (46) The case of Jane demonstrates the clinical use of decentering.

Jane sought treatment for weight loss. She understood her struggle with food as eating too many "bad" foods during the week. She further described that she could not bear to be fat. In fact, the reason why she was now separated from her husband was because he could not bear her "fatness," as well. She described her marital relationship as "close" when she was thin and "distant" when she was fat. Thus, using Jane's reasoning, the primary problem in her life was one of being "fat," and not one of perhaps marrying a man who did not love Jane at the level of her vulnerable core. Indeed, Jane's struggle with food is penetrating and likely indicates a more serious struggle with her sense of self, her sense of differentiation, and her sense of worthiness, respect, and esteem.

A dietitian working with Jane might recognize the depth of her pain, actively work toward establishing a trust and rapport not based on "diet," but based on the human contact between Jane and the dietitian. This would help Jane to develop awareness that people can indeed like her and develop a mutual relationship with her for reasons other than her weight. The dietitian, therefore, would be educating Jane on her other attributes which are desirable, her strengths. Thus, it may be apparent that techniques are not used in isolation. This last example demonstrates reattribution, as well as decentering.

Once rapport is developed, the dietitian might gently begin to explore Jane's ideology of "fat and goodness." Where did it come from? What was the most salient life experience that taught her to believe this? What role model in her life demonstrated this ideology to her? Under what conditions might this ideology not be true? When had this ideology perhaps not held true for Jane in the past? Through gentle, understanding, and empathic confrontation, the dietitian can create a level of ambiguity within the client's ideology. Once formed, this ambiguity can be molded and transformed to more rational thinking in terms of oneself, one's relationships, and one's problems.

PSYCHOEDUCATIONAL TREATMENT STRATEGIES

Techniques that involve both a cognitive component and a behavioral component are called psychoeducational techniques. Many dietitians already use psychoeducational techniques in their counseling practices, although they may not name them as such.

This portion of the chapter explores psychoeducational techniques in four ways: first, the word is explored; second, the techniques are differentiated from both behavioral and cognitive techniques; third, clinical utility is discussed; and fourth, sample techniques (distraction, delay, and parroting) are explored and modeled.

Root Words

The root "psycho" generally implies of the mind or mental processing. Freud was the first to describe such processing. (53) Relative to psychoeducational techniques, "psycho" implies physical and mental impulses or urges. Included under this category are states of being (i.e., hunger, fullness, mood), and physical sensations (i.e., bodily feelings).

The suffix "educational" suggests knowledge, which is acquired through a process of teaching and learning. Thus, psychoeducational implies a process of learning about oneself, self-understanding (one's physical and mental impulses, instincts, and/or patterns of behavior), and gaining new knowledge (i.e., the number of grams of fat in a teaspoon of butter), and learning to regulate one's behavior in accordance with some standard.

Differentiation

Guerney, Stollak, and Guerney (54), initiators of the psychoeducational movement, describe this technique as a method not focused on "curing," but rather, on "managing" physical and mental impulses appropriately. Thus, through psychoeducational technique a client develops greater self-understanding of impulsivity, temperament, hunger cues, and other bodily sensations, and learns to regulate behavioral responses in accordance with need, societal ideals, or some standard.

It may be apparent to the reader that psychoeducational techniques are indeed different from both behavioral and cognitive techniques. They differ from behavioral ones in that behavior change with psychoeducational techniques occurs because of a two-fold process. First, one's level of self-awareness and understanding must be increased, and second, the client is then trained how to manage his or her temperament and/or impulse.

Psychoeducational techniques differ from cognitive techniques in that the cognitive ones focus primarily on one's system of attitudes and beliefs. Further, cognitive techniques do not employ a procedural component directed at understanding one's impulses, temperament, and/or bodily sensations.

Clinical Use

Psychoeducational techniques are suitable for a variety of dietary problems. They may be used in cases of anxious eating, depressive eating, and unintentional eating. A client who suffers with anxiety might use food to manage this state of being. However, the client may not be aware of the function food serves in this situation. Through a process of exploration, the dietitian might help the client identify ways in which food functions in his or her life.

Some clients use food to manage depressive states of being. Often people who are depressed complain of an "empty" feeling. Sometimes this feeling of "emptiness" is framed (described) as hunger. It may be that a person's internal states of hunger and depression become confused. (8) Psychoeducational techniques might help a client become physically and mentally aware that emptiness and hunger are, in fact, two different states of being, and thus must be treated differently.

Finally, some eat for unknown reasons. These clients are simply not in touch with their physical and mental processes. Both exploration and education are necessary to help this client increase his or her level of self-awareness so that eating might be better managed.

Psychoeducational techniques may be helpful, therefore, when a client requires both behavioral change, as well as cognitive change. In addition, a client might benefit from "self awareness" training. These techniques are outlined by Garner, Rockert, Olmsted, Johnson, and Coscina in their chapter on *Psychoeducational principles in the treatment of bulimia and anorexia nervosa* (30); however, they have applicability with other dietary related problems. Their focus is such that one may manage an urge to eat, to the degree that the desire to eat might be extinguished. This may be accomplished with three techniques: distraction, delay, and/or parroting.

Three Sample Treatments
The author often uses these techniques with a weight reducing population. One client, Gretchen, who went from 469 pounds to 350 pounds over a period of seven months, described her success strategies as distraction, delay, and parroting. Below are explanations and examples of each technique. Further, clinical utility of these techniques will be illustrated with the case of Gretchen, a forty-year-old female who sought weight loss to a healthier, undetermined, weight.

Distraction. This technique may be used as a first line of defense against urges to eat unnecessary calories or to avoid any behavior that seems somehow undesirable. Well before the urge is experienced, the client must first compile a list of alternate behaviors that may help distract the client from the urge. Gretchen used distraction often. She described experiencing cravings to eat usually in the evening. During her workday she experienced few, if any, urges to eat. The list Gretchen compiled to cope with these urges included riding her stationary bike, removing herself from the kitchen to her bedroom to read a book or watch television, calling a friend on the telephone, or writing a letter. Gretchen often found reading in her bedroom quite effective; however, on occasion this was not sufficient to defend against the urge to eat. When the urge outlasted the defense, Gretchen tried delay.

Delay. Many clients complain of intense urges to eat. Moreover, they describe this urge as a state other than hunger. Still, they feel compelled to eat, and sometimes do. When eating does occur, clients are at risk of being drawn into such old thinking patterns as, "Oh I blew it; I might as well finish the package. I'll start my diet tomorrow." The single eating episode may result in increased eating for a variety of reasons. Delay, used by itself or in combination with parroting, may prevent this automatic response.

The author has often heard clients remark, "If I wait ten minutes, often the urge to eat goes away." Indeed, this is true for many clients. But how might a dietitian use this technique and with what type of client? Delay might be used as a scheduled homework assignment. The dietitian might assign the client the following task.

Dietitian: When you feel like eating tomorrow you might try to delay eating. It might be helpful to think of this as your homework, and we can talk about your success at our next appointment. Tomorrow when you feel the urge to eat, you may try repeating to yourself, "I will not eat for fifteen minutes" (a parroting technique). At the end of fifteen minutes you might reevaluate your need to eat. Often the urge to eat goes away after ten or fifteen minutes. I feel it is important that you try this technique, if only to learn that you can indeed *bear* this urge without acting on it. You don't have to eat simply because you feel the urge to eat. How does this sound to you?

Client: It sounds reasonable to me. But I never tried to stop eating once the urge came over me. I just ate. But what if I cannot stop my urge to eat?

Dietitian: What do you imagine it might be like for you to feel this urge to eat and not act on it? (imagery) Can you describe for me what you might think and feel?

Client: Well, I might feel anxious. I might begin to think, "I need to eat this chocolate. I might not be able to stop myself from eating. "

Dietitian: What do you imagine this chocolate might do for you? (imagery) How do you imagine feeling maybe thirty minutes after eating the chocolate? What do you think the chocolate might be doing for you at that moment that another behavior cannot accomplish for you?

The dietitian and client may continue the conversation using the technique, delay, as a forum to explore the client's experience of eating, while at the same time revealing irrational thinking, and educating the client on more appropriate ways of thinking and eating. The process is an evolutionary one, in that it may occur over a period of weeks, and may require continual reinforcement on behalf of the dietitian and others. A counseling goal for both the dietitian and client might be to substitute the dietitian's role of reinforcing and exploring for another person who regularly communicates with the client. In doing so, reinforcement will be more available. The client will, therefore, have a forum to more regularly reinforce more appropriate ways of thinking and behaving with regards to food.

Gretchen often found delay to help defend against eating urges. She often combined delay with distraction. She might first read in her room, then acknowledge that she would wait ten more minutes, and become engrossed in some activity. At times, however, Gretchen found herself still craving to eat after the ten-minute period had elapsed. When this occurred, Gretchen used parroting techniques.

Parroting. As the name implies, parroting is a technique where the client repeats certain phrases to himself or herself in an attempt to dissipate and extinguish eating urges. To be most effective, these statements should be written well in advance of an eating urge. When the urge occurs, a client is often too vulnerable to strategize and is more at risk of responding to the urge rather than defending against it. While the ultimate result of parroting is that the irrational urge is disputed and abated, a more profound change may occur within the client's belief system. Parroting provides clients a forum to reprogram previously held maladaptive beliefs. These beliefs can only be reprogrammed when new, more adaptive statements are practiced and repeated frequently. Gretchen found parroting quite effective, especially when combined with distraction and delay. She regularly used the following statements:

"Come on Gretchen, you're not hungry. You just ate dinner."
"Go find something else to do Gretchen; you already ate your allotted four hundred calories."
"This is not hunger you are feeling; it is boredom. Go to sleep."
"Don't go in the kitchen right now, that will put you at risk. You're not hungry."
"One bite will make a difference. You don't need it."
"I often get the urge to eat when I feel depressed; but, this does not mean my body needs food."
"Food will not help me feel less depressed and/or less anxious."
"If I always do what I've always done, I will always get what I've always gotten."

Gretchen's parroting statements all focused on eating urges; but, this technique may help to manage other behaviors as well. Some clients complain of excessive urges to exercise, not to exercise, to smoke, or to weigh themselves.

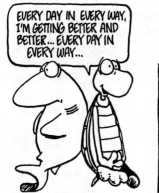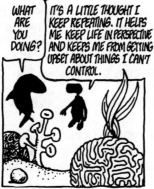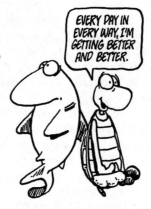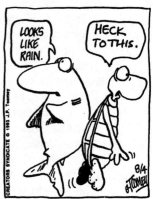

SHERMAN'S LAGOON by J.P. Toomey   Used with permission of J.P. Toomey and Creators Syndicate.

You can be instrumental in helping your clients develop parroting statements. First, explain to your client the purpose and utility of such statements. Second, provide examples from your own life or another client's of how parroting was both helpful and effective. Groups may be especially useful in this regard. Group members may model and role-play the way in which they use parroting techniques to cope with unwanted eating urges. Finally, provide continued support to clients who feel they cannot control their urge to eat, by giving them permission to eat when techniques do not work. Often, merely knowing that one has permission to eat makes the urge somehow less shameful and more manageable.

CLINICAL IMPLICATIONS AND CONCLUSIONS

The cognitive-behavioral model of counseling draws on such methods as self-monitoring, stimulus control, imagery, role playing, real-life performance-based, self-reinforcement, modeling, systematic desensitization, delay, disputing, decentering, reattributing, distraction, and parroting. Indeed, these are efficacious methods; in addition, their use is well supported with empirical research (2-5).

> **Further research is beginning to focus on identifying which treatment is most effective with which individual, with what problem, at what time. Clinicians are not merely slaves to their intuition. (2-5)**

While it is well established that cognitive-behavioral programs help *some* individuals achieve their desired health goals, these methods are not a panacea for changes in weight, eating, cholesterol, blood sugar, hypertension, and/or cigarette smoking. Indeed, some individuals seem to exhibit no improvement.

Many dietitians have worked with clients who spend months at the same weight, with the same eating problems, without significant changes in laboratory values or anthropometric data. Despite your most insightful advice, a most creative diabetic calculation, or a most perfect dietary formula, by clinical standards an individual *may fail* to recover. It may indeed be a discouraging experience to work with such individuals. Should you focus solely on physical recovery as a source of professional reinforcement, you may be left feeling ineffectual. One might look deeper for evidence of improvement.

Individuals may benefit from other relational factors, which are not overtly apparent to either you or the client. For example, perhaps you created a relationship based on trust, where it had not been previously experienced. Perhaps the client experienced a greater degree of mutuality in relationships outside of counseling because of the mutuality that was modeled and experienced between you and your client. Perhaps the client simply feels a greater sense of significance, because of the unconditional respect and warmth given by you. These are factors, which may not be accounted for in lost weight, lowered blood pressure or blood sugar. These are human factors, which may be experienced even if you do not *prescribe* a diet, *provide* an educational handout, or *calculate* exchanges. These factors are perhaps less well measured and less well explained; however, these factors exist.

It is the author's contention that a client's emotional condition is equally as important as a change in one's physical condition. Dietitians may indeed be sources of *normative* relational experience. This is indeed important, and sufficiently so, to the degree that a dietitian and client may dedicate an entire session to the discussion of how trust was developed between them. The implications of such trusting situations are profound.

According to Erik Erikson, trust is the basis of one's personality, religious, emotive, and ideological experience. (53,54) Dietitians may consider their counseling appointments, therefore, in developmental terms.

> **Trust is the basis of one's personality, religious, emotive, and ideological experience.**

The challenge for dietitians then is, perhaps, not method and not even technique, but rather, staying attuned to the human and relational factors of nutrition therapy. It is the author's contention that these factors are often ignored because dietitians feel uncomfortable focusing on relationship and the *individual* within. Rather than focusing on *technique*, dietitians might focus on the *relationship* created between dietitian and this person. It is perhaps this relationship that is most therapeutic.

References
1. Minuchin S, Fishman HC. *Family Therapy Techniques.* Cambridge, MA: Harvard University Press; 1981.
2. Corey G, Corey MS, Callanan P. *Issues and Ethics in the Helping Professions,* 4th ed. Pacific Grove, CA: Brooks/Cole; 1988.
3. Corey G. *Theory and Practice of Group Counseling,* 6th ed. Pacific Grove, CA: Brooks/Cole; 2000.
4. O'Leary KD, Wilson GT. *Behavior Therapy: Application and Outcome,* 2nd ed. Englewood Cliffs, NJ: Prentice-Hall; 1987.
5. Ivey AE, Ivey MB, Simek-Downing L. *Counseling and Psychotherapy: Integrating Skills, Theory, and Practice,* 2nd ed. Englewood Cliffs, NJ: Prentice-Hall; 1987.
6. American Psychiatric Association. *Diagnostic and Statistical Manual of Mental Disorders.* Washington DC; 1994.
7. Brownell KD, Foreyt JP, eds. *Handbook of Eating Disorders: Physiology, Psychology, and Treatment of Obesity, Anorexia, and Bulimia.* New York: Basic Books; 1986.
8. Bruch H. *Eating Disorders: Obesity, Anorexia Nervosa, and the Person Within.* New York: Basic Books; 1973.
9. Reiff DW, Reiff KKL. *Eating Disorders: Nutrition Therapy in the Recovery Process.* Washington: Life Enterprises; 1997.
10. Wilson GT, Pike KM. Eating disorders. In: Barlow DH, ed. *Clinical Handbook of Psychological Disorders: A Step-by-Step Treatment Manual,* 3rded. New York: The Guilford Press; 2001.
11. Glanz K, Snelling A, Payne D, Semenske AR. Strategies for modifying behavior to reduce cardiac risk. In: Kris-Etherton PM, VolzClarke P, Clark K, Dattilo AM, eds. *Cardiovascular Disease: Nutrition for Prevention and Treatment.* Chicago, IL: The American Dietetic Association; 1990: 224-247.
12. *Report of the Expert Panel on Blood Cholesterol Levels in Children and Adolescents.* Washington D.C.: U.S. Department of Health and Human Services; 1990.
13. Report of the Expert Panel on Population Strategies for Blood Cholesterol Reduction. Washington D.C.: U.S. Department of Health and Human Services; 1990.
14. Rabb C, Tillotson JL, eds. *Heart to Heart.* Washington, D.C.: U.S. Department of Health and Human Services; 1983.
15. *Report of the Expert Panel on Detection, Evaluation, and Treatment of High Blood Cholesterol in Adults.* Washington D.C.: U.S. Department of Health and Human Services; 1989.
16. Remmell PS, Gorder DD, Hall Y, Tillotson JL. Assessing dietary adherence in the Multiple Risk Factor Intervention Trial (MRFIT). *J Amer Diet Assoc.* 1980; 96: 351.
17. Williams AB. Behavior Modification. In: Holli BB, Calabrese RJ. *Communication and Education Skills: The Dietitian's Guide.* Philadelphia: Lea & Febiger; 1986: 81-102.
18. Brownell KD, Kramer FM. Behavioral management of obesity. *Medical Clinics of North America.* 1989;73(1): 185-201.
19. Perri MG, Nezu AM, Patti ET, McCann KL. Effect of length of treatment on weight loss. *Journal of Consulting and Clinical Psychology.* 1989; 57(3): 450-452.
20. Perri MG, McAllister DA, Gange JJ, Jordan RC, McAdoo WG, Nezu AM. Effects of four maintenance programs on the long-term management of obesity. *Journal of Consulting and Clinical Psychology.* 1988; 56(4): 529-534.
21. Wadden TA, Stunkard AJ, Liebschutz J. Three year follow-up of the treatment of obesity by very low calorie diet, behavior therapy, and their combination. *Journal of Consulting and Clinical Psychology.* 1988; 56(6): 925-928.
22. Graham LE, Taylor CB, Hovell MF, and Siegel W. Five year follow-up to a behavioral weight loss program. *Journal of Consulting and Clinical Psychology.* 1983;51(2):322-323.
23. Westover SA, Lanyon RI. The maintenance of weight loss after behavioral treatment. *Behavior Modification.* 1990; 14(2): 123-137.
24. Kayman S, Bruvold W, Stern JS. Maintenance and relapse after weight loss in women: Behavioral aspects. *Am J Clin Nutr.* 1990; 52: 800-807.
25. Wing RR. Behavioral treatment of severe obesity. *Am J Clin Nutr.* 1992; 55: 545S-551S.
26. Brownell KD, Wadden TA. Etiology and treatment of obesity: Understanding a serious, prevalent, and refractory disorder. *Journal of Consulting and Clinical Psychology.* 1992; 60(4): 505-517.
27. McDonald LS, Woolsey M, Murray A. Weight management. In: Kris-Etherton PM, Volz-Clarke P, Clark K, Dattilo AM, eds. *Cardiovascular Disease: Nutrition for Prevention and Treatment.* Chicago: American Dietetic Association. 1990; 175-189.
28. Buckmaster L, Brownell KD. Behavior modification: The state of the art. In: Frankle RT, Yang Mei Uih, eds. *Obesity and Weight Control: The Health Professional's Guide to Understanding and Treatment.* Rockville, MD: Aspen Publishers; 1988:205-224.
29. Morton CJ. Weight loss maintenance and relapse prevention. In: Frankle RT, Yang Mei Uih, eds. *Obesity and Weight Control: The Health Professional's Guide to Understanding and Treatment.* Rockville, MD: Aspen Publishers; 1988: 315-332.
30. Garner DM, Rockert W, Olmsted MP, Johnson C, Coscina DV. Psychoeducational principles in the treatment of bulimia and anorexia nervosa. In: Garner DM, and Garfinkel PE, eds. *Handbook of Psychotherapy for Anorexia Nervosa & Bulimia.* NY: The Guilford Press; 1985: 513-572.
31. Fairburn CG. Cognitive Behavioral treatment for bulimia. In: Garner DM, Garfinkel PE, eds. *Handbook of Psychotherapy for Anorexia Nervosa & Bulimia.* NY: The Guilford Press; 1985: 160-192.
32. Garner DM, Bemis KM. Cognitive therapy for anorexia nervosa. In: Garner DM, Garfinkel PE, eds. *Handbook of Psychotherapy for Anorexia Nervosa & Bulimia.* NY: The Guilford Press; 1985: 107-146.
33. Fairburn CG, Marcus MD, Wilson GT. Cognitive Behavioral therapy for binge eating and bulimia nervosa: A comprehensive treatment manual. In: Fairburn CG, Wilson GT. *Binge Eating: Nature, Assessment, and Treatment.* NY: The Guilford Press; 1993: 361-404.
34. Egan G. *The Skilled Helper: A Systematic Approach to Effective Helping,* 3rd ed. Monterey, CA: Brooks/Cole; 1986.
35. Williams R, Long J. *Toward a self-managed life style.* 3rd ed. Boston: Houghton Mifflin; 1983.
36. Linehan M, Bootzin R, Cautela J, London P, Perloff M, Stuart R, Risley T. Guidelines for choosing a behavior therapist. *Behavior Therapist.* 1978; 1(4): 1820.
37. Eysenck HJ. Behavior Therapy. In: Eysenck HJ, Martin I, eds. *Theoretical Foundations of Behavior Therapy.* NY: Plenum Press; 1987; 335.

124

38. Watson JB. *Behaviorism.* Chicago: University of Chicago Press; 1930.
39. Mineka S. A primate model of phobic fears. In: Eysenck HJ, Martin I. *Theoretical Foundations of Behavior Therapy.* NY: Plenum Press; 1987; 81-111.
40. Levey AB, Martin I. Evaluative conditioning: A case for Hedonic Transfer. In: Eysenck HJ, Martin I. *Theoretical Foundations of Behavior Therapy.* NY: Plenum Press; 1987; 113-131.
41. Wilson GT. Behavior Therapy. In: Corsini RJ, et al. *Current Psychotherapies,* 6th ed. Itasca, IL: F.E. Peacock Publishers; 2000.
42. Lowe CF, Horne PJ, Higson PJ. Operant conditioning: The Hiatus between theory and practice in clinical psychology. In: Eysenck HT, and Martin I. *Theoretical Foundations of Behavior Therapy.* NY: Plenum Press; 1987; 153-165.
43. Heiby EM. Assessment of frequency of self-reinforcement. *Journal of Personality and Social Psychology.* 1983;44(6): 1304-1307.
44. Miller JB. *What Do We Mean By Relationships?* Wellesley, MA: Stone Center; 1986.
45. Bandura A. *Social Learning Theory.* Englewood Cliffs, NJ: Prentice-Hall; 1977.
46. Rose, SD. Group counseling with children: A behavioral and cognitive approach. In: Gazda GM, ed. *Basic Approaches to Group Psychotherapy and Group Counseling,* 3rd ed. Springfield, IL: Charles C Thomas; 1982.
47. Brown TA, O'Leary TA, Barlow DH. Generalized anxiety disorder. In: Barlow DH, ed. *Clinical Handbook of Psychological Disorders: A Step-by-Step Treatment Manual,* 2nd ed. NY: The Guilford Press; 1993; 137-188.
48. Ellis A. Rational-Emotive therapy. In: Corsini RJ, et al. *Current Psychotherapies,* 6th ed. Itasca, IL: F.E. Peacock Publishers, Inc.; 2000.
49. Piaget J. Piaget's theory. In: Mussen PH, ed. *Manual of child psychology,* 3rd ed. NY: John Wiley & Sons; 1970; 703-732.
50. Ginsburg HP, Opper S. *Piaget's Theory of Intellectual Development,* 3rd ed. Englewood Cliffs, NJ: Prentice-Hall; 1988.
51. Selman RL. The child as a friendship philosopher. In: Asher SR, Gottman JM, eds. *The Development of Children's Friendships.* Cambridge, MA: Cambridge University Press; 1981; 242-273.
52. Elkind D. *All Grown Up and No Place to Go.* Reading, MA: Addison Wesley; 1997.
53. Freud S. A *General Introduction to Psychoanalysis.* Garden City, NY: Doubleday; 1943.
54. Guerney B, Stollak L, Guerney L. The practicing psychologist as educator: An alternative to the medical practitioner model. *Professional Psychologist.* 1971; 2: 276-282.
55. Erikson EH. *Childhood and Society.* NY: W.W. Norton & Company; 1993.
56. Erikson EH. *Identity and the Life Cycle.* NY: W.W. Norton & Company; 1994.

Chapter 10

Inpatient Counseling
and the Continuum of Care
Bridget Klawitter, PhD, RD, FADA

After reading this chapter, the reader will be able to:
- ♦ Recognize the changes, as well as continued value of nutrition counseling, in today's acute care environment.
- ♦ Identify regulatory standards applicable to the nutrition counseling process.
- ♦ Discuss the components of a nutrition plan of care.
- ♦ Discuss applications of the Nutrition Care Model.

BENEFITS OF CLINICAL NUTRITION SERVICES IN ACUTE CARE

We all know that well-nourished individuals are more resistant to disease and infection; are better able to tolerate other therapies; and recover better from acute illness, surgical interventions, and trauma. Inadequate nutritional intake can precipitate disease or increase its severity. Early detection of nutrition-related problems and appropriate nutrition interventions are effective in helping the patient recover more quickly and decrease the number of days requiring hospitalization.

Registered dietitians and registered dietetic technicians are critical members of health care teams. Medical nutrition therapy, coordinated by a registered dietitian, is an integral part of disease prevention, treatment, and recovery, and is necessary to maintain quality of care and achieve cost savings. It involves two phases: 1) assessment of the patient's nutritional status, and 2) treatment, which includes diet therapy, counseling, or the use of specialized nutritional support.

Changes in Healthcare Climate and Clinical Practice
At The American Dietetic Association's Future Search Conference in 1994, speakers stated that health care in America in the year 2000 would not look anything like it did at that point in time. (1) As predicted, healthcare has been increasingly affected by regulatory changes, increased market competition for patients, and hospital mergers and affiliations. The U.S. economy is facing a new world of medicine driven by technology and the needs of a graying population. Our jobs look different, too. Concerns about escalating costs and limited services in managed care, coupled with consumers' expectations not being met, created a growing concern about the quality of patient care. Hence, quality assessment and cost benefits of nutrition services have taken on new significance.

> **Already the U.S. spends approximately 14% of its gross domestic product on medical care and may increase to 17% within the next decade. (2)**

The opportunities to provide inpatient nutrition counseling continue to decrease as patients are discharged from acute care settings sooner and sicker. At the time of discharge, patients are often not ready for comprehensive nutrition counseling nor is the typical hospital environment conducive to lengthy individual counseling sessions. The rapid turnover, patient cognitive condition, and short lead times limit a clinical dietitian's ability to identify specific counseling needs, provide counseling, and evaluate the patient's knowledge and understanding prior to discharge.

Despite the above circumstances, patients and physicians expect (and accrediting agencies require) that appropriate nutrition education take place, if possible, in the hospital setting so the patient and his or her family do not aggravate, but instead encourage continued improvement of the patient's physical state. "Survival" nutrition counseling may include basic types of foods to limit or avoid, portion sizes, and meal frequency. The majority of dietitians now seem to agree that it is most appropriate to counsel patients on survival or "need to know" information during brief hospitalizations, and to refer patients for more comprehensive nutrition counseling in the outpatient setting. The majority of patients receives abbreviated nutrition intervention in the hospital setting and is increasingly referred to outpatient counselors for more comprehensive instruction or follow-up. Diabetes care often is more structured. For example, the rapid expansion of diabetes self-management training (DSMT) programs recognized by the American Diabetes Association, expansion of Medicare nutrition counseling coverage for select diagnoses, and a growing number of private practice dietetic practitioners have provided expanded continuity of care options to the discharged patient and their families.

Value of Screening in Cost Containment

> **Clinical dietetic practitioners should use a comprehensive nutrition-screening program to zero in on patients who possess co-morbid nutritional conditions so that physicians can formally diagnose and together we can more adequately address patients' needs.**

Nutrition screening results can also provide a basis for communication with physicians. Screening data can help establish the need for medically appropriate, cost-effective nutrition interventions, including counseling. An increasing trend in pre-admission screening to improve medical and nutrition status prior to admission has led to more formal pre-admission nutrition screening protocols. (3) In the inpatient setting, computer linking between departments such as nursing, pharmacy, lab, and the clinical dietetic department allows dietetic practitioners to obtain the clinical nutrition data to facilitate the identification of patients who are at nutritional risk. A nutrition-screening program is an inexpensive method to streamline clinical nutrition care and identify those patients at nutritional risk who are most likely to benefit from special nutrition intervention during their hospital stay. See Chapter 7 for a more in-depth review of screening and assessment.

A growing body of evidence in the literature points to protein-energy malnutrition (PEM) as a complication that can potentially increase morbidity, mortality, and mean length of stay. (4,5) Malnutrition causes deterioration in physical and psychological function, as well as general well being. There is also considerable evidence that nutritional intervention reduces morbidity and mortality. (6,7) Because PEM cuts across diagnostic and treatment categories, traditional methods of identifying high-risk patients may need to be more sensitive in order to detect nutritional risk.

Many third party payments to healthcare providers are based on the average cost of caring for patients classified by diagnostic related groups (DRGs). DRGs were developed as the foundation of the Medicare reimbursement system for individual inpatient reimbursement. The DRG categories are based on diagnoses, treatment, and anticipated length of stay. Claim classifications consider a number of factors including principle diagnosis, secondary diagnoses (called "complications" or "co-morbid conditions"), surgical procedures, and the patient's age and sex. (8) Several studies (9,10) have confirmed that declines in the nutritional status of hospitalized patients are associated with increased complication rates and significantly higher hospital costs. The development and implementation of a basic nutrition screening program, coupled with a standardized nutrition assessment form, can ensure that dietetic practitioners seize every opportunity to provide early interventions for patients at nutritional risk.

The clinical dietetic practitioner can control costs. For example, focusing nutrition therapy efforts on high and moderate nutrition risk patients can concentrate efforts on those patients who may benefit most from nutrition interventions in the acute care setting. By monitoring the use of high-tech nutrition therapies, including parenteral nutrition, substantial savings can be realized when enteral feedings are substituted for parenteral nutrition. (11) Clinical dietitians can also play an essential role in ensuring the most cost-effective enteral products are used without sacrificing quality nutrition care through their evaluation of the enteral formulary. (12)

CONSIDERATIONS FOR INPATIENT COUNSELING

When Time Is Short

When time is not a factor, inpatient counseling can follow the guidelines discussed in other chapters. The typical abbreviated, but essential, "need to know" information used in inpatient counseling involves:

1. Establishing behavioral diagnoses
   - Distinguish between behavioral and nonbehavioral causes (for example, weight gain due to decreased activity versus as a result of taking corticosteroids).
   - Define behaviors in relation to condition (such as less physical activity coupled with increased calories leads to weight gain).
   - Rank behaviors in order of importance (increased activity versus decreased calories).
   - Assess ability for behavior change (easier to decrease portion sizes than find time for exercise).
   - Prioritize behaviors based upon importance and ability to change.

2. Assessing what client wants to learn
   - Perceive these as immediate needs. (How many calories do I need? or Why do I need to limit sodium?)
   - Acknowledges client's independence in decision-making.
   - The adult patient must acknowledge there is a problem (see Chapter 3 for more information on the needs of adult learners).

Practice Guidelines, Protocols, and the Nutrition Care Process

Nutrition practice guidelines provide systematically developed assistance to dietetic practitioners. (13) These guidelines should be based on a synthesis of scientific literature, expert opinion, and clinical practice. By developing and using practice guidelines and protocols (or critical pathways or care maps) that standardize practice in order to produce positive outcomes, you better ensure efficiency and effectiveness in your delivery. In 1998, the American Dietetic Association formed the Health Services Research (HSR) Task Force to investigate the current research state of medical nutrition therapy effectiveness and outcomes. The Nutrition Care Model (Figure 10.1) identified the components of what dietetic practitioners do (or should do) in the Nutrition Care Process (Figure 10.2). (14) Several of the components directly impact the identification of knowledge deficits and opportunities for nutrition counseling.

Dietitians should evaluate the outcomes of nutrition interventions so that cost effectiveness and cost benefits can be delineated. The disease-specific (Medical Nutrition Therapy Across the Continuum of Care) MNTACC protocols and practice guidelines are an excellent resource for coordinating counseling efforts with the specific disease and measurable outcomes. (15-18)

Many patients in acute care settings require comprehensive nutrition plans of care when they are discharged to promote continuity of care and prevent early re-hospitalizations. Discharge planning should start the day of admission and be designed to provide continuity of care and allow for a smooth transition for the patient from one care setting to another. This means systems must be set up to facilitate the transition to outpatient nutrition services in the home, clinic, community, or in other institutions. To facilitate the transition back to home, a family-centered approach (to assess the involvement and the needs of family members) can impact long-term compliance and success with lifestyle changes. Discharge planning is a multidisciplinary process and should be considered a priority by dietetic professionals.

Locations for Counseling Have Been Changing

As hospital stays become shorter, clinical dietitians need to plan to change *where* they counsel patients. Murray discusses the philosophy of nutrition therapy and the need to take a more client-centered approach. (19) Recognizing the shrinking lengths of stay, key counseling points should be introduced or reinforced in the inpatient setting in conjunction with processes to promote follow-up counseling in the pre- and post-hospitalization continuum of care. For example, inpatient dietetic practitioners can be key players in facilitating the completion of referrals to outpatient or private practice nutrition counseling locations.

Figure 10.1 Nutrition Care Model

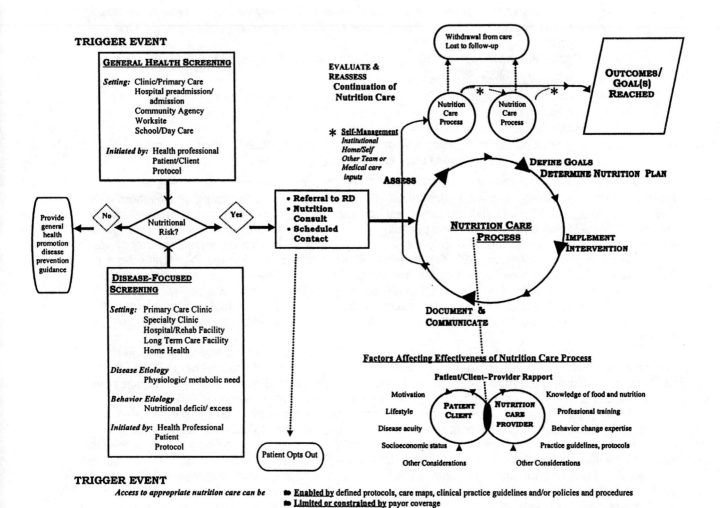

Source: Splett P, Myers EF. A proposed model for effective nutrition care. *J Amer Diet Assoc.* 2001; 101(3):357-363.
Copyright 2001, The American Dietetic Association. Used with permission.

Figure 10.2 Nutrition Care Process

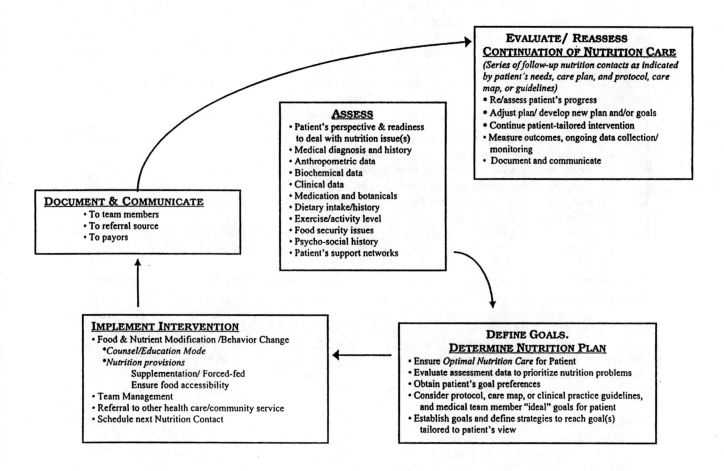

Several other factors also have contributed to shifts from inpatient acute care to outpatient ambulatory care. Factors to be considered are the aging population, advances in medical technology, increased health care costs, increased focus on prevention and wellness, the AIDS epidemic, and the coexistence of malnutrition with chronic diseases. (1) Additional trends identified by the American Dietetic Association include an individual's value changes regarding health, the challenges of the modern lifestyle, working, food systems, and the increasing cultural and ethnic diversity of the population. (20) Consequently, an increased need for expanded nutrition counseling services in the outpatient, ambulatory, and private practice settings has been identified.

QUALITY IMPROVEMENT

Continuous Quality Improvement (CQI) is the process of continual information feedback, evaluation, and improvement of delivery systems and outcomes based on objectively measured quality parameters. Quality management is synonymous with a commitment to continuous improvement. Ongoing CQI should be an integral part of inpatient, as well as outpatient, services with the focus on outcomes as a result of counseling interventions. Dietetic practitioners are critical to accelerating and supporting practice change towards evidenced-based practice (EBP). See Chapter 22 for more information on the implications of EBP to our profession.

Three terms are important to understand: (21)
- *Quality* **assessment** measures the level of quality care at some point in time but does not connote any effort to change or improve that level of care.
- *Quality improvement* is customer driven and emphasizes coordinating and integrating various health care professionals in the assessment of processes that affect patient outcomes.
- *Continuous Quality Improvement* (**CQI**) is a more proactive and all encompassing concept, which includes the measurement of the on-going level of care provided, and when indicated, the attempt to continually improve it.

Quality improvement can be determined from *structure,* process, or outcomes: (22)

Structure consists of tangible or organizational components involved in patient care (i.e., facilities, equipment, personnel, or organizational structure). The program review process may include reviewing current nutrition counseling programs and assessing the need for other programs like group diabetes or breastfeeding classes. Structure indicators (an *indicator is* an index used to monitor the stability or change in a designated process) may also review the policies that guide patient education and counseling, or review the accuracy and appropriateness of nutrition educational materials.

Process denotes what actions are carried out in the provision of care (i.e., interventions, counseling, or treatment). Patient education process indicators target the delivery of patient teaching and may include counselor effectiveness, documentation, and the flow of the counseling.

Outcomes are the effects on the health status of the patient. Outcome indicators evaluate behavioral changes in the patient by measuring knowledge and skills at the time of the counseling and often after discharge. The process of continuing quality improvement (CQI) is dependent upon linkages between structure and process, and between process and outcomes. For example, the availability of adequate clinical dietetic staff to conduct nutritional counseling and decrease the number of re-admissions for uncontrolled blood sugars in a child with diabetes.

IMPACT OF REGULATORY REQUIREMENTS

Dramatic changes in the overall healthcare marketplace have occurred over the past 25 years as hospitals have transitioned to a more ambulatory and community-based model of care. (23) The basic functions of external controls (by government or private agencies) in health care are to:
- Offer formal standards
- Survey the providers of care (hospitals, mental health and addiction programs, long-term care facilities, rehabilitation centers, etc.)
- Assess the degree of compliance with those standards
- Impose sanctions or incentives in response to reported deviations from the standards

OBRA and Long-Term Care

The 1987 Omnibus Budget Reconciliation Act (OBRA) requires the inspection of nursing homes and other skilled nursing facilities receiving Medicare and/or Medicaid funds from the federal Health Care Financing Administration (HCFA). Each state also has long-term care licensure requirements, which are usually similar to the federal guidelines but may be more rigorous. OBRA requires states to conduct inspections with a focus on the needs of individual residents and the quality of services being offered to them. (24)

Residents' needs may range from denture problems and multiple medications to too much gas or brittle bones. Many have a keen interest in food and nutrition. It is important to document any discussions with the resident in regards to the prescribed diet, choices regarding meals, snacks, and activities, and care or treatment. Surveyors will also look for a comprehensive multidisciplinary care plan with measurable objectives and a timeline to meet identified needs. See Chapter 7 for an overview of the requirements for long-term care.

Joint Commission on Accreditation of Healthcare Organizations (JCAHO)

The "Joint Commission" or JCAHO is a peer review organization that evaluates healthcare facilities and ranks their compliance with established standards. Its mission is to improve the safety and quality of care provided to the public using accreditation as a tool to motivate health care organizations to improve systems and processes that most influence client care and outcomes. (25) An accreditation survey assesses the level of an organization's compliance with applicable JCAHO standards. The survey includes written and verbal evidence of compliance and on-site observations by the survey team. The JCAHO also serves to assist organizations in education and consultation regarding compliance to standards.

With the most recent annual Accreditation Manual for Hospitals (AMH), JCAHO reiterates that its new approach will require hospitals to shift their thinking away from a checklist of "things to do" towards a more thoughtful "did it work" approach. Beginning in 2004, JCAHO will implement a new, improved accreditation process called, "Shared Visions—New Pathways." This initiative is to ensure and enhance the relevance of the standards to the health care setting and contribute to quality care. The JCAHO standards base accreditation on measured outcomes and actual improvements in patient care, a direction it feels all health care organizations must take. American businesses came around to this realization of accountability many years ago, and healthcare adopted this approach more diligently in the last 10-15 years.

Standards Related to the Care in the Inpatient Setting
Standards and processes for nutrition care are similar to those of other disciplines. In the new 2004 proposed standards, many of the discipline-specific references have been removed, instead focusing on general statements with broad applicability across the various disciplines potentially providing care. Elements contained in the proposed 2004 still address the coordination of care and continuing treatment, assessment and reassessment of patients, education and training specific to the patient's needs, and competency of staff providing care.

"Top 10" JCAHO Survey Items
• Screening
• Equipment temperature
• Staffing
• Assessment and reassessment
• Staff competency
• Drug-nutrient interactions
• Cultural and ethnic needs
• Food and enteral nutrition safety
• Patient/family education
• Patient safety and health care errors

Source: Pavlinic J. *De-stressing the JCAHO Survey.* Roundtable presented at CNM Symposium 2003, Charleston, SC.

Originally, the implementation of the standard regarding nutrient-drug counseling was the responsibility of dietetic services, but it has been recognized that a multidisciplinary approach is needed. Much controversy had centered on this aspect of the standards and it had been rated less effective than other standards in its ability to improve patient care. (27) There is a lack of agreement over which drug-food interactions are clinically important, but monoamine oxidase (MAO) inhibitors are most frequently mentioned followed by anticoagulants, tetracycline, Coumadin, and diuretics. Ideally, each patient should be counseled on all clinically relevant drug interactions. However, limitations in time, resources, and personnel do not always make this possible. Those patients at greatest risk for substantial nutrient-drug interactions should be targeted for counseling. Other patients should at least receive written materials (i.e., computer print-out with the pertinent information) at the time of discharge. Eventually, as more hospitals go to paperless charting and dietitians carry portable handheld computers, it will not be as difficult to have drug-nutrient information available at bedside.

Surveyors encourage multidisciplinary collaboration in the care of patients. This includes such disciplines as physicians, dietitians, nurses, pharmacists, therapists, and social workers. Collaborative care teams and critical pathways are more common now in response to this area of emphasis by surveyors. Dietetic practitioners in the acute care settings need to become involved in clinical nutrition and education committees whenever possible to represent the nutritional aspects of total patient care and facilitate these multidisciplinary approaches for the provision of nutritional care.

The standards for the education function illustrate the three areas that impact the patient: the organization's focus on education; the direct impact of education on the patient and his or her family; and the program evaluation in relation to patient outcomes. The primary goal of the standards for education is to provide clients with knowledge of their condition/illness and their treatment, so they may learn behaviors and skills that will promote recovery and improve function. Client education and counseling should be specific to the needs, abilities, and readiness of the individual patient as appropriate to the length of stay. This includes counseling on potential nutrient-drug interactions, nutrition interventions, and/or modified diets as appropriate.

Organizations must provide the resources to systematically assess and meet the educational needs of the patient and family in a coordinated, multidisciplinary way. The education standards themselves, located in the (JCAHO) Provision of Care chapter, have remained essentially unchanged from prior standards, except for a continued emphasis on patient and family responsibility for the patient's ongoing care needs. This includes the recognition that active participation in one's treatment is an important factor in a patient's outcome, as well as, the use of medications and medical equipment, potential nutrient-drug interactions, counseling on diet modifications, and how/when to obtain further treatment if indicated. Health care organizations do have flexibility on how they comply with the education standards. The standards, for example, do not dictate which profession(s) will be responsible for an educational process. This could mean, however, that dietitians might not be consulted for diabetes, breastfeeding, or other nutrition-related educational consults, unless they have established their expertise and value to others on the multidisciplinary team.

The standards also compel providers to share discharge instructions with the organization or individual(s) responsible for the continuation of care. (26) This includes the assessment of patient needs, ensuring that they are smoothly transitioned from one care setting to another, and the provision of information to patients, family, or other providers of care who are receiving the patient. These standards are often referred to as the framework for case management. The standards concerned with the continuum of care advocate that based on an initial assessment of the patient, the most appropriate plan of care is to be developed.

Components of the standards related to continuity of care require a process or system to ensure clinical continuity and communication between providers of care as patients move from one care setting to another. The ultimate goal is continuous, appropriate, and well coordinated care—a "seamless" provision of services.

> **The focus of the JCAHO standards is progressively shifting toward outcome evaluation, which may necessitate changes in the methods used by some institutions to chart.**

DOCUMENTATION OF PATIENT CARE

Institutions, as well as various departments within institutions, use a variety of forms and formats to document clinical care provided to patients. The primary purpose of documentation is to direct the care of the client, especially when multiple disciplines are involved, and to record the client's status or response to the interventions. Routine interventions are generally formulated into standards of care, while client-specific interventions are formulated into a plan of care. The documentation process is also crucial to the review and evaluation function of total quality management—the process of ensuring high quality output to enhance customer service and improve customer satisfaction. (28) In some cases, documentation serves as the justification for reimbursement.

Traditionally, such regulatory agencies as JCAHO or the Department of Health and Human Services do not have specific charting formats for documentation delineated in the regulatory standards; however, the standards do identify documentation requirements. Institutions can define their own documentation formats as long as they are in compliance with all legal, accreditation, and professional standards. See Chapter 22 for more specifics on documentation methodology.

Nutrition Plan of Care

The nutritional plan of care for a client should identify a priority set of problems for that individual, as well as communicate what to observe, to teach, or to implement in order to achieve certain outcome criteria within an anticipated time frame. The plan of care also serves to identify specific interventions for the client, family, or specified disciplines to implement. The typical components of the plan of care include:

- Problem statements
- Outcome criteria/goals
- Interventions
- Evaluation

Many facilities integrate multiple disciplines into the care of each individual client. A primary responsibility of these multidisciplinary groups is to continually assess and improve patient care through the development of clinical care pathways and/or protocols.

The nutrition **problem** statement is a statement of concern (other than the medical diagnosis) for which the nutrition staff provides intervention that can be evaluated. Problem statements can often be prefaced with the statement, "Alteration in .... as related to ...." as is often seen in the nursing documentation process. "Alteration in oral intake related to poor dentition," or "Alteration in bowel elimination related to low fiber intake" are examples dietetic practitioners may want to consider.

Outcome *criteria* (or goals) should be statements describing measurable indices or behavior of the client/family denoting a favorable response (changed or maintained) after implementing the plan of care. In effect, the outcome criteria serve as standards for measuring the effectiveness of the plan of care. When outcome criteria are not being achieved, the diagnosis should be reevaluated and the plan of care and/or goals revised. Collaboration among disciplines is instrumental in designing an effective nutrition plan of care.

Interventions are autonomous actions by each discipline involved in the client's care, based on scientific rationale, and executed to benefit the client in an anticipated way related to their diagnosis and outcome criteria. Interventions may either be independent (i.e., discipline-specific prescribed treatment) like a dietitian prescribed diet order or delegated (i.e., physician prescribed diet order with monitoring by another discipline to determine compliance or effectiveness). Interventions may be either activities that are performed for or with the client, like monitoring oral intake or assisting with daily menu completion using exchanges, or may be activities such as assessments to identify new problems or determine the status of existing problems. Whenever possible, interventions should provide for active participation by the client with a goal of maximizing their ability to self-manage their health.

Evaluation of the client's status compares it to the outcome criteria anticipated from the plan of care. Continuous evaluation allows each discipline, either individually or collaboratively, to determine if the client is progressing as planned. **Summary evaluation statements** for each anticipated outcome should specifically address what the client has accomplished or is able to do, to verbalize, or perform. The evaluation phase should be continual from the time the plan of care is implemented to the termination of care and any referrals made.

Progress notes, regardless of where in the medical record they may be located, serve to document significant data or events in the care of the client. Each notation should be specific to the diagnosis, interventions, and outcomes of nutrition therapy.

Discharge planning is an important component of the plan of care. As mentioned previously, the discharge planning process should begin at the time of admission. Discharge planning may include:

- Written nutrition instruction materials
- Follow-up outpatient visits
- Referrals to other home care or community resources

At times, referrals to sources outside the immediate area may be indicated and early discharge planning allows time for the appropriate arrangements to be made and all discharge summary documentation to be completed.

WHY CHARGE FOR INPATIENT CLINICAL SERVICES?

Diagnosis-specific coding for reimbursement is vital to documenting alterations in nutritional status. Although dietetic specific codes have been proposed, current systems in the majority of acute care settings dictate that documentation by dietetic practitioners use medical-specific coding. (29)

Cost reduction activities such as restructuring and staff reduction have been common practices in healthcare, and dietetic practitioners have not been immune from the process. (30) The American Dietetic Association has recognized these challenges faced by its members and recommended dietetic practitioners focus on patient satisfaction and cost effectiveness of their services. (31,32) Dietetic practitioners must be prepared to answer some tough questions from hospital administrators. The lack of specific nutrition billing codes often makes it difficult to track the fruits of dietetic services, specifically:

- Improved patient outcomes and satisfaction
- Reduced number of re-admissions through effective nutrition counseling and outpatient follow-up
- Increased DRG nutrition-related revenue
- Increased potential revenues from inpatient and outpatient counseling and other clinical nutrition services

The increase in capitated plans and inpatient DRG payments make the issue of revenue generation a difficult discussion to support, but the benefits of disease prevention and health promotion are even stronger. However, in an analysis of 1601 nutrition intervention case studies compiled by the American Dietetic Association, it was revealed that the average annual cost savings for patients could equal thousands of dollars, for example, $10,538 for gestational diabetes; $6,556 for a tube/IV feeding; $2,496 for hypercholesterolemia; and $2,178 for type 2 diabetes. (33) So often, administrators consider clinical dietetic services as "insignificant" revenue sources. This makes it all the more important that you market what you provide. (34)

In the past, many dietetic practitioners have been hesitant to charge for inpatient and/or outpatient nutrition services such as assessments and nutrition counseling. Changes in third party payer mixes, as well as reimbursement policies, have had a dramatic effect on acute care billing for clinical nutrition care. Clinical nutrition departments now must differentiate routine services from nonroutine services. Nonroutine services are generally physician-ordered and provided to selected at-risk patients. Examples of basic nutrition care may include:

- Screening of patients identified at nutritional risk
- Obtaining food preferences or determining allergies
- Menu distribution process
- Quality control: meal rounds, tray assessments, and surveys
- 3 meals per day and nonpharmaceutical nourishments and snacks
- Phone consultations
- Resolution of patient satisfaction issues

All other services are often considered specialized and billable. If you charge for services, charge fair fees and promote the value of your services, not just the revenue potential. Following are the reasons many hospitals charge for nonroutine nutrition services:

- Provides financial accountability for dietetic services.
- Promotes fair distribution of clinical staffing by prioritizing clinical nutrition services.
- Provides cost benefits in relation to decreased LOS (length of stay) when nutrition intervention is involved.
- Improves quality of patient care through early intervention and preventive nutrition.
- Assigns value to clinical nutrition care.
- Enhances professional image.

Nutrition Education in a Typical Pathway
Susan DeHoog, RD

When patients are admitted to the hospital our role and responsibility is to provide medical nutrition therapy and education to the patients, along with providing nutritional expertise and education to the interdisciplinary health care team. In accordance with the changes of the Joint Commission on Accreditation of Hospital Organization (JCAHO), the emphasis has shifted to interdisciplinary patient care. We must demonstrate verbally and in writing that we have conferred with the other health care professionals regarding the education of the patient and/or significant other.

Therefore, we need a functioning mechanism designed to standardize and communicate nutrition care approaches and processes in both the inpatient and outpatient areas. One element of this mechanism can be part of the clinical pathways developed by the facility. Clinical pathways track patients' interventions and outcomes throughout their hospital stay. Pathways are established to ensure processes are standardized and result in a defined positive outcome. Each day of hospitalization has identified interventions and outcomes. Clinical pathways can start in the outpatient department; be implemented inpatient, and conclude back in the outpatient area.

All assessments are based on the average length of stay for the disease state. For example, nutritional status hospital day one (HD #1) with intravenous Cisplatin, the outcome is for the patient to maintain 50% of nutritional needs with or without antimetics. By HD #4, patient/family education needs to be completed (Average length of stay is six days). Discharge planning usually begins when the patient enters the hospital.

All hospital clinical dietitians should be active in your hospital's education and nutrition committees. The nutrition committee, whose members usually include medicine, surgery, nutrition, pharmacy, and nursing promotes the optimal use of nutrition resources for patient care. The education committee, which can include the same disciplines, oversees all educational mechanisms. This could include all nutritional instructions and all potential food/drug interactions. The process should include follow-up care either to a nutrition clinic, private practice dietitian, or a dietitian at the referring facility. Diseases such as heart disease, kidney disease, cancer, diabetes, hypertension, and other leading causes of death where lifestyle impacts the disease process all need nutrition education intervention.

Inpatient Counseling
Your inpatient process of nutrition counseling could be as follows:
1. The dietitian assesses the patient's learning ability and readiness for learning, comprehension, and the ability to implement changes. Consideration is given to literacy, cognitive limitations, religious food-related practices, family beliefs, values, and culture. When indicated, an interpreter will be used.
2. The patient and/or significant other receive education specific to the patient's diagnosis, assessed need and abilities.

The dietitian assesses the patient's and/or significant other's comprehension and ability to implement changes. Learning needs may need to be prioritized.

Discharge
JCAHO standards require that any discharge instructions given to the patient are also provided to the facility or individual responsible for the patient's continuing care. A copy of the discharge summary and instructions should also be forwarded to the patient's primary care provider. The nutrition discharge summery should contain the following information:
1. Pertinent information on weights, labs, food intake, calculated needs, medications
2. Summary of nutritional problems and therapies
3. Outcome of nutritional therapies
4. Statement of patient education to include:
   - patient and/or significant other has been instructed on prescribed needs,
   - expected adherence to prescribed diet,
   - comprehension of nutrition information and self-care, and
   - drug/nutrient interaction education, if appropriate.
5. Statement on expected "progress"
6. Recommendations for follow up
7. Continuum of care plans
8. Statement that indicates other members of the health care team are advised of the education provided to the patient and/or significant other.

FOR FURTHER READING
Grant A, DeHoog S. *Nutrition Assessment, Support and Management,* 5th ed. Seattle WA; 1999.

SUMMARY

The healthcare marketplace is a dynamic environment driven by consumer empowerment and the increasing demands of the aging baby boomer population. (35) Effective admission nutrition screening is crucial to identify those patients at nutrition risk or in need of nutrition counseling to promote lifestyle changes for improved health. Dietetic practitioners have had to shift their primary counseling efforts in acute care to "need to know" information and establish referral mechanisms to outpatient and community-based dietetic practitioners for continued counseling. Current regulatory standards recognize this important shift in providing care along the continuum of care.

Learning Activities

1. For each of the following admitting diagnoses or situations, describe your approach for inpatient nutrition care and "survival" nutrition counseling components you would address. Role-play the counseling session with a peer.
   - Post-cardiac bypass
   - Uncontrolled type 2 diabetes admitted with diabetic ketoacidosis (DKA)
   - Peptic ulcer disease, admitted with a GI bleed
   - Acute pancreatitis with a history of alcoholic cirrhosis
   - Pneumonia with a recent weight loss of 10% in the past month

2. Using the Nutrition Care Model, discuss implications and applications for:
   - Hospital-based inpatient dietetic practitioners
   - Hospital-based outpatient dietetic practitioners
   - Private practice dietitians
   - Dietitians who are certified diabetes educators

References
1. Brook RH, Williams KH, Davies Avery A. *Quality* assurance *in the 20th century: will it lead to improved health in the 21st?* Santa Monica: Rand Corporation; 1975: 5530.
2. Hutte P. Getting a reading on lending to surgery centers. *RMAJ.* 2002; 85(4).
3. Schwartz DB, Gudzin D. Preadmission nutrition screening: expanding hospital-based nutrition services by implementing earlier nutrition intervention. *J Am Diet Assoc.* 2000; 100(1): 81-87.
4. McWhirter JP, Pennington CR. Incidence and recognition of malnutrition in the hospital. *BMJ.* 1994; 308 (6934): 945-948.
5. Sullivan DH, Bopp MM, Roberson PK. Protein-energy undernutrition and life-threatening complications among the hospitalized elderly. *J Gen Intern Med.* 2002; 17(2): 923-932.
6. Green CJ. Existence, causes and consequences of disease-related malnutrition in the hospital and community, and clinical and financial benefits of nutrition intervention. *Clin Nutr.* 1999; 18 (Supplement 2): 3-28.
7. Sullivan DH, Sun S, Walls RC. Protein-energy undernutrition among elderly hospitalized patients: a prospective study. *J Am Med Assoc.* 1999; 281 (21): 2013-2018.
8. Donabedian A. The quality of care: how can it be assessed? (Chapter 2). In: Graham NO, ed. *Quality assurance in hospitals: strategies for assessment and implementation.* Rockville: Aspen Publishers; 1990: 1430.
9. Gallagher-Allred CR, Voss PC, Finn SC, McCarnish MA. Malnutrition and clinical outcomes: the case for medical nutrition therapy. *J Am Diet Assoc.* 1996; 96(4): 361-366.
10. Braunschweig C, Gomez S, Sheehan PM. Impact of declines in nutritional status on outcomes of adult patients hospitalized for more than 7 days. *J Am Diet Assoc.* 2000; 100(11): 1316-1322.
11. Hedberg A, Laron DR, Aday LA, Chow J, Suki R, Houston S, Wolf JA. Economic implications of an early post-operative enteral feeding protocol. *J Am Diet Assoc.* 1999; 99(7): 802-807.
12. Bell SJ, Stack JA, Forse RA, Delfierro C, Wade E, Burke P. Generic enteral formulas: a new idea for the 1990's. *Nutr Clin Prac.* 1995; 10(6): 237-241.
13. Monk A, Barry B, McClain K, Weaver T, Cooper N, Franz M. Practice guidelines for medical nutrition therapy provided by dietitians for persons with non-insulin dependent diabetes mellitus. *J Am Diet Assoc.* 1995; 95(9): 999-1006.
14. Splett P, Myers EF. A proposed model for effective nutrition care. *J Am Diet Assoc.* 2001; 101(3): 357-363.
15. *Medical Nutrition Therapy Across the Continuum of Care* (MNTACC), 2nd ed. Supplement 1, the American Dietetic Association and Morrison Health Care. Chicago IL: American Dietetic Association; 1998.
16. *The American Dietetic Association: Nutrition Practice Guidelines for Type 1 and Type 2 Diabetes Mellitus.* Chicago IL: The American Dietetic Association; 2001.
17. Wiggins K. *Guidelines for Nutrition Care of Renal Patients.* 3rd ed. Chicago IL: The American Dietetic Association; 2002.

18. *Medical Nutrition Therapy Evidenced-Based Guides for Practice: Hyperlipidemia medical nutrition therapy protocol.* Chicago IL: The American Dietetic Association; 2001.
19. Kiy AM. The philosophy of nutrition therapy. *TICN.* 1998; 13 (2): 51-62.
20. Jarratt J, Mahaffie JB. Key trends affecting the dietetics profession and the American Dietetic Association. *J Am Diet Assoc.* 2002; 102(2): 1821-1839.
21. Oakland J, Morris P. *Pocket guide to TQM.* Oxford: Butterworth-Heinemann; 1998.
22. Splett PL. *Developing and Validating Evidence-Based Guides for Practice: a tool kit for dietetic professionals.* Chicago IL: The American Dietetic Association; 1999.
23. Goldsmith J. A look back, a look ahead: operation restore human values. *Hosp Hlth Networks.* July 5, 1998: 65, 74, 76.
24. Consultant Dietitians in Healthcare Facilities. *Steps to Success for Consultant Dietitians.* Chapter 6: Federal and State Regulations (pp 6-1 -6-11). Chicago IL: The American Dietetic Association; 1998. www.jcaho.org/ Accessed June 11, 2003.
25. *JCAHO hospital crosswalk: current 2003 standards to the revised 2004 standards provision of care chapter.* http://www.icaho.org/accredited+organizations/hospitals/standards/new+standards/pc hap xwalk.pdf Accessed 7/12/2003.
26. Wix AR, Doering PL, Nalton RC. Drug-food interaction counseling programs in teaching hospitals. *Amer J of Hlth Promotion.* 1992; 49:855-860.
27. McDonald SC. Total quality management (TQM) in healthcare. *J Can Diet Assoc.* 1994; 55:12-14.
28. Kight MA. Chapter 9: Nutritional diagnostic codes and measurable outcomes. In: Helm KK, Klawitter B, eds. *Nutrition Therapy: Advanced Counseling Skills.* Lake Dallas TX: Helm Seminars; 1995: 163-165.
29. Dodd JL. Look before you leap—but do leap! *J Am Diet Assoc.* 1999; 99(4): 422-425.
30. Laramee SH. Nutrition services in managed care: new paradigms for dietitians. *J Am Diet Assoc.* 1996; 96(4): 335-336.
31. Position of the American Dietetic Association: nutrition services in managed care. *J Am Diet Assoc.* 2002; 102(10): 1471.
32. Holmes V, ed. How you can promote the value of your services. *ADA Courier.* 1994; 33:2.
33. Sweeney KC. The malnutrition initiative: results of a program enhancing dietitian impact on revenue generation. *J Am Diet Assoc. Suppl* 1999; 99(9); A130.
34. Coddington DC, Fischer EA, Moore KD, Clarke RL. *Beyond Managed Care: How consumers and technology are changing the future of healthcare.* San Francisco CA: Jossey-Bass; 2000.

Chapter 11

Group Therapy
Kathy King, RD, LD

After reading this chapter, the reader will be able to:
- ♦ List the six components of the group process.
- ♦ Describe the steps (dimensions) of the group process.
- ♦ Identify at least two advantages of group counseling.
- ♦ Identify at least two disadvantages of group counseling.
- ♦ Define the roles and responsibilities of the facilitator.

Working with clients in groups can be challenging as well as rewarding. Traditionally, nutritionists have used groups when teaching multiple clients about a nutrition topic like diabetes, sports nutrition, breastfeeding, or weight loss. Group instruction to learn new skills, such as low fat meal preparation or stress management, can be as effective as individual instruction, if careful attention is given to classroom plans and *sufficient practice in the skill* being taught to attendees is provided. (1,2,3) Group instruction can also be a useful preface to individual counseling. This allows the general information to be given to a group followed by more focus and implementation in individual therapy. Counseling a group of clients is different than teaching a group or counseling one-on-one.

When teaching a nutrition topic, interchange of information between the leader and participants usually is limited and traveling in one direction—from the leader to the group. The information usually is the same for all group members with only abbreviated comments to members with different needs.

Counseling in a group setting is timesaving when compared to individual counseling. You can see ten patients in little more time than it takes to counsel one person. It is cost effective in that you can generate more revenue in a shorter period of time, and your patients usually save money because they pay less for a group meeting than for individual counseling. Group settings are more social with more opportunity to have various viewpoints and problem-solving opportunities.

In case it sounds easy to make more money by seeing patients in groups, counselors will tell you it's not. Acting as a group facilitator is not a job that should be taken lightly. The facilitator's effectiveness depends on adequate, and frequently, extensive preparation, careful diagnosis, planning, knowledge, and always, consideration of alternatives. (4)

Group members often arrive with very different expectations, different behavioral and psychological needs, and different communication styles. Instead of having one person to help, and one personality and family problem to deal with, you may have ten. One member may feel as facilitator, you pay too much attention to other members. Another may feel your questions or the discussion is too personal. One person in the group may refer all his or her friends to your program, and another in the same group may drop out after the second session due to disappointment.

Brownell reported that group therapy (in behavioral weight loss programs) was more successful than individual counseling in helping patients achieve their goals. (5) Some people and problems, such as those that need social acceptance and peer support, respond well in groups if the group is a good match. However, other people need and respond to the individual support and close rapport established with their personal therapist. Human dynamics make it hard to generalize about something so complex.

GROUP THERAPY

Group therapy is where individuals with similar nutrition-related problems come together to work through those problems. Instead of the therapist working with only one client at a time while the others look on, the group becomes a means for testing reality, a taste of the real society, an accumulation of the personalities and problems that occur on the outside. (4) Many of the components used in nutrition education lectures like basic physiology, diet therapy, food changes, and taste testing may be incorporated in therapy sessions, but often they do not constitute the majority of the program.

Group therapy members discover that the group has the capacity to support and love, and to provide a release for anger or problem solving. Group therapy usually attracts a population less severely disturbed or at less nutritional risk than those that require intense, individualized care. As a therapist, you may decide that for some patients, joining a nutrition support group may be an important part of their therapy, especially for patients with eating disorders who have pulled away from interaction with other people. For some patients, the group involvement may come after seeing a nutrition therapist individually or it may be suggested as the first mode of treatment.

A *confrontation group* is a type of group therapy used to confront group members with honest views about themselves, which can be disconcerting and even traumatic for some individuals. This approach began as an alternative with hard-core drug addicts and alcoholics, where unless change occurred immediately, a self-destructive cycle of events would continue. The confrontation approach is based on the assumption that a person needs to be shaken out of previous patterns, awakened from his lethargy, and made to face his own self-created realities. (4) Taken to an extreme, this type of therapy can be terrorizing for the therapist and members. Once a person recognizes his misperceptions, there must be follow-up to make sure new, more positive behaviors are internalized. Using this type of therapy exclusively is highly controversial, but if one works in drug and alcohol rehabilitation centers, you may see patients who have recently gone through a similar experience. As you might guess, this therapy is only for trained counselors.

Group Process

Good group process is the series of actions or operations that lead toward growth (or success) in a group therapy setting. It is aided by humor, as well as sensitivity, participation, experience, risk and openness. (3,6)

- **Humor** breaks the tension and helps people share common pleasurable moments. Clients remember things more easily that occur in humorous settings. (3)
- **Sensitivity** to the needs and feelings of others in the group. While it is part of the group process to challenge and to probe, this must be done in a nonthreatening or nonderogatory manner.
- **Participation** by every member of the group is the backbone of good group process.
- **Experience** is the key to learning in the small group setting. It is not the experience that each person brings to the groups, but instead, what each person learns and practices.
- **Risk** should be minimized. A successful group experience means the group members feel support as they try new, potentially uncomfortable ways of thinking and acting. They may risk changing relationships, comfortable habits, and familiar ways of eating.
- **Openness** should be encouraged. Group members must be willing to be open with each other, to admit their deficiencies, to share their ideas, and to let the group profit from their knowledge and experience.

Group therapy involves the same basic dimensions as the one-on-one approach, including the following dimensions of group process: (1, 7)

Step 1 Establish a productive counselor/participant relationship.

This includes establishing rapport with warmth, empathy, and an atmosphere of genuineness. There must be a feeling of trust in order to promote openness and interpersonal communication. Sessions might start with humor, an open-ended question, or an interesting shared experience. Initially, the facilitator should plan some "get acquainted" exercises to help group members know each other.

It is important to establish the "ground rules" for the group in the first session. Some facilitators prefer to come up with the rules as a group, others informally offer suggestions, and others pass out a written list that they ask members to commit to and sign. Rules usually consist of such things as: effort will be made to attend every class, all group conversation and sharing will be kept confidential, members agree to participate in discussions, and so on.

Step 2 Balance the facilitator generated and group generated information.

This step includes balancing the didactic nutrition information offered by the facilitator with problem-identification and real-life challenges identified through collaboration and interaction with group members. The facilitator helps members explore the causes and contributing factors to problem behaviors and thoughts. Together, group members and the facilitator may help another member confront irrational beliefs.

Step 3 Design problem-solving strategies.

The facilitator must limit use of directive statements (telling members what to do to solve their problems) and use more nondirective statements (facilitating members to decide for themselves what to do). Group members should be encouraged to become sources of problem-solving ideas. Use role-playing solving typical scenarios, personal experiences, and exploration to come up with ways to take care of old problems.

Step 4 Provide the opportunity for group members to practice new skills.

In Step 3 the person develops a cognitive understanding of the new skills or behaviors. Real learning occurs during the practice sessions. Practice should first take place in the group setting to assure that everyone understands what to do (for example, what to say or do the next time his favorite high calorie snack is offered). The facilitator can ask members to pair off or divide into whatever size group is most appropriate in order to practice the new skill. As each person practices what to say, the other group members offer suggestions, and learn along with him. At subsequent meetings, group members report back on their successes and new challenges encountered while using the skill in "real life."

Step 5 Use positive role models and good pacing to keep the group motivated.

Because the purpose of the group session is to help people overcome their problem thoughts and behaviors, the facilitator should sufficiently acknowledge the positive changes that all members are making. It is not unusual, however, to have someone in a group who reports trying hard but still can't succeed (at losing weight, controlling blood sugar level, or whatever).The facilitator should acknowledge the problem and spend approximately the same time with that person as with anyone. If the person is in denial or obviously needs more time, the facilitator should ask the person to stay later for more personal attention (so the class can continue for the benefit of the majority). This suggestion will usually satisfy the person and keep the rest of the group from getting frustrated.

Step 6 Ask for evaluation and feedback.

This step should be an ongoing process whenever the facilitator tries a new strategy or technique with a group. He or she might ask, "Did it work for you to role play today?" or "What have you learned since we started that has helped you the most (or least)?"

Advantages of Groups

Clients usually rank peer support as the most helpful aspect of groups. A group can help its members feel accepted, loved, and "not alone" in facing whatever common nutrition-related concerns they have. The shared experiences and problem solving may help a member cope, or change thoughts and behaviors more than didactic information does. Groups provide an economical way for clients to afford long-term therapy.

From the therapist's point of view, groups are often dynamic and stimulating, which can add challenge and professional satisfaction. They are a good way to reach a larger number of clients in a shorter time and to generate good revenue for the time invested.

Disadvantages of Groups

Group therapy is not for everyone and group process is not always effective. Group members are sometimes uncomfortable disclosing personal information in a group setting. It's easier to "get lost" in a group and never really deal with your problems because the facilitator's time is limited. While trying to help one or more members, a lot of time can be spent on topics and problems unrelated to the needs of others in the group.

In an individual consultation, the patient and therapist only have one other person to establish rapport with in order to progress into the therapy process. Group members have the opportunity to develop multiple alliances, which can be positive or stressful, depending upon who is in the group. In the group setting even one very negative or overbearing member can make the group sessions trying for everyone.

ROLE OF FACILITATOR

Facilitating a nutrition therapy group is often challenging and it sometimes tests your inner strength. It may call upon your best counseling and interpersonal skills. The person in this position is expected to serve several well-defined roles like meeting organizer, contact person, interactive facilitator, and at times, nutrition authority, but most importantly the person is expected to exercise good judgment.

The facilitator is responsible for the following: (6,7)

- organizing the group and establishing a comfortable atmosphere;
- keeping the group focused and productive;
- monitoring the discussion and keeping any records;
- stimulating exploration and self-discovery by group members;
- offering strategies for cognitive and behavioral change;
- acting as a nutrition resource for food choices, menu planning, new food products, and diet therapy questions;
- maintaining control of the therapy situation, which may include keeping interaction between participants nonthreatening(emotionally or physically), making sure participants act and speak civil to one another, or removal of a disruptive participant.

Although some facilitators demand food records and perfect attendance as requirements for adult group participation, this philosophy is not consistent with adult learning principles because it treats the adult as a child. Keeping food records and regular attendance are considered very effective behavior change tools, but establishing and maintaining rapport and respect are far more important. By showing concern for a client and his or her needs, the facilitator reinforces that the person is more important than his or her weight or other problem. Through mutual problem solving and breaking tasks into smaller steps, the person feels supported, empowered and in return often commits to the process and the group effort.

A facilitator should not take it personally if a group member uses the group as a social outlet, as long as he or she isn't disruptive to the progress of the group. It may be that the group serves other needs for that person.

Group members often look to the facilitator as a role model. Therefore, the group will watch closely how the facilitator handles stress, how he or she sets boundaries, how situations that demand assertiveness or flexibility are handled, and whether the facilitator practices what he or she preaches.

ROLE OF GROUP MEMBERS

The members have the responsibility to participate actively in the discussions of the group. However, a member may say at any time, "I don't have anything to add," or "I want to listen longer before I comment." Members must be willing to both give and accept constructive criticism, and be willing to practice new skills outside of class time.

Members assume many roles in a group therapy setting. Three types of roles surface as the group handles different problems: task roles, group maintenance roles and individual roles. (4)

***Task roles* help a group achieve its explicit goals for action:**

- The "initiator" person discusses what could be done, or how to approach a problem.
- The "information source" may add what others have tried or what he has tried.
- The "opinion" person may agree or disagree with what is being offered.
- The "elaborator" will take what has been said and add new insights.
- The "coordinator" will clarify the various suggestions and prioritize them.
- The "critic" or "evaluator" will question facts and assess whether the task is feasible.
- The "energizer" will prod the group to action.
- The "procedural technician" knows where and how to find resources to complete the task.

As a group member at times yourself, it may be easy to recognize yourself in many of these roles. As mentioned earlier, these roles are used to complete a group task.

Group maintenance roles **focus on the personal relations among members in a group.** They help a group work together: (4)

- The "encourager" may ask for additional examples or ask if others have similar opinions.
- The "supporter" may agree with others and offer commendations.
- The "harmonizer" may attempt to mediate differences between members or points of view, or relieve tension with a joke.
- A "gatekeeper" may ask someone who has not spoken in a while if he or she has anything to add.

Individual roles **meet only that person's needs,** which are irrelevant to any group task or in helping the group work as a unit. Individual-centered behavior may be aside jokes, personal attacks, bragging about something not related to what the group is working on, and so on. This behavior often induces similar behavior from other group members, which may disrupt the group process.

Some strategies for dealing with disruptive members include: (7,8)

- Use of reflective listening skills: you might say, "Jim, something about the topic of eating meals at home as a child seems to make you uncomfortable and want to change the subject."
- Use of assertiveness skills by the facilitator: you might say, "Marie, before you take the discussion in another direction, let's give other group members a chance to speak about their experiences."
- Encouraging all group members to return to the discussion at hand: you might say "OK, OK, that was a great joke, but I want us *all* to return to our topic of how you handle stress without eating."
- Removal of the disruptive participant from the group (a very last resort—do this privately).

Why People Join or Leave Groups

Some of the factors that increase the attractiveness of a group: (4)

Cooperation. A cooperative relationship is more attractive than a competitive one.

Interaction. Increased interaction among members may increase the attractiveness of the group. People usually want to make friends and hear other points of view, not just sit in a group listening to a lecture.

Size. Smaller groups are usually more attractive than very large ones. In a smaller group that is still large enough to function well, people become closer, support the cause better, and have a sense of being a significant participant. Six to twelve people are usually the range for more effective group participation.

Success. Members are more inclined to join groups or continue in groups that are successful or prestigious. The more prestige a person has within the group, or may attain while in the group, the more attractive the group.

It stands to reason that the factors people often cite for leaving a group are the opposite of those listed above. Also, the member's needs or his perception of the group may change, or a close friend in the group may stop coming. Usually as long as there is more attraction for the group than negative force against it, the person will stay.

SETTING THE STAGE FOR SUCCESS

It is very important when you plan a therapy group you take into consideration a number of factors:

- *Choose a location that is convenient for the members.* Consider going to a community center with ample parking if your hospital's meeting room is down a maze of hallways in a basement or parking is expensive. In private practice, ask to use a conference room or waiting room *after hours* when no one else is there, if your office is too small.
- *Consider the target group's characteristics when determining the time for the class.* If most of the members are retired, a daytime class may be more convenient. If the class

will be mostly working people, an evening class or maybe early Saturday morning might work. If you don't know which time of day is best, ask the people who call to sign up for the class. If *everyone* wants Tuesday night and you don't want 25 people in the group, consider offering an early group from 5:30-6:30 PM and another from 7:00-8:00 PM on Tuesday.

- ***Ask for the class fee by the first session with no refunds.*** This practice will ensure better attendance on the part of the members, and better attendance is often equated with better compliance and outcomes. A deposit may be paid in advance to secure the place in the group with the balance paid at the first session. If the therapist takes credit cards, debit slips may be signed in advance to pay for the group in three equal payments. For on-going groups, practitioners usually ask for a monthly payment in advance, and some offer a discount if the person pays for three months or so in advance.

- ***Don't allow your classes to be too large.*** In an informal survey of dietitians who work with groups, six to twelve people is the maximum number they usually allow in a therapy group. Nutrition education groups to teach new skills and a body of information with limited interaction may have 15 to 50 people.

- ***Consider assessing and/or instructing each member on an individualized regime before the group begins in order to better meet each member's needs.***

- ***Don't allow new members to join a week or two late,*** or if you do, take the time to nurture them and bring them into the group so they feel comfortable.

- ***Dietitians are not interchangeable.*** Each has different skills and abilities. Do not let whoever is working late on Tuesday run the groups. Choose the best person for the job. Group members do not like rotating facilitators. Market the person for the job and let that person become known for being the best on that topic.

- ***It is a misconception to believe that your one-hour class gives you rights to a member's whole evening or afternoon.*** Start the groups on time (within 5 minutes of the scheduled time) and end the sessions within 5 minutes of the scheduled time unless you ask for permission to continue some important issue. Members appreciate facilitators who are organized and on time.

- ***Make sure the environment is as conducive to good group process*** as if you were counseling one-on-one. There should be sufficient sturdy, comfortable chairs, usually placed in a circle (with or without a table); good temperature control; adequate lighting; and beverage service, especially if an exercise component is offered before or after therapy.

- ***Always prepare for the group sessions and be responsive.*** If you offered to look something up at the last session, follow through on your word. If you offered to speak to members in between sessions, or if they call your office, return the phone calls.

Interactive Techniques to Try
There are a number of techniques to try that will increase member involvement or learning. It often helps to ask members to break into smaller groups to give time to problem-solve or practice a new behavior.

Posting on a flip chart or blackboard is a good way to show the results of small group interaction or group brainstorming. Having each member number his or her top five choices can prioritize options. It can help increase idea visibility, stimulate discussion, and focus attention. This method can be overused, however, and it will never save a poorly prepared or unskilled facilitator. (4)

Role-playing is most effective in helping participants experience reality instead of just talking about it. They may use scripts, so time must be allowed for becoming familiar with the words, getting into character, and practicing with the other actors. The advantage of using scripts is roles can be replayed with different interpretations. Observers are asked to take notes and gather details to be used in later discussion. After the scene is played, the discussion enlarges from individual player's reactions to implications or alternatives for that situation. (4) Then observers are asked to comment.

Sociodrama or psychodrama is acted out without formal written scripts. In a **sociodrama,** group members will be asked to act as people in a social situation, i.e., a working mother, a father, and a teenage daughter discussing how each can contribute to making meals more nutritious and less time-consuming. In a **psychodrama,** group members volunteer problems they want to work on, such as how to better handle a spouse's temper at mealtime or a boss who always offers food in the lounge at work. The member who suggests the problem may play a part, or he or she may choose just to observe. Members who observe may offer suggestions or act out alternative solutions. Both techniques can help members see new alternatives to handling old or anticipated problems.

Replay drama is like those above, but it differs in that group members replay a real situation or incident that did not go well in order to explore what could have been said or done instead.

Role reversal is used to illustrate how well one person perceives and understands another. Group members may be asked to assume the mannerisms and point of view of the person across the table, or on the other side of an argument. It is ideal for opening stalled communication and/or when two people see each other as being totally wrong on an issue.

The Buddy System can be used to improve the commitment to exercise. Whether or not group members live close enough to walk together, they can still call the buddy to encourage and check to see what activity the person has done or plans to do.

POTENTIAL PROBLEMS WITH GROUPS

Although many problems and their solutions have already been discussed, here are a few others: (6,8)

- **The sluggish group.** Sometimes groups just don't know where to begin or how to work together. As the facilitator, resist stepping in and carrying the whole conversation. Try asking more open-ended questions to stimulate conversation, or use more "get acquainted" exercises, like interviewing a partner and reporting interesting information back to the group about that person.
- **The hostile group.** Sometimes individuals in a group blow up at each other or more subtly, allow distrust or anger to fester, which may show up as one or more members withdrawing from group participation. When hostilities occur, the air must be cleared, either in front of the group if that is appropriate or in private with the involved parties. *Don't proceed with business as usual because it won't happen. Deal with the problem in a nonjudgmental way. Don't take sides or become personally involved.*
- **The timid member.** A more timid or submissive member may have the most to contribute to the discussion but be unwilling to fight for equal time. The facilitator should be alert to members and how often they contribute to the discussion. A simple statement like, "Jane, do you have anything to add from your experience?" will give the member a chance to speak.
- **The domineering member.** A certain amount of dominance by one or more members is common in any group, but if the person assumes the authority role for the group, the group process fails. A facilitator may encourage challenges by other members to what is being said, or ask other members if they have had similar experiences or other solutions, in an effort to draw them back into the discussion.
- **Silence serves a purpose.** Don't jump in and break each period of silence. Sometimes everyone needs time to reflect upon what they have just heard, or to formulate new thoughts. Stay patient and relaxed. Periods of silence do not reflect poorly on the facilitator. You are not there to keep the troops entertained!

SUMMARY

If a group actively supports its members while they seek new behaviors and answers, the group process is considered successful. Group therapy can be challenging, stimulating, and productive. It takes practice, supervised training, and experience to act as a facilitator and do it well. If you want to conduct groups, join other therapy groups and see how other facilitators handle the group dynamics and process. If you have a lot of individual counseling skill, consider co-conducting a therapy group with another therapist with group experience (psychologist, psychiatrist, psychiatric social worker, nurse specialist, health behaviorist, etc.). When considering all of the components of successful group process, don't lose sight of the ultimate goal: to help group members achieve outcomes that improve their health and quality of life.

Residential/Group Center for Weight and Health Management

Marsha Hudnall, MS, RD, Nutrition Director, Green Mountain at Fox Run, Ludlow, VT

Residential centers for health management have been popular since the Roman Empire days when people visited hot mineral spring baths. Today, these places are called spas, or fitness, health, or wellness retreats. Some cater to overworked executives or overweight individuals, while others cater to individuals looking for new lifestyle philosophies and behaviors.

In the past, most centers' programs concentrated on lots of exercise and healthy cuisine. Today, many programs also offer counseling and programs for the mind so that changes learned during a week or two at the center are better maintained when the person returns home to "real" life. One residential group program for weight and health management is unique in that it was started 30 years ago by a Registered Dietitian, and it's philosophies and programs are now more timely than ever before. The market has finally caught up with what Thelma Wayler, MS, RD, knew all along.

Green Mountain at Fox Run

The diet boom had just begun in 1973 when Ms.Wayler started a weight management center based on a revolutionary concept—diets don't work. Three decades ago, when Thelma told women that one brownie never made anyone fat, and encouraged women to start exercising, she made waves with both her nutrition colleagues and the public. These waves got her national attention, including a full-page feature in the *New York Times* and appearances on programs such as *The Donahue Show*. Now, 30 years later, most practitioners in the weight management field embrace her message.

Today, Thelma's education-based program, Green Mountain at Fox Run in Ludlow, Vermont (now directed by her son Alan H. Wayler, PhD, a nutritional biochemist) continues to offer cutting-edge information and a practical, take-home experience to women from all over the world. They come because they're tired of dieting. Rather than give up on health altogether, they seek a lifestyle approach to weight and health management that offers a livable means by which to feel well, look good, and stay that way.

Program

Participants may attend one, two, four, or more week sessions beginning on specific starting dates. This ensures a sequential and structured format for imparting information in a consistent fashion. The program day is comprised of a mix of workshops, behavior groups, physical activity, and stress management classes. Along with the professional staff of Registered Dietitians, exercise physiologists, and behavioral specialists, Green Mountain employs massage therapists, most of whom are registered nurses.

Sessions are limited to 42 women to ensure a highly personalized experience. We use a group-based approach for workshops and behavior sessions to take advantage of the powerful educational dynamic it offers. Additionally, participants can meet one-on-one with professional staff in private counseling sessions.

Summary

Dietitians, physicians, psychological therapists, nurses, and other health specialists refer clients, and use Green Mountain as an adjunct to their ongoing treatment program. Residents receive a broad and intensive treatment experience away from the distractions of everyday life to permit focus on establishing priorities for weight and health goals. The resident begins or reinforces the process but returns home to the support of a professional where the ongoing work of reeducation and counseling continues. Our message is that successful weight and health management is an ongoing process that requires periodic reinforcement.

Learning Activities

1. Observe a group nutrition counseling/education session with at least ten participants.
   a. What roles/responsibilities did the facilitator exhibit?
   b. Identify the "group maintenance roles" you observed.
   c. What interactive techniques were observed?
   d. How would you improve this particular group session?

2. Interview a group nutrition counselor/facilitator.
   a. What/how are the ground rules established?
   b. What are his/her expectations for group member participation?
   c. What do they perceive as their role in the group process?
   d. How are groups planned?
   e. How are groups evaluated?

REFERENCES

1. Ivey A, Authier J. *Microcounseling.* Springfield, IL: Charles C. Thomas; 1978.
2. Hearn M. Three modes of training counselors: A comparative study. Unpublished dissertation. London, Ontario: Univ. of Western Ontario; 1976.
3. Curry J. Facilitating Small Group Learning in Problem Based Learning, in *The Facilitator's Guide to the Small Group Process,* Ohio State University College of Medicine.
4. Napier R, Gershenfeld M. *Groups: Theory and Experience,* 6th ed. Boston: Houghton Mifflin Company; 1999.
5. Brownell K. The psychology and physiology of obesity: Implications for screening and treatment. *J Am Diet Assoc.* 1984; 4:406-413.
6. Snetselaar L. *Nutrition Counseling Skills,* 3rd ed. Gaithersburg, MD: Aspen Publishing; 1997.
7. Raczynski J. *The Latest in Nutrition Counseling.* Presentation at ADA Annual Meeting, Orlando, FL October 20, 1994.
8. Corey G, Corey MS, Callahan P, Russell JM. *Group Techniques*, 3rd ed. Wadsworth Publishing; 2003.

Chapter 12

Teaching Developmental Skills

Alanna Benham Dittoe, RD

After reading this chapter, the reader will be able to:
- Identify different components of a comprehensive counseling needs assessment.
- Describe seven developmental-behavioral skills.
- Identify seven components to include in a food plan.
- Apply the Problem Solving Model to counseling practice.

If we can successfully teach clients the life skills or developmental skills to change behavior, we will have exponentially greater impact than if we only instruct them on a food or fitness plan. Not only will our clients be more successful but they will also perceive our services at a higher level. In addition, we will achieve more professional satisfaction by completing cases and maintaining long-term relationships with clients. Over the last fifteen years, I have developed and implemented a skill-based approach to counseling adults, which uses many assessment tools and visuals. My consultation services cover four phases:
- Identifying needs through a comprehensive evaluation process
- Investing Time and Money for Health: Developing plans
- Teaching developmental-behavioral skills
- Developing long-term resource and referral support

This approach can be applied to numerous conditions, including obesity, diabetes, hypercholesterolemia, eating disorders, pregnancy, sports nutrition, and family and corporate health. In designing this approach, I took into consideration overall consumer needs and trends such as the need for personalized service, the need for various options to solutions, and the need for self-management. I found these considerations increase the perceived value of the service, thus ensuring adequate client caseload.

Identifying Needs Through A Comprehensive Evaluation Process

Assisting clients identify their needs is one of the most important tasks we can provide. It will determine clients' future independence. The ultimate goal is to allow the clients to eventually manage their nutritional health on their own (i.e., self-management). The comprehensive evaluation process will identify clients' needs at multiple levels. During this process, we are modeling for clients how the needs identification works so they can do it for themselves in the future. An in-depth approach is necessary to extract and clearly identify needs. Our evaluation accomplishes the following:

1. Identifies specific problems and needs.
2. Identifies general as well as specific solutions and communicates them in a concrete fashion to the clients through dialogue and visuals.
3. Explores the pros and cons around various treatment options.

As a result, the client and nutrition therapist create a mutually agreeable treatment plan to allow enough structure for learning, but enough flexibility to experiment with ideas and to build skill base.

This process begins with the initial client contact, which is usually the phone call to schedule the appointment. I spend up to 10 minutes briefly listening to the client's concerns and discussing the need for a comprehensive evaluation. The initial consultation lasts 1-1/2 to 2 hours, depending upon the complexity of the case. The key is being flexible. No two clients give the same level of information nor do they go through the process in the same manner. (Historically, dietitians have been too anxious to educate so they abbreviate the evaluation process. This sends the wrong message to clients about the complexity of the change process.)

After the first session, the client should be given a complete overview of the treatment process including how their goals and needs will be met. A client will be more receptive to follow-up having a clear picture. So clients feel they are active participants in the evaluation process, a written "needs assessment" packet is sent home with the client to gather more information on:

- Culinary preferences
- Fitness needs
- Actual food intake, including assessing hunger regulation and volume status
- Habit inventory assessing twenty different eating habit categories using 80 scored statements

The Culinary Assessment tool asks clients to list their favorite foods, as well as how much and how often they usually have the item. Favorite foods at particular meal times and special occasions/ holidays are also listed. This assessment tool also asks what types of restaurants the client frequents (including ethnic preferences), and the kinds of foods they like to order.

The Fitness Assessment tool contains a listing of various exercises and asks the clients to circle the ones they find most interesting. The evaluation also assesses their preference of time/day, location, and weather conditions.

The Habit Inventory tool assists clients with identifying problem areas that may need work. See Appendix 12-A for this tool.

A vital part of the evaluation is diagnosing the problems and showing clients exactly what problems are occurring, why they are occurring, and more importantly, what can be done about them. Visuals are invaluable. We use a Food Patterns visual that explains three typical ways we see people eat: from semi-starvation and bingeing (stuff and starve), to more moderate fluctuations in intake but adequate calories, and finally, to severe dieting with inadequate calories and deprivation.

During the evaluation, we assess seven developmental-behavioral skills. The following will give a brief description of how we assess the client's ability in each skill.

1. **Active listening** is easily assessed through the conversation style of the client. If clients are having difficulties in this area, they are easily distracted and interrupted. They have difficulty answering questions and following directions correctly. Although this skill is so obvious, it is easily overlooked.

2. **Determines needs** is assessed by inquiring about clients' health, family, career and personal goals. Their responses will give insight as to how in tune they are with their own needs.

3. **Decision making skills** will be apparent when you ask a client what changes he or she would propose to make. The classic symptoms of poor decision-making are when the client: a) has difficulty generating options, b) vacillates between options, c) becomes "stuck," and/or d) denies there is a problem.

4. **Separation skills** will be identified when clients easily take the load of others, distracting them from taking care of their own needs. External forces often drive clients' thoughts and actions, or they confuse their needs with others. They generally show excessive worry about others.

5. **Delegation skills** are necessary when the client takes on too much. They could benefit from asking for assistance and/or help. Clients often express feelings that are out of control or overwhelming.

6. **The level and intensity of questioning by the client can assess assertiveness skills**. A more assertive person will be more active in the counseling process. A less assertive person often will be more agreeable and accepting of any suggestions made by the therapist. A

passive-aggressive person may be agreeable on the surface, but may have no intention of following through.

7. **Limit-setting skills** will be indicated if clients have a lot of chaos in their lifestyles, feel overwhelmed, and show signs of just "letting things happen." Lack of the skill shows when the client cannot find time for assignments and appointments designed to improve his or her health, the stated goal.

At the end of the evaluation, the client will leave with a concrete idea of what is happening, and what will be occurring in the future in therapy. Overall skill levels become more apparent as treatment progresses, and clients try working through problems and changes in behavior. Evaluation continues through the entire treatment process because the client's needs and skills also will evolve from analyzing and experimenting with ideas. Treatment will be adapted as the client changes. It is essential the client understands this from the very beginning.

Investing Time and Money for Health: Developing Plans

The average consumer lacks an appreciation for the amount of time, effort, and money that it takes to make behavioral changes. They are clearly aggravated by health care providers who do not address this issue directly. There is every indication in the marketplace that consumers are willing to spend time and money on health as indicated by the money spent on books, videos, weight management programs, fitness clubs, and lite food products. We need to "market" the benefits of our services to our customers, to health care insurers, and managed care providers. In our practice we found that if we impress clients with how the skill-based process will meet their needs better, there is a greater willingness on clients' part to invest time, money, and effort into the process.

We work with clients to help them allocate adequate time for addressing health issues. Some clients have this figured out before they arrive for the first visit, but others start from scratch. With our help, clients identify the various steps in freeing time to work on health, and then to figure actual time allotments for office visits, exercise, and meal preparations. Some may need to deal with identifying scheduling problems or conflicts.

We created a "Phasing Treatment" visual that illustrates our stages of therapy. It shows that as skills improve, treatment visits are less frequent. The phasing concept shows timing flexibility, encourages self-improvement, and shows that treatment will not go on indefinitely. Some individuals have concerns regarding this, and discussing it assists in giving structure and appropriate expectations.

Designing A Food Plan

A client benefits by helping design his or her own food plan. A Food Plan worksheet identifies various needs to consider prior to making decisions on what to eat.

> **Calorie needs** is an estimate of needs; we use an abbreviated version of the Harris-Benedict equation.
>
> **Culinary preferences** give clients permission to include all food preferences, which assists clients in moving away from the "dieting" mode.
>
> **Volume needs** identify satiety and the volume of food a client's body needs to feel satisfied. Internal cue regulation will be discussed later.
>
> **Lifestyle needs** are straightforward and need to be addressed in detail at this stage and in the future. More specifically, clients need to anticipate challenging situations, create solutions, and practice them in your office before experiencing them (e.g., dining out, traveling, a holiday party, etc.).
>
> **Transition needs**, like holidays and schedule changes, magnify existing problems and issues. Clarity and confidence, not to mention a change in attitude, are often derived from handling an event well. One of our goals is to teach clients to "think on their feet." Experience is often the most effective facilitator, and the counselor supports this through a neutral but optimistic attitude.
>
> **Structure** is needed in food, fitness, and health management plans. Clients know what to do when they leave the office, but plans are flexible enough to allow them to experiment with ideas. It is important to assess how much structure individual clients need.

Nutrient supplementation is based upon what the client realistically is unable to consume through his or her diet. Recommendations are not made until the food plan is developed because we often see improvement in nutrient density.

A "Sample Menu" is developed that incorporates the following concepts:
- Structure
- Food preferences
- Experimenting with decreasing fat
- Identifying true hunger and volume needs
- Increasing nutrients through better food choices

The overall goal is to allow adequate time to experiment with these concepts to clarify needs in all areas, which usually takes several weeks. Food plans need to be continually updated with a client.

Internal Cue Regulation: Hunger and Satiety
We have discovered that addressing hunger and satiety are two of the most effective self-monitoring tools used for long-term food control. They allow clients to move away from external monitoring tools such as diet records and food plans. While addressing this issue, many feelings may surface that effect food intake.

Figure 12.1 Volume Needs

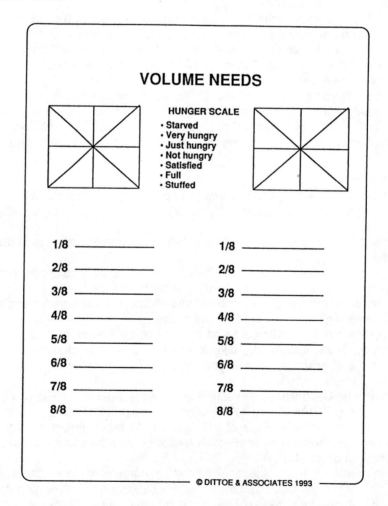

The "Volume Needs" hunger scale (Figure 12.1) represents every possible option from starvation to stuffed. Have the client take a standard sandwich and divide it into eighths. The client should begin the experiment at a comfortable hunger level, not starved, as it will distort his or her volume needs. The client should eat 1/8 at a time slowly, experiencing the different levels until satiety is reached. The experiment may need to be repeated a second or third time until the client is able to internalize the appropriate volume. The majority of clients state it takes anywhere from 6/8 to a full sandwich to feel satisfied. Ninety percent of the time this is less than they commonly eat. Clients' volume needs will vary slightly from meal-to-meal and day-to-day, but this will make them consciously aware of how much food makes them feel physiologically satisfied. They will begin to distinguish between physical and psychological hunger. It is reasonable to expect hunger again in several hours, and people will vary when they feel it. Be sure to encourage clients to use this test at the time they eat the food. Recall is too inaccurate.

Acquiring Developmental-Behavioral Skills

We find the majority of our clients with eating and health problems have difficulty with many of the developmental-behavioral skills mentioned earlier in this chapter. Acquiring these skills will have an enormous impact on a client's ability to achieve more complex problem solving. It is our experience that a dietitian's ability to teach these skills is limited by that person's own emotional growth and familiarity using the skills.

Dietitians can be taught these skills through formal education and training, such as getting a master's in counseling or taking Laurel Mellin's *ShapeDown* weight management certification (1), *The Solutions Program* (2), and *Pathways Program* (3). Other methods are to experience psychotherapy supervision or therapy with a competent licensed counselor, psychologist, or psychiatrist.

If a client is having continued difficulty with basic problem solving or compulsive/addictive behavior, it is very appropriate to refer him or her to a mental health counselor. We find that by using a collaborative approach with clients, their long-term outcomes are very successful. We use developmental-behavioral skills to improve our clients' nutrition and food-related outcomes.

Active listening

It is very appropriate to discuss this skill "head-on" with clients. Give clients examples of how to listen more actively such as concentrating on the concepts instead of each word the other person is saying, maintaining eye contact (when culturally appropriate), keeping hands and feet still, and avoiding listening to or thinking about anything but the immediate conversation. There is an accumulative effect as treatment progresses. Poor listening skills usually stem from a deficit early in life either genetic (e.g., Attention Deficit Disorder), a learned behavior, or possibly from a hearing or learning impairment.

Decision-making

To help clients improve their ability with this skill, begin with simple decisions around scheduling appointments, deciding on food plans, and meeting schedules where they are likely to have guaranteed success. Ask the client to generate an option or decision first. If the client gets stuck, ask it again, rephrase it, or come back to the question later. This will force the client to start thinking on his own. For example, "It appears you have a need for quick dinners; what are your options?" Walk through the pros and cons of each option until he/she discovers a reasonable one.

Ask, "What are your fitness options on the weekends, during the week, and during the winter?" Have clients draw from both past and projected experiences. When you walk clients through this detailed process, they will be able to create decisions, determine their needs, and build on them later. If clients are coached in a gentle way; their progress is acknowledged; and they are encouraged to do it more often; their confidence will grow.

Separation skills

We help clients improve in this skill by encouraging them to become more neutral and less effected by the views of others. We ask clients to comment on others' behaviors and then walk them through the "so what" process. It allows clients to see the absurdity of the other individual's behavior, the significance of it, or how their own behavior is judgmental. This concept is called "grounding." It provides a foundation for protecting clients' own needs, and therefore, separating from others. It also is effective to walk clients through the impact of their decisions, which generally translates into conflict and causes anxiety for clients. As a result, they need to learn to tolerate others' anger and inappropriate feelings in order to hold onto their own decisions. By explaining this on a practical level and using humor, it helps clients grow through the process. As mentioned earlier, if clients have a prolonged struggle in this area, a referral to a mental health professional is appropriate.

Delegation skills

This skill gives considerable leverage and freedom to a client. In our world of juggling many roles, learning to delegate can relieve stress created by a pressured schedule. To help clients, have them create a list of all tasks and situations they ideally would like to delegate. Discuss the pros and cons of each, and determine which ones could be delegated. Often we get a better understanding why clients aren't delegating through this process. Walk the client through the list starting with the easiest task first. Clients will again build upon their successes and hopefully, continue the process after nutrition intervention is over.

Assertiveness

The lack of assertiveness is a common problem for clients having difficulties with food issues. When a person is not assertive, he often feels lack of control except in one area—what and how he chooses to eat. Becoming assertive allows clients to ask for help when they need it, set limits on others' inappropriate behavior, and ultimately improve their self-esteem. We initially help clients define aggressiveness and passiveness, then we explore the middle ground with assertiveness. It helps to point out times when they are assertive on an issue, and congratulate them for it. Role-playing through "lifelike" examples suggested by the client or created by the nutritionist allows the client to acquire confidence and experience. Start on less emotional examples to build the client's confidence, and then move on to more "emotionally charged" issues when he or she is ready. Continue to work on the skill through several sessions, if necessary. We stress that being assertive usually means speaking in a reasonable tone, stating needs in a reasonable fashion with confidence, and including some room for flexibility.

Setting limits

This task involves setting limits on tasks, individuals, and situations to allow adequate time to become healthier. Many times this process raises conflicts that are difficult for clients. By exploring these conflicts, you will get an idea of how complex the client's problems are, and again a referral may be in order.

The next step is to walk clients through past food-related scenarios that were a problem, and rework them. This will give them lifelike experiences before they tackle anticipated problems. For example, doing too much on the weekend is a classic issue with many clients. Have clients set priorities so they can incorporate some fun and let less important tasks go (or delegate them)! A second common example is having too much to do after work. Have clients learn to set limits on phone calls or tasks that interfere with their ability to unwind and relax. Have them ask family members for help with dinner or to run errands for them. Again, walk them through solutions so they can build confidence in this skill.

Developing Long-Term Resource and Referral Support

Resources help you design options. The more resources you can offer, the greater the chance for success for both the client and the nutrition counselor. Consider multiple types of resources. They require time and effort but will be great leverage to your clients. Here are a few ideas:

- Health care providers (especially specialists)
- Personal trainers (including yoga, massage, physical therapists)
- Financial resources (accountants, financial advisors, and strategists)
- Psychiatric services (pediatric, adolescent, and adult)
- Rehabilitation services (chemical dependency)
- Travel resources
- Culinary resources (take out, dining out, private chefs, catering, food products)

PROBLEM SOLVING MODEL

The Problem Solving Model (Figure 12.2) will give you visual guidance on how to problem-solve with your clients.

Figure 12.2

PROBLEM SOLVING MODEL

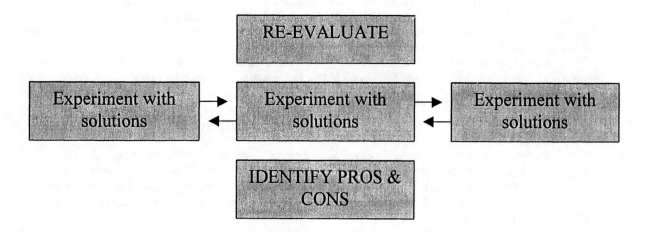

MIDDLE GROUND OPTIONS

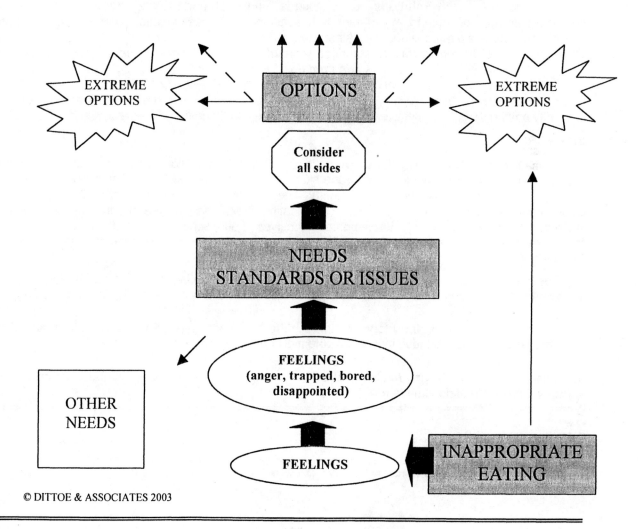

Feelings. Begin at the bottom of the model with the feelings box. Assist the client in identifying the feelings that result in inappropriate eating. These feelings can be positive or negative. Clients will vary on their ability to access feelings, and there will be a correlation between your own ability to access feelings and being able to assist clients.

Needs/Standards/Issues. Give your clients the opportunity to identify what their true needs, standards, or issues are. This should evolve from identifying feelings, and is a critical step in problem solving. Be certain to have them separate their needs from those of others. Clients are often confused between the two. Examples: Is the need to have more time for themselves? Is the need to have a certain quality of work? Is the need to feel closer to someone?

Consider All Sides. This step is essential before options are designed. There are many sides to issues. This is called "abstract thinking." Many individuals are quick to react to a situation prior to really thinking it through. Spend adequate time with clients on this aspect. For example: The need is to spend more time alone. To consider all sides, one would consider the following: what time is available now, what conflicts might arise, the discomfort in taking time for oneself, the demands of the family, or there is too much to do, etc.

Options. There are many options to solutions. Clients may find it easier to start with the extreme options. Often they are familiar with these options and some clients might immediately identify with the absurdity of it too. This step is also critical in generating middle ground options (reasonable, balanced, and fair options). Middle ground options give hope. The dietetic practitioner needs to be very creative in this area.

Identify Pros and Cons. This step will assist you in making better decisions about which solutions to try. This type of analysis is often missed in the highly reactive client or the client that has difficulty abstracting his or her thinking.

Experiment with Solutions. Experience is "king." You need to encourage clients to take a significant amount of time to experiment with solutions. The best solutions will be derived from experience. There is a famous quote by Albert Einstein:

> *Pure logical thinking cannot yield us any knowledge of the empirical world; all knowledge of reality starts from EXPERIENCE and ends with it. Propositions arrived at by purely logical means are completely empty of reality."*

Reevaluate. This step is an ongoing process. After clients experiment with different solutions; they may have different perspectives on the problem. They find it easier to create a solution.

SUMMARY

The cumulative effect of learning the above developmental skills will allow clients to problem-solve at a higher level. By counseling clients using the skills and the suggested tools, clients understand their problems better and the solutions more clearly. They get to the root of many of their long-standing behaviors and thoughts that have been complicating their lives for years. As a result, nutrition intervention can become a major turning point in the lives of our clients.

Learning Activities

1. Observe an initial counseling session with a client (or a role-play). How are needs determined? What client problems are identified? Can the client verbalize why these problems are occurring?

2. Administer the Habit Inventory to three different individuals. For each individual, what patterns/trends can you identify? What potential counseling areas can you identify?

3. Using the Problem Solving Model, analyze a challenging behavior change you are contemplating for yourself. What do you learn?

References
1. www.shapedown.com
2. Mellin L. *The Solution: For safe, healthy and permanent weight loss.* New York: Regan Books (HarperCollins); 1998.
3. Mellin L. *The Pathway: Follow the road to health and happiness.* San Anselmo, CA: Balboa Publishing Company; 2002.

Chapter 13

Exercise Resistance, Obsession, and Recommendations

Karin M. Kratina, PhD, MPE, RD

After reading this chapter, the reader will be able to:
- ♦ Identify factors that can precipitate exercise resistance.
- ♦ Distinguish between daily physical activity and exercise.
- ♦ Identify characteristics of exercise dependence.
- ♦ List strategies to counsel the exercise dependent client.

Most dietitians recommend physical activity to their clients at some time during a consult. We know that physical activity can improve health. But, as with nutrition counseling, individuals come to see us with a myriad of issues that can interfere with a sound program of physical activity. Exercise is actually a subcategory of physical activity and exercise is not always the goal (see side bar). Since dietitians encounter many clients who are unable or unwilling to follow a moderate exercise program, it is crucial to understand and have solutions for exercise resistance and dependence or obsession. This chapter will also cover the specifics of exercise prescription.

Physical Activity versus Exercise Bridget Klawitter, PhD, RD, FADA

"Physical activity" and "exercise" are terms that describe different concepts. However, they are often confused with one another, and the terms are sometimes used interchangeably in the literature. Physical activity is defined as any body movement produced by skeletal muscles that result in energy expenditure. Casperson and colleagues suggest five categories of physical activity: occupational, sports, conditioning, household, and other activities. (1) Exercise is a subset of physical activity that is planned, structured, and repetitive and has as a final or an intermediate objective the improvement or maintenance of physical fitness by requiring a relatively high percentage of maximal aerobic capacity over a prolonged period of time.

Characteristics that contribute to physical fitness include cardiovascular-respiratory fitness, muscular strength and endurance, body composition, and flexibility. The quantity and quality of exercise needed to attain health-related benefits is significantly lower than that which is recommended for fitness benefits. (2)

OVERCOMING EXERCISE RESISTANCE

"I know I would feel better if I just got some exercise, but I can't seem to get motivated. If I could just lose a little weight first, it would be easier...besides, I don't want this fat turning into muscle because I would be just as heavy."

"I don't like to sweat, it makes me feel gross. Three years ago I exercised for six months and it felt good, I'm not sure why, but I did lose 24# then. If only I could get motivated, but I get angry sometimes when I think about exercise... I just don't want to... Forget it, I don't even have the time to do it."

Many people know that more activity would be good for them, but they can't seem to get motivated. Even when they know they will feel better with an exercise program, the excuse list is extensive: "I am just too heavy, too old, too uncoordinated, too self-conscious," etc., etc. These individuals often start exercise programs but quit soon after initiating them, even when they report enjoying the exercise. Many say they hate to exercise. Others are interested, but resist moving their bodies with the assumption they'll "get to it some day."

Resistance to exercise must be approached carefully, as it can arise for a variety of reasons. An individual may not understand how to do the exercises or may feel intimidated by equipment and/or fancy moves in aerobics. Others may be so overwhelmed by the demands of life that making time for exercise seems impossible. Still others are resistant to exercise on a much deeper level. While the excuse list is similar, the true resistance arises from a much different place. Presenting an exercise prescription may motivate these individuals initially, but invariably unless the exercise resistance is dealt with, the prescription is useless. Counseling needs to focus on determining the source of the resistance and overcoming that resistance.

According to Glasser (3), exercise resistance can develop when:

1. **Exercise is associated with dieting.** Exercise is often connected with dieting, which has a 95% failure rate. Most people will fail on their diet and quit their exercise program with a resultant negative attitude towards exercise. They often see exercise as a necessary evil.
2. **Exercise is used to change the body into a culturally accepted shape.** "For many women, quitting exercise is connected with a despair over societal sex role stereotyping, which encourages women to get in shape as a means of increasing their personal value by becoming more sexually attractive. Men and women who try to change their body with exercise are often disappointed in themselves, as well as with the exercise when they don't become that ideal shape." (3)
3. **Exercise is used as an external measure of self-worth.** In our culture, "exercise is revered as something that supposedly reflects on an individual's inner character, a testimony to their strength and inner worth." (3) Rebellion is common when exercise is used this way. "If there has been a history of sexual abuse, especially if the perpetrator was male, the rebellion is even stronger. It can reflect a refusal to participate in a sexist or demeaning system." (3)
4. **Exercise is used as punishment.** Exercise can be used to punish oneself when goals such as a limit on food intake or weight loss are not accomplished. They view their bodies as bad and self-indulgent.
5. **Sexual abuse has occurred.** Moving the body can "bring up body memories of the abuse. Exercise can trigger flashbacks of repressed abuse while exercising. It can stimulate old thoughts due to the movement of the body, being warm or sweating, or simply because the abuse took place in the body and in some way, the trauma is stored there." (3) Exercising is often curtailed after abuse begins, at puberty, or at some point when being sexually objectified.

Any exercise with the goal of weight loss, competition, or perfection will need to be explored. A move must be made to exercise with a focus on pleasure, nurturance, self-fulfillment, movement, social and psychological benefits, energy boost, and a sense of self-mastery in order to help clients move away from exercise resistance.

The decision to exercise needs to come from deep within. False starts with exercise occur because individuals begin for externalized reasons, such as "I should do it for my health," "I need to lose this weight," "My partner really wants me to." The decision to exercise is about reconnecting with the body. Making a commitment to becoming more physical "will have a deep impact on the individual's internal experience. Effective motivation will need to speak to the inner life of the individual and promise an improved experience of living. Emphasis needs to be placed on the way exercise makes one feel in one's body, emotionally and spiritually. The changes in external body shape are a side effect, and if viewed as the main goal, will sabotage the healing mind/body connection." (4)

TREATING EXERCISE RESISTANCE

Treating exercise resistance must be accomplished individually. Initially, I often ask clients to commit to no activity at all. This pleases some and some are upset, wondering how they will lose weight...all are surprised. When they ask why they shouldn't start/increase exercise, I explain I don't believe they are ready to change physical activity patterns and that it will be counter-productive if they attempt to do so.

I usually will not address exercise again for the initial six to eight weeks of nutritional counseling or until the client broaches the topic. At this point, the client is given assignments related to exercise attitudes, but is still asked for a commitment to no prescribed exercise. Assignments are limited only by the imagination. Some ideas are to ask the client to:
1. Interview ten people to determine why they like to exercise.
2. Interview ten people to find out if their exercise focus is to move the body or to change the body. (Which group seems to enjoy exercise more?)
3. Watch children play for 30 minutes and record your observations in a journal.
4. Play with a child where the child has freedom to move around.

While ideas are endless, *the goal is to bring the client to an awareness of the joy of movement.* Many have never experienced, as an adult, the joyful pleasure and sense of self-mastery that can come with moving. Reconnecting with this experience is at the core of overcoming exercise resistance. Discuss these assignments in a counseling session. Help the client form a vision for their relationship with physical activity.

> **The goal is to bring the client to an awareness of the joy of movement.**

Differentiate between exercise used to change the body and that used to move the body. Exercise resistance is typically fueled when changing the body is a goal. (This motivation also fuels eating disorders.) Ask your clients to select two physical activities, one with a goal of exercise, the second with a goal of movement and joy. What is their attitude towards them? Ask them to do these activities and record their experience. In another assignment, clients make two lists: one of exercises they believe would change the body, and the other, activities that focus on movement. Again, discuss in a counseling session.

During this time, challenge cognitive distortions concerning health, fitness, and exercise. Most people don't realize how little physical activity is needed to be healthy, that it doesn't have to involve an exercise prescription or routine, and that it can be a part of day-to-day life. Fitness should be pleasurable, and unfortunately, popular health advice often ignores less intense, more enjoyable forms of physical activity. "Because of the hype, many people feel discouraged; they can't achieve the ideal prescription of vigorous exercise sessions, and the sleek look of the sinewy models glowing out of magazine covers somehow evades them. So they do nothing." (5)

One long-term study found that health benefits began for those who burned up as few as 500 calories a week. This could be accomplished with a 15-minute walk each day or two hours of bowling. Death rates declined by 20%, even with this small amount of activity. (Death rates dropped another 10 to 20% when using 2000 calories for activities each week.) (6) Just getting moving is enough to give substantial benefit to a "couch potato."

Exercise should be undertaken in a noncompetitive environment with activities that will nurture self-esteem. The biggest mistake is to push too hard too soon, so a slow and gentle start is important. Initially, it is best not to concentrate on goals or fitness. Help clients think of pleasurable activities that can be done in the course of the day, as part of life, and preferably without structure. "For example, gardening-hoeing, digging, pulling weeds, and pushing a lawn mower--can increase heart rates by 20 to 25%; for a sedentary person, this may be enough of a boost to improve health." (4) An occasional swim, bouncing up and down in a swimming pool, a wild dance, batting a tennis ball back and forth with a friend, hitting a racket ball against a backboard, bowling, playing catch or Frisbee with a friend are good ideas. Walk the dog. Take an extra spin around the mall when shopping. Carry all the groceries from the car rather than asking for help. Take a dance class. Play with the children or dog. Rake leaves, shovel snow, push a lawn mower. Make love. Garden..." Gardening gets you outside, and instead of running nowhere, you end up growing something new, something alive." (5) Walk with a goal that has nothing to do with exercise. For instance, pick flowers along the way and plan to come home with a little bouquet of flowers for your dining room table. Plan some new landscaping by looking for ideas along the way. Be the judge of a contest to pick the house in the neighborhood with the best grass, cleanest windows or prettiest walkway.

Our clients need to know that every bit of activity counts and adds up to better health, especially in the beginning.

"Encourage your client not to expect improvement overnight. In fact, don't expect anything." (7) Have them compare, and possibly journal about, "their mind and body state before and after exercise. Pay attention to the sensations in the body. Hot, sweaty, breathless—these are all natural results of physical activity. With time they can learn to tolerate and even enjoy these feelings." (7)

Work with the client to adjust activity so that it meets their needs. Talk them through the specifics of their activity to visualize what they will be doing. For instance, if walking has been selected...where will they walk, with whom, what will they wear, what will they do when it rains, can they incorporate a walk when they shop at the mall, etc.? If playing ball with a child is the activity planned...when, where, what ball, what time of day?

Encourage the use of affirmations such as "I feel my strength when I move," "I like myself and feel easy in my body" during exercise. *Do not compliment a weight loss client based on physical size or shape.* When congratulated for weight loss, what does that mean when weight is regained? Most inevitably do gain and feel worse about themselves as a result. When somebody says, "I lost weight" a good response could be "How do you feel about that?" Rather than telling someone they are shaping up, you might say, "You look more content since you have been exercising."

Avoid talking about fat, burning calories, losing weight, or about appearance. Also, avoid talking about exercise for example:

As punishment, "Walk an extra mile to help burn off that brownie."

As a cure, "Some extra sit-ups will help get rid of that pudge," or "If you exercise, you can have the body you want."

"Remember that fatness does not preclude fitness. Thin people aren't always fit, nor heavy people necessarily unfit. The great dancer Isadora Duncan was a "big woman" and 200 pound Virginia Zucci, of the Russian Ballet, was famous for her pirouettes." (5) Lynne Cox, who swam the English Channel, broke the women's record by three hours, the men's record by one hour, is 5'6" and 180# (and 33% body fat). The winner of the 1994 Nike Fitness Leader of the Year Award was a large woman named De Dast-Hakala who teaches step aerobics and champions the cause of large women. Heavy women need to and can move as much as anyone else.

EXERCISE OBSESSION/DEPENDENCE

You may know her. She arises each morning at 5:30, hitting the pavement before most people are even awake. She doesn't feel ready to face her day unless she does her brisk three miles. She does it, rain or shine. At work she looks forward to her lunchtime trip to the fitness center, where they have a special 45-minute workout for people on their lunch break. She's glad that she can get that workout in and be back to work in just a little over an hour. After work she goes to another health club, this one closer to home. She completes one-hour aerobics, a half-hour on the Stairmaster, and also a half-hour on the Lifecycle. If, for any reason, she wasn't able to get her lunchtime workout in, she'll take another aerobics class. She knows everyone at the gym and she engages in conversations during her workouts. From the outside, she appears to be a motivated, fit, and happy person. Actually, she's too exhausted to go out with her friends and is increasingly alone and lonely. Her legs ache constantly, but she continues to work out despite her shin splints. Her doctor is confused by her refusal to slow down; she's usually a very compliant patient. At one point, her doctor forced her to stop exercising for a week. Her depression and anxiety were so overwhelming, she was virtually immobilized until she could get back to her workout.

Men and women such as this are coming to counseling in increasing numbers. They tend to present, not because they want to stop the compulsive activity, but because they cannot continue. If these exercisers were willing to take a look at what they are doing, they would find that their activity is not about performance or reshaping their bodies, but about dealing with life. They would find exercise is essential to them to provide a feeling of mental well being, to release their tension and anger, and even relieve anxiety and depression. They also would find they have few other strategies to cope with these feelings.

162

While there are many terms in the literature used interchangeably with compulsive exercise, "exercise dependence" is the author's preferred term, as it does not refer to a particular sport (dependence can occur to any sport), and because it classifies this behavior with other compulsive behaviors. In 1987, de Coverly Veale proposed diagnostic criteria for exercise dependence using the core features of a dependence syndrome: (8)

1. A narrowing of repartee, leading to a stereotyped pattern of exercise with a regular schedule, once or more daily;
2. Salience with the individual; giving increased priority over other activities to maintain the pattern of exercise, obviously giving up other things in life so that they can maintain their exercise;
3. Increased tolerance to the amount of exercise performed over the years;
4. Withdrawal symptoms related to a mood disorder, following cessation of the exercise schedule;
5. Relief or avoidance of withdrawal symptoms by further exercise;
6. Subjective awareness of a compulsion to exercise;
7. Rapid reinstatement of the previous pattern of exercise and withdrawal after a period of abstinence.

Associated features:

1. Either the individual continues to exercise despite a serious physical disorder known to be caused, aggravated, or prolonged by exercise, or is advised as such by a health professional;
2. The individual has argumentative difficulties with his partner, family, friends, or occupation;
3. The self-inflicted loss of weight by dieting is as a means towards improving performance.

According to de Coverly Veale, "primary exercise dependence" occurs when an individual meets all of the proposed criteria and anorexia nervosa and bulimia nervosa are ruled out. (8) Pure exercise dependence is found most often in middle-aged men in their 40's and 50's. Weight loss by dieting is seen in primary exercise dependence as a means to improve performance; however, if weight loss is too drastic, performance would be impaired, so typically weight is not allowed to drop too low.

Excessive exercise directed towards weight loss or balancing caloric intake is regarded as "secondary exercise dependence." Most often, this kind of activity involves individuals who have a primary diagnosis of an eating disorder.

The prevalence of exercise dependence is not known. Some researchers believe a relatively small percentage of men and women have a severe dependence; others feel that as many as 7% of committed exercisers are dependent on exercise. The author postulates that at least 50% of people with anorexia and bulimia deal with some form of exercise dependence.

A core feature of any dependency is the experience of negative affect when the object of dependence is removed. Glasser described the negative effect that runners experience when they are forced to forego running. Symptoms he found were: depressed mood, irritability, fatigue, anxiety, impaired concentration, sleep disturbance, guilt, tension, and vague sense of discomfort. These symptoms were relieved when running was resumed. (3)

There are no conclusive studies as to why these affective withdrawal symptoms occur. Some believe these exercisers are addicted to endorphins, the morphine-like hormones secreted by the body under stress, and that withdrawal from endorphins creates the symptoms. It is the endorphin release that is thought to cause what is commonly referred to as "runner's high."

Another theory regarding exercise dependence is that exercise has become a means of coping. A person may exercise to deal with feelings (tension, stress, anger, guilt, anxiety, loneliness, etc.). Often unaware of the feelings, the dependent person simply acknowledges the drive to exercise that pushes down these feelings. Without exercise, the thoughts and feelings that have been avoided and denied flood back. Essentially, the dependent exercisers have been working out their bodies rather than their problems. Without effective coping mechanisms, they become overwhelmed and are compelled to exercise again to control unwanted feelings. What begun as the pursuit of pleasure had become the avoidance of pain.

Treating The Exercise Dependent Client

Typically, compulsive activities are a source of shame and embarrassment. Not so with exercise dependence. This is not a shame-based activity. The exercisers like what they are doing. Exercise dependent clients typically present to treatment because they no longer are able to continue the exercise. Possibly their doctors require therapy due to injury, or their partner or spouse threatens to leave if therapy is not initiated. These clients tend to be extremely resistant to exploring issues around their exercise.

If the purpose of exercise dependence is to avoid and deny the underlying feelings, anxiety, and/or depression, the recovery involves identifying and dealing effectively with these feelings. Without effective coping skills, it is difficult to endure the uncomfortable feelings that arise when exercise is curtailed. An understanding friend, a skilled dietitian or exercise physiologist, or a therapist may aid in the process.

Some may be ready to make changes in their exercise patterns, while others may need to stay at their current level of exercise while therapy is initiated. Their relationship with exercise will need to be challenged. An option is to ask them to make changes in their exercise program. I asked one client to wear sandals rather than walking shoes when she power-walked. She returned with a very different perspective of her walking, and thereafter, used her ability to "chose sandals for her walk" (and go for a more relaxing walk) as an indication of the intensity of her feelings. The possibilities are endless for the creative dietitian, especially one who understands that most dependent exercisers have repetitive exercise patterns. For example, ask the client to:

- Go the opposite direction. Run clockwise instead of counter-clockwise.
- Change the order of the activities. Do weights first rather than last.
- Switch activities. Swim instead of run; use free weights for biceps rather than a machine.
- Take a different aerobics class.
- Wear different gear. Run in torn gym shorts rather than sleek running shorts.
- Quit counting. How do they know when to stop?
- Express feelings during exercise. Instead of pushing a feeling down, stay present to it while exercising. Move in such a way that the feeling is expressed. A form of aerobic dance, NIA (Non-Impact Aerobics) uses feelings expression. (2)

Frequently, the intensity, frequency, or duration of exercise must be reduced. This reduction can occur over time, or can be "cold turkey." Since withdrawal symptoms are usually most intense 36 to 48 hours after ceasing exercise, I challenge clients to omit exercise for three days. I explain what they most likely will experience and help them set up a support system. This intervention often allows the client to see the impact exercise has on their lives and creates openness to pursue these issues.

Exercise-dependent individuals will need to examine their belief system around exercise, health, and fitness in order to unravel cognitive distortions. The client will need to understand and accept that training daily is counterproductive, that a low percent of body fat does not necessarily make them healthier, that they will not get out of shape if they take off a day or two, that muscles need days without exercise to recover and refuel, that calories eaten will replace depleted glycogen stores which will help them perform better, or even that minimal movement can contribute to health and be considered exercise.

For instance, in a group I facilitated, a client, "Debbie," was expressing difficulty getting in touch with her feelings. A group member challenged her saying, "Well, you exercise all the time anyway" (inferring that it is difficult to get in touch with feeling when exercising frequently). Debbie disagreed with her stating she exercised "20 minutes a day." I said, "I'm confused because you come to my aerobics class, and that's a 45-minute class. Do you leave before we're finished?" "No," she said "twenty minutes. The other stuff, the sit-ups, push-ups, and other stuff are not really exercise." I asked her, "What is exercise?" She said, "Exercise is when you get your heart rate up." Someone else said, "You walk all the time, you walk to the store and everywhere." Debbie said, "Walking is not really exercise, because I don't get my heart rate up." We explored her beliefs, but she steadfastly maintained that she exercised only 20 minutes a day. Later, she described another group member as a person who "exercised all the time." I said, "Why is walking exercise for her, but not for you?" She laughed at this inconsistency in her thinking and was willing to discuss it. Thereafter, she began to open up and explore her own relationship with exercise.

Alternative coping methods must be strengthened. Clients will need to explore a variety of coping strategies to find those in which they are comfortable. A consultation with an exercise physiologist familiar with exercise dependence may be helpful to outline a sound exercise program. Relaxation tapes and writing in a journal can help with feelings and anxiety that may arise. Help clients learn to enjoy movement (see section on exercise resistance).

As exercise is decreased, clients will have more time on their hands. Help your clients plan activities that are nurturing and relaxing (movies or dinner with a friend, adopt and train a pet, maintain an aquarium, garden, take a slow walk on the beach, sit and watch the sunset, read a good book) to take the place of goal directed exercise.

Recovery involves learning to trust relationships, to vent feelings, to be assertive, to take risks, and to meet personal needs. Underlying conflict, previously avoided and denied, will need to be confronted and worked through. Self-image and self-esteem will need to be built in areas other than exercise. Ultimately, clients will need to learn to trust and depend on other people in their lives in order to move beyond exercise dependence.

PRINCIPALS OF EXERCISE PRESCRIPTION

An exercise prescription is a "recommended regimen of physical activity designed in a systematic and individualized manner." (9) The prescription includes frequency, intensity, and duration of training, the mode of activity, and the initial level of fitness. Optimally, fitness level would be determined with an exercise test in which heart rate, electrocardiogram (ECG), arterial blood pressure, and functional capacity are objectively evaluated. However, as will be discussed, in most people, an exercise test is usually not required before starting an exercise program. In any case, careful consideration should be given to the individual's health history and risk factor profile. As a nutrition therapist, if you have not taken a course in fitness evaluation or exercise physiology, consider referring your clients to an exercise physiologist or hire one to work with your clients. (See Figure 13.1 for a typical client interview in sports nutrition.)

Target Heart Rate Range

The target heart rate range is only a guideline to follow in prescribing exercise (See Table 13.1). An individual's response to the exercise must be evaluated and the intensity altered to provide for the participant's comfort and safety while achieving a training effect. Counting the pulse for ten seconds immediately after exercising and multiplying by six gives a good estimate of the exercise heart rate.

Table 13.1 Calculating Target Heart Rate Range				
		Lower Limit		Upper Limit
		220		220
Age of individual (for example, age 40)		-40		-40
Age-adjusted maximal heart rate		180		180
Individual's Resting heart rate		- 60		- 60
Heart rate reserve		120		120
Conditioning intensity (60-80% HR range)		x.60		x.80
		72		96
Resting heart rate		+ 60		+ 60
Target heart rate range		**132**	to	**156**

Figure 13.1

Typical Sports Nutrition Consultation
Kathy King, RD, LD

The client is a 17-year-old female named Mandy. She is a senior at Central High School and the best player on the girl's basketball team. Last year she blew out both knees and has spent the remainder of the time in rehabilitation under the supervision of a personal trainer. Mandy has the ability to get a college scholarship in basketball if this year goes well for her. Her mother called for an appointment because Mandy gained about 30 pounds this past year and needs to get it off without jeopardizing her basketball season, which opens in four weeks.

Mandy is 5'5" at 174# and 27% body fat. She appears stocky and solid in build. She is an only child and her father was a good athlete and professional football player. He has been her coach since she was four years old, but now they argue too much for him to coach her. Her mother is overweight, but very conscious about what to prepare for meals. She wants to support Mandy and yet put the responsibility to eat well on Mandy's shoulders. Mandy is an honor student.

Mandy has a personal trainer who has helped her regain her strength and agility since her injuries. She works out six days per week, usually for 2-4 hours total in a variety of aerobic, flexibility, and strength routines.

Mandy goes to basketball practice an hour before school starts and can't practice with breakfast in her stomach. School lunch is either the hot meal, which she seldom eats, or a salad bar with 3/4 cup of dressing and 4 crackers. Afternoon snacks are usually with team members at a fast food restaurant and consist of burritos, hamburgers or pizza, fries, malts or colas. The evening meal is lighter because she works out three nights per week for two hours with her trainer and works out on her own or with team members the other two evenings. Weekends are "pig-outs" with her friends.

Therapist: "Mandy, I am really proud of you and what you have accomplished. By working together we can help you lose weight and still stay strong for basketball. Are you willing to change how you eat if we make it reasonable?"

Mandy: *"Sure. I've had a really hard year mentally and physically. This time last year the doctor said I'd never play again and I knew I'd prove him wrong. But I went through hell last spring when my second knee went out. I didn't know if I could handle the pain again, but I did. I ate too much when I couldn't exercise, and I've only lost 6# since starting with my trainer."*

Mandy's mom: "We really pulled back and let her make up her own mind about everything. She wants to play basketball again and her doctor and trainer say she's stronger than before. I think I buy the right foods at home, but she doesn't always eat at home."

Therapist: "I agree. Her food records show she eats well at home. Mandy, it's common for athletes to gain weight when they stop exercising. Later, when you started rehab and working with your trainer, weight from increased muscle mass could cover up weight loss from burned off fat. Tell me, have you ever had to lose weight in the past?"

Mandy: *"The people in our family are not petite. I've always been a jock, so I never had to worry about gaining weight. So this is my first official 'diet.' "*

Therapist: "Instead of calling it a 'diet,' think of it as learning how to eat again. You have to eat enough calories to support the training you do each day, but you will be eating less than you used to, so you will be losing weight. Let's start with breakfast. What are you willing to eat after practice but before school starts?"

Mandy: *"I don't have time then, but I have study hall first hour and I can eat there."*

Therapist: "Are you willing to try a granola bar, dry cereal, fruit, or little box of juice? You need more liquids and carbohydrates after practice."

Mandy: *"I can do that."*

Therapist: "Lunch is a really good time to get more food and liquids stored for afternoon practice. It's no wonder that you are starved later on and overeat with just a salad for lunch--and a very high-fat one at that. What kind of lunch are you willing to bring from home?"

Mandy: *"I will eat a peanut butter sandwich or ham. That's about it."*

166

Therapist: "What about fresh fruit? You mentioned yogurt on your food record. Will you take yogurt or drink low-fat milk?"

Mandy: *"I can buy milk there or I can take yogurt with a sandwich."*

The discussion continued until Mandy had identified what she would eat on school days. During basketball season, Mandy often skipped meals on the weekend and slept in or ate out. She was willing to eat more regularly at home in order to better maintain her energy and fluid intake while she loses weight.

Therapist: "Mandy, your mom seems to know what to buy and how to prepare lower fat meals. That's what an athlete needs: a diet high in fruits, vegetables, grains, and fluids; lower in fat; and moderate amounts of protein. Your diet has been very high in fat. I will give you this sheet where I've written down what we've agreed upon for meal ideas, but can you give me an idea of what you plan to eat each day?"

Mandy remembered what to eat and even added a few new selections.

Therapist: "That's great! I want you to keep a written record for me and bring it next week along with your training schedule. We'll talk about how to eat on the day of competition next week. Please call me if either of you have any questions before we meet again."

Mandy: *"My basketball coach has some muscle building powder he wants me to take, but mom wants you to see it first."*

Therapist: "No problem. Either drop the product information by this week or bring it next time. This week I want you to do the best you can. You will be getting yourself ready for this year's basketball season through your efforts. Time is short right now, but I don't want you to be too rigid with yourself. I want you to enjoy eating, but just change some of what you eat. How does that sound?"

Mandy: *"I can live with that. My dad just took a job out of town, so I think it will be easier to do this now. He won't be back until Thanksgiving."*

Therapist: "Is your dad concerned about your weight?"

Mandy: *"He makes fun of overweight women. He always yells at me when I come off the court when I play a game because he wants me to play better. I'm already the best player on the team."*

Mandy's mom: "Her dad is getting better. I tell him that if he loves Mandy and me, he will love us no matter what size we are, and he agrees. In fact he is getting a stomach himself."

Therapist: "You said earlier that your dad was an athlete and professional ball player. That could make him overly concerned about looking fit. By the time he sees you in several months, your season should be in full swing and your weight will be coming down. You appear to be relaxed and confident. Is that true?"

Mandy: *"I feel a lot older than I did last year. Kids are coming to me for advice. The quarterback had to go through a similar operation to mine a month ago and I called him up to tell him what to expect. We're sort of friends now."*

Therapist: "You never know how life works, but it sounds like you have really grown from your knee experience. You sound like you will be OK whether basketball is your life or not."

Mandy: *"I didn't believe I was important without basketball, but now I do."*

Mandy's mom: "We've become much closer after this year.... Thank you for seeing us."

Therapist: "I have thoroughly enjoyed myself and I look forward to seeing you next week."

Increased intensity of exercise is associated with increased cardiovascular risk, orthopedic injury, and decreased compliance. Therefore, programs with low to moderate intensity with longer duration are recommended. Heart rate fluctuates during exercise, so intensity is prescribed in a range as in the above example. Signs and symptoms of coronary artery disease (CAD) or other diseases may require exercise intensity being maintained at levels below those calculated. If cardiovascular problems are suspected, the client should be referred to his or her physician before beginning any exercise.

Duration of Exercise Sessions

The conditioning period may vary from 20 to 60 minutes, excluding warm-up and cool-down. The conditioning response is a result of the product of the intensity and the duration of the exercise. Significant cardiovascular improvements have been realized with five to ten minutes of exercise that is at 90 percent of functional capacity. However, since high intensity, short duration sessions are not desirable for most participants, better results are obtained with low intensities and longer duration. Such programs may also have a lower risk of orthopedic injury and have a higher caloric expenditure.

Frequency of Exercise Sessions

"The recommended frequency varies from several daily sessions to three to five periods per week according to the needs, interests and functional capacity of the participants." (2) For some individuals, sessions of five minutes duration several times a day may be desirable. Typically however, participants should exercise at least three times a week on alternate days. "The amount of improvement in VO2 max tends to plateau when frequency of training is increased above three days per week. The value of the added improvement found with training more than five days a week, is small to not apparent in regard to improvement in VO2 max. Training of less than two days a week does not generally show meaningful change in VO2 max." (2)

Rate of Progression

How quickly an individual progresses in the exercise program depends on their functional capacity, health status or age, and needs or goals. Initially, exercise should include light calisthenics and low level aerobic activities, where there will be a minimum of muscle soreness and avoidance of injuries or discomfort. Initially, the aerobic conditioning phase should be at least ten to fifteen minutes. This initial stage usually lasts from four to six weeks, depending on the rate of adaptation of the participant. Somebody with a low fitness level may take as many as ten weeks in this initial phase.

Over the next four to five months, intensity is typically increased to the target level with the duration increased every two to three weeks. Cardiac patients and less fit individuals should have more time to adapt at each stage. They may initially use discontinuous aerobic exercise and progress to more continuous aerobic exercise. The duration of exercise for these participants should be increased to 20 to 30 minutes before an increase in the intensity. After the first six months of training, the participant usually achieves a satisfactory level of cardio-respiratory fitness. Continuing the same workout schedule will enable them to maintain fitness, although further improvement is minimal. At this point, the program can be reviewed and goals altered.

Body Composition

We know that excess body fat is harmful to health, but there are many misconceptions about the assessment and interpretation of body composition. Thinness has become a national obsession with dieting and exercise used to meet this cultural ideal. Some believe that professionals may contribute to the extreme concern with thinness by encouraging the "thinness = health" equation and by allowing those that will never be thin to believe they can become thin by following "the formula." This ignores research that indicates that people come in all shapes and sizes and that some people are genetically loaded to be larger than "normal."

Unfortunately, "professionals have frequently established targets for body composition that are unrealistically low, in terms of health benefits. Thinner is not necessarily healthier, evidenced by similar mortality risk across a wide range of body composition values. Health risk increases significantly only at the upper end of the body composition distribution." (10)

The American College of Sports Medicine states that, "we should tolerate a broad range of body composition values as normal" and recommends that "intensive intervention of weight loss should be implemented in persons at the upper end of the distribution."(9) Additionally, it recommends that clinicians "should be aware of the wide range of normal values, and not encourage all participants to achieve a particular value." (9) In light of this information, we need to interpret each person's body composition individually, taking into account his or her clinical status and other risk factors. We may need to be more comfortable aiding our heavier clients to become healthier.

Muscular Strength and Endurance

The goal of muscular strength and endurance training is to increase the strength and endurance of the muscles so that they become more efficient in dealing with every day demands placed on them, such as mowing the grass, carrying groceries, or moving luggage. Strength is defined as the amount of force exerted by a muscle group for one movement. Endurance is the ability of the muscle group to maintain continuous repetitions over time. The American College of Sports Medicine recommends strength training two times a week, consisting of eight to ten exercises with the major muscle groups, a minimum of one set of eight to twelve repetitions.

Muscular strength and endurance are developed by the overload principle. Muscular strength is best developed by using heavy weights (that require maximum or nearly maximum tension development) with few repetitions and muscular endurance is best developed by using lighter weights with a greater number of repetitions.

While increased frequency of training and additional sets and/or repetitions "elicit larger strength gain, the magnitude of the differences is usually small." (10) One study compared training two-days-a-week with three-days-a-week for an 18-week time period. (11) The subjects performed one set of seven to ten repetitions to fatigue. The two-day-a-week group showed a 21 percent increase in strength compared to a 28 percent increase in the three-day-a-week group. In other words, 75 percent of what could be attained in a three-days-a-week program was attained in a two-day-a-week program.

HERMAN

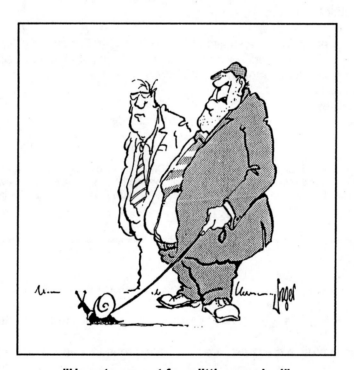

"He gets me out for a little exercise!"

Flexibility

Any exercise program should include activities that promote maintenance of good flexibility, particularly at the lower back. Stretching exercises are designed to improve and maintain range of motion in a joint or series of joints. These exercises should be performed slowly with a gradual progression to greater ranges of motion. Participants should move into the stretch slowly, hold for 10 to 30 seconds and repeat three to five times. They should not stretch to a point of significant pain. Stretching exercises should be performed at least three-times-a-week and can be included in the warm-up and cool-down periods around the aerobic conditioning phase.

Warm-Up and Cool-Down

Each exercise session should include a warm-up of five to ten minutes and a cool-down of five to ten minutes. The warm-up period gradually increases the metabolic rate from the resting level to that level required for conditioning and may include walking or slow jogging, light stretching exercises and calisthenics or other types of muscle conditioning exercises. The cool-down includes exercises of diminished intensity, such as slower walking or jogging, stretching and in some cases, relaxation activities.

EVALUATION OF PARTICIPANTS PRIOR TO EXERCISE PARTICIPATION

It is important to evaluate individuals prior to exercise testing or exercise participation. Individuals are divided into three risk classifications: (2)

1. Apparently healthy—those who are asymptomatic and apparently healthy with no more than one major coronary risk factor (Table 13.2).
2. Individuals at higher risk—those who have symptoms suggestive of possible cardiopulmonary or metabolic disease (Table 13.3) and/or two or more major coronary risk factors (Table 13.2).
3. Individuals with disease—those with known cardiac, pulmonary, or metabolic disease.

Table 13.2 Major Risk Factors (2)

1. Diagnosed hypertension or systolic blood pressure $\geq$ 160 or diastolic blood pressure $\geq$ 90 mmHg on at least 2 separate occasions, or on antihypertensive medication
2. Serum cholesterol $\geq$ 6.20 mmol/L ($\geq$ 240 mg/d)
3. Cigarette smoking
4. Diabetes mellitus *
5. Family history of coronary or other atherosclerotic disease in parents or siblings prior to age 55

* Persons with insulin dependent diabetes mellitus (IDDM) who are over 30 years of age, or have had IDDM for more than 15 years, and persons with non-insulin dependent diabetes mellitus who are over 35 years of age should be classified as patients with disease and treated according to the guidelines for those people who fit in Table 13.3.

Table 13.3
Major symptoms or signs suggestive of cardiopulmonary or metabolic disease** (2)

1. Pain or discomfort in the chest or surrounding areas that appears to be ischemic in nature
2. Unaccustomed shortness of breath or shortness of breath with mild exertion
3. Dizziness or syncope
4. Orthopnea/paroxysmal nocturnal dyspnea
5. Ankle edema
6. Palpitations or tachycardia
7. Claudication
8. Known heart murmur

**These symptoms must be interpreted in the clinical context in which they appear, since they are not all specific for cardiopulmonary or metabolic disease.

RECOMMENDATIONS

"No set of guidelines on exercise testing and participation can cover every conceivable situation." (9) The American College of Sports Medicine provides the following recommendation in an attempt to provide some general guidance: (9)

Apparently Healthy Individuals

Apparently healthy individuals can begin moderate (intensities of 40 to 60 percent VO_2 max) exercise programs (such as walking or increasing usual daily activities) without the need of exercise testing or medical examination, as long as the exercise program begins and proceeds gradually and as long as the individual is alert to the development of unusual signs and symptoms. (10) To classify moderate exercise, it must be within the individual's current capacity and be able to be sustained comfortably for a prolonged period, for example, 60 minutes.

Prior to beginning a vigorous exercise program, men over 40 and women over 50 should have a medical examination and a maximal exercise test. Vigorous exercise (intensity greater than 60 percent VO_2 max) is defined as exercise intense enough to represent a substantial challenge and results in significant increases in heart rate and respiration. Usually, untrained individuals cannot sustain this level of intensity for more than 15 to 20 minutes.

Individuals at Higher Risk

An exercise stress test prior to beginning a vigorous exercise program is desirable for higher risk individuals of any age. Individuals at higher risk are those with two or more major coronary risk factors (Table 13.2) and/or symptoms suggestive of cardiopulmonary or metabolic disease, or who fit the diabetes guidelines. For those without symptoms, an exercise test or medical examination may not be necessary if moderate exercise is undertaken gradually with appropriate guidance and no competitive participation. Maximal exercise tests in patients at high risks should be physician supervised.

Individuals with Disease

Persons of any age with symptoms suggestive of coronary, pulmonary, or metabolic disease should have a medical examination and a physician supervised maximal exercise test prior to beginning an exercise program.

SUMMARY

Recommendations should be made in the context of a participant's needs, goals, and initial abilities. In this regard, a sliding scale as to the amount of time allotted and intensity of effort should be carefully gauged for both the cardio-respiratory and muscular strength, and endurance components of the program. An appropriate warm-up and cool-down, which would include flexible exercises, is also recommended. The important factor is to design a program for the individual, to provide the proper amount of physical activity and to attain maximal benefit at the lowest risk. Emphasis should be placed on factors that result in permanent lifestyle change and encourage a lifetime of physical activity.

"Exercise should be done neither as a punishment for looking bad nor as a necessary evil for looking good. It's a gift you give yourself because you need and deserve it. So start playing to play, instead of to win, and you'll find yourself in a no-lose situation. Dinah Shore once said, "I've never thought of participating in sports just for the sake of exercise, or as a means to lose weight . . . or because it was a social fad. I really enjoy playing. It's a vital part of my life." (5)

References

1. Casperson C, Powell KE, Christensen GM. Physical activity, exercise, and physical exercise: definitions and distinctions for health-related research. *Public Health Reports.* 1985; 100 (2): 126-130.
2. American College of Sports Medicine. *The Recommended Quantity and Quality of Exercise for Developing and Maintaining Cardiorespiratory and Muscular Fitness in Healthy Adults.* Position Stand. Indianapolis: 2003.
3. Glasser W. *Positive Addiction.* New York: Harper & Row; 1976.
4. White F, White T. *Treating Overweight and Emotional Overeating Disorders.* Santa Barbara, CA: Handouts from workshop; Sept. 1994.
5. Ornstein R, Sobel D. *Healthy Pleasures.* New York: Addison-Wesley Publishing Company; 1989.
6. Leon AS, Connett J, Jacobs DR, et al. Leisure time physical activity levels and risk of coronary heart disease and death. *J Am Medical Assoc.* 1987; 258: 2388-2395.
7. Freedman R. *BodyLove: Learning to Like Our Looks and Ourselves: A Practical Guide for Women.* New York: Harper & Row; 2002.
8. de Coverley Veale DM. *Exercise Dependence. British Journal of Addiction.* 1987; 82(7):735-740.
9. American College of Sports Medicine. *Guidelines for Exercise Testing and Prescription.* Philadelphia: Lea & Febiger; 2000.
10. McArdle WD, Katch FI, Katch VL. *Exercise Physiology: Energy, Nutrition, and Human Performance,* 5th ed. Philadelphia: Lippincott Williams & Wilkins; 2001.
11. Braith RW, Graves JE, Pollock ML, Leggett SL, Carpenter DM, Colvin AB. Comparison of two versus three days per week of variable resistance training during 10 and 18 week programs. *Int. J Sports Med.* 1989;10: 450-454.

ADDITIONAL READING

(Out of Print, but copies available on Amazon.com)

Benyo R. *The Exercise Fix.* Champaign, IL: Human Kinetics; 1990.

Gavin J. *The Exercise Habit.* Champaign, IL: Leasure Press; 1992.

Prussin R, Harvey P, DiGeronimo T. *Hooked on Exercise.* New York: Fireside/Parkside: Simon & Schuster; 1992.

Yates A. *Compulsive Exercise and the Eating Disorders.* New York: Brunner/Routledge, Inc.; 1992.

Chapter 14

The Challenge of Maintaining Change

Idamarie Laquatra, PhD, RD

After reading this chapter, the reader will be able to:
♦ Identify four motivational processes that may enhance maintenance of a skill.
♦ Describe at least two external situational variables that may decrease skill maintenance.
♦ Identify maintenance skills that clients can utilize to minimize long-term relapse.

Maintaining lifestyle and eating changes has been an area of intense interest and concern to practitioners. Why do many clients have such a difficult time maintaining dietary changes in their lives? Although problems with maintenance seem to be publicized more frequently in the area of weight control, the truth remains that any dietary change faces maintenance challenges. For example, most individuals who suffer a myocardial infarction have little problem altering their behaviors to accommodate a low-saturated fat and low-cholesterol eating pattern. As health returns, however, their priorities often change, causing them to lose their focus and backslide to old behaviors.

Maintenance of diet change once treatment is discontinued does not occur naturally. (1) The skills needed to change behavior differ from those required to maintain the change. Individuals who do extremely well during the treatment phase may or may not have success at maintaining new behaviors. In fact, some therapists feel more concerned about those clients who have no problems of adherence during treatment, because the clients may not have been confronted with situations to "test" their coping strategies.

Maintenance of any skill involves an interaction of motivational processes within the client with situational variables in the post-treatment environment. In other words, dietitians need to know what's going on inside and outside of their clients in order to foster the maintenance process.

Internal Processes

Kelman (2) described three motivational processes: compliance, identification, and internalization. Self-sabotage is also an internal process, but it may be triggered by a high-risk external situation.

Compliance, a low-level process, refers to participation in a program to avoid punishment or to gain rewards. Compliance examples include clients who change their eating behaviors because they fear another heart attack, derive all their reinforcement from a change in their scale weight, or dread an insulin reaction. Maintenance of change is not likely to occur if the motivational process remains at the compliance level.

A higher level of motivation, *identification,* occurs when clients do things for the counselor. Clients learn what is required to maintain a satisfying relationship with the counselor, and so they alter their behaviors accordingly. They want to be liked by the counselor. Unfortunately, clients backslide once in the post-treatment phase, when the counselor becomes less available.

Internalization ranks as the highest level of the motivational processes. In this stage, the rationale for change agrees with the client's value system (he/she becomes functional—see Chapter 1), and performing the behaviors becomes intrinsically rewarding. During the treatment phase, external reinforcement comes easily and often for the client. It can be a lower blood pressure or cholesterol reading, a comment from a co-worker about how great the client looks, or a better controlled blood glucose. After treatment, when the external reinforcement wanes, the need for an internal reward system becomes apparent. The chances of maintaining behaviors will be much greater when clients internalize the motivation for change. It's easy to spot clients who internalize the motivation for change: *they don't follow a diet; they've modified their lives.*

Clients do not always pass through each level of motivation. Some clients you counsel may internalize right away. Other clients grow through the counseling process and pass through one or more levels. You may find that some clients may get "stuck" in the compliance or identification level. Counselors need to be prepared to gently confront clients to encourage the internalization process.

Self-sabotage can be a common problem during maintenance when the clients experience negative self-talk. It can occur when clients focus on the immediate perceived benefits of an action versus the delayed benefit. For example, faced with an urge for a high-fat food, a client may think: "Oh, it would taste so good" and lose sight of how it will impact the total fat content of the diet or the self-recrimination that may follow once the food is eaten. It must be pointed out that high-fat foods can have a place in an overall healthy diet, and that eating a high-fat food does not necessarily mean that self-recrimination will follow. Unfortunately, clients who have a problem with self-sabotage often develop consistent behavioral patterns. They usually do not balance eating high-fat foods with low-fat foods and self-loathing results when behaviors occur outside of their self-specified limits.

Self-sabotage also occurs when clients repeatedly deceive themselves into thinking that "one time won't hurt me." While it is absolutely true that exceptions do not derail maintenance efforts, when exceptions become the rule, self-sabotage may be at work. Rationalizing behaviors, such as eating high-sodium foods because there just wasn't time to prepare an appropriate meal, or dealing with stress by eating can also sabotage efforts. Finally, clients who think negatively about their abilities or who take comfort in the victim role may deliberately set themselves up to fail, thinking, "I knew I couldn't do it."

Situational Variables

Factors outside the client may have an influence on whether or not a new behavior will be maintained. Clients must be skilled to make the appropriate food choices in many different environments and under varying conditions.

High-risk situations test the abilities of clients. How often have you heard "I was doing so well until ..." High-risk situations include social events, such as weddings, office parties, and eating out. They extend to negative life events such as divorce or changing jobs. High-risk situations also include negative emotional states such as depression, anxiety, anger, and stress. Clients who deal successfully with high-risk situations build confidence. Those who fail can torpedo their maintenance efforts, resulting in lapse, relapse and collapse. (3)

A *non-supportive environment* makes maintenance of any behavior difficult, especially if clients have not internalized the change process. A nonsupportive environment can be a spouse who complains about the food being served or a work cafeteria where lower fat food options do not exist. Dietitians must recognize that maintenance of skills requires a supportive environment. New skills are fragile at first, and need to be nurtured to grow strong. When you first work with new clients, try walking them through a typical day and explore where they get support for their new lifestyle decisions; role play how clients can ask for support or how they can deal with negative comments and lack of support. *(ed. For years I have used a parable called "Weed out the garden of your life" to help clients visualize how to deal with unpleasant things they can't keep from happening. They learn that they can control how they react and no longer allow it to be a problem. K King)*

Relapse

Throughout the treatment phase and maintenance process, relapses often occur. Relapse should be understood as a process rather than an outcome. (3) Marlatt and Gordon (4) describe the process of relapse as a specific series of cognitions and behaviors. Their relapse model integrates internal and external factors: cognitive function, self-efficacy (defined as an individual's expectation concerning his or her capacity to cope effectively with whatever it is that the present situation demands)(5), environment and situational variables. For example, the person is depressed and feeling sorry for himself (cognitive), then the person doesn't feel confident that he has the ability to handle new stresses at this time (self-efficacy), and finally, a high-risk situation presents itself (environmental/situational). The person may return to old behaviors briefly and take the relapse in stride while determining other ways to handle depression or his response to it. Or, he may choose to believe that the return to old behaviors was out of his control or inevitable, given his internal weakness or flaws.

A person is most vulnerable to relapse when he or she is angry, depressed, upset, or feeling sorry for him/herself. Following are six steps to take to better control the relapse event: (6)

1. **Stop the behavior EARLY**
2. **Stay calm**
3. **Renew eating vows**
4. **Analyze what's happening**
5. **Take charge**
6. **Ask for help**

It is said that the relapse itself is not the problem; it is how clients deal with the relapse that determines the ultimate outcome. Often, people who try to change their behaviors expect perfection of themselves. When they slip, self-recrimination occurs, and they view their failure as a character flaw. Called the *Abstinence Violation Effect,* this type of thinking sets the individual up for a downward spiral of deteriorating behaviors. (6) Danish has suggested instead that we encourage our clients to think of maintenance of change like a basketball game--no one expects 100% of the shots to make it through the hoop—so, a strategy for handling rebounds is part of the game plan. (7) You can help your clients understand that learning to rebound is part of what must take place for change to be maintained.

As individuals begin the journey towards lifelong maintenance, they need to expect to encounter difficulties. They must be counseled to learn the strategies that work for them when faced with high-risk situations. When they do relapse, they need to remove the moral overtones. (It is not the end of the world and they are not bad people; they just ate some food. That's all.) It helps when clients view changing eating behaviors as an ongoing learning process because learning involves testing boundaries, making mistakes, and growing from them. As clients practice their new eating skills in different environments, they may make errors in judgment, but continued practice will build self-confidence to deal with even the most challenging situations. Relapse prevention is a self-control process that combines training in coping skills, cognitive interventions, and lifestyle changes. (6)

> **It is not the end of the world and they are not bad people; they just ate some food. That's all.**

Maintenance Skills

While most of the research on maintenance skills was completed with individuals who lost weight, each of the principles can be generalized to any dietary change. Although exercise seems more related to weight loss and maintenance than to other dietary issues, it is actually vital to every person's health maintenance, as well as for recovering from illness or injury. Research supports that individuals who incorporate exercise into their lives appear to be able to maintain their weight loss better than those who do not exercise. (6) The exercise not only increases calorie expenditure, but it also seems to facilitate other positive maintenance behaviors.

Other maintenance skills that have been identified include self-monitoring, planning, setting goals, setting boundaries, and developing coping skills.

Self-monitoring refers to an awareness of eating behaviors. Clients need to be conscious of what they eat. During the treatment phase, keeping written records or oral accounts (through audiotapes) of eating behaviors help clients increase their understanding of what, where, when and how much they eat. During the maintenance phase, it becomes easy to lose track of eating as other priorities surface. Dietitians must help clients stay focused enough to retain treatment gains.

Planning refers to meal-planning and strategy development for high-risk situations. Haphazard eating can derail the best intentions, and allow the environment to control the client. Skills in meal-planning and developing strategies for high-risk situations such as social occasions or negative emotions (depression, anxiety) give clients concrete plans to use rather than entering situations blindly, hoping for the best.

Setting goals, a critical life skill, was described in Chapter 8. Clients can often be so vague about what they want to achieve that they never know when they have achieved anything. Goals need to be specific, realistic, and under the client's control.

Clients should *set boundaries* that have meaning for them. For example, a client concerned with weight control may set a boundary of five pounds or fitting into a particular piece of clothing. Individuals trying to maintain a low-cholesterol, low-saturated fat eating style may set boundaries in terms of types of foods. Still other boundaries may have to do with quantities of food (protein amounts on a restricted protein diet, for example). Boundaries should be salient so they can trigger the client to take action when nudged.

A common factor in everyone's life continues to be stress. Learning how to cope with stress and with other life problems without turning to food or backsliding will be vital during the maintenance phase. Clients may need to learn to be more assertive, to deal with problems head on, or to learn how to relax. *Coping skills* will differ with each client. The counselor must actively listen to understand the client well and to help design appropriate strategies. (See side bar "What do you say when a client calls at 10PM?")

What do you say when a client calls at 10PM to say she is eating everything in sight?
Kathy King, RD, LD

Marge, a 46-year-old divorced CPA with grown kids, has lost 30# the last seven months through increased exercise, a lower fat diet, and a lot of psychological support by the nutrition therapist. Marge and the nutrition therapist, Laura, have a close professional relationship. This is the first time Marge has ever taken Laura's offer to "call if you need me."

Marge: *"Hi, Laura, I hope I'm not calling too late."*
Laura: "No, that's just fine. How are you doing?"
Marge: *"I'm getting really depressed and I'm putting food in my mouth just to have it there. I can't still be hungry, I've eaten too much."*
Laura: "Ok. Let's talk this through. Are you feeling OK otherwise? *(yes)* Can you tell what lead you into this? What has changed?
Marge: *"It's the craziest thing. This week I started wearing my new clothes and I was in a good mood, and everyone at work started telling me how great I looked. They could finally tell how much I had lost."* (both client and therapist laugh)
Laura: "So, the attention is new and scary for you? *(yes)* You know that it was bound to happen when you finally stopped wearing your baggy clothes. Thirty pounds is a lot to lose. What about it made you so scared?"
Marge: *"I started to feel anxious because I've lost weight before and then couldn't keep it off. I didn't want it to happen again this time."*
Laura: "You didn't want to regain your weight like before, so you started overeating to help calm your nerves? (both laugh) Would you rather gain the weight back instead of dealing with the attention?"
Marge: *"I can't gain the weight back because I'd have to go back on the blood pressure medicine and my chemistries will go back up."*
Laura: "There are other very important reasons besides your appearance to keep the weight down. So what can you do to deal with the comments?"
Marge: *"I can do something besides say, 'Oh, thank you,' become embarrassed and leave the room."*
Laura: "Your answer is fine, but is there something you could do besides becoming embarrassed and leaving?"
Marge: *"I could remember the other reasons why I needed to lose the weight. I may not tell them why. I may just say, 'I feel so much better now.' "*
Laura: "That's good. You need to remember all the other changes you have accomplished besides weight loss. Let's remember what they are. Your cholesterol..."
Marge: *"My cholesterol dropped from 250 to 202; my triglycerides are down from 455 to 230, and I don't have to take blood pressure medicine anymore, so I don't have all the side effects from that."*
Laura: "Great! It puts all of this in perspective better doesn't it? (yes) Is your anxiety the only thing you are dealing with when they compliment you? Are you proud of yourself?"
Marge: *"Yes, I feel proud, but then I feel pressure to succeed, and then I feel anger."*

At this point, Laura can tell that not all of the issues have been explored. She could take more time at this stage to identify and work through the new issues, or suggest that Marge think about her anger and write it down so they could discuss it at the next visit. Laura chooses to continue while the discussion is flowing.

Laura: "What are you angry about?"

Marge: *"Just for a moment I feel angry because people who haven't talked to me in months are now taking the time to tell me two or three times in a week how nice I look."*

Laura: "It angers you that people treat you differently because of your weight. That's understandable. Our society has an obsession about weight. Let me ask you this though. You said in the beginning that you were in a good mood this week. You bubble when you look good. I don't know if you have ever noticed it?"

Marge: *"I know I do. I know what you are getting at. It wasn't just my weight. I wore my new clothes, I felt good and looked good, so people started saying things to me."*

Laura: "Would you rather that they didn't talk to you or didn't say that you looked nice? (both laugh) You know, in a little while people will be used to your appearance and won't say anything. Then will you miss it?"

Marge: *"Of course, that's how I am."*

Laura: "Are you feeling better? *(yes)* Do you want to go eat now?"

Marge: *"I've eaten enough. But it doesn't interest me now at all. I wasn't eating because I was hungry; I was eating because I was stressed out and I didn't know how to cope."*

Laura: "Do you deserve to lose weight and look good? *(yes)* What are you going to say and do the next time someone tells you that you look so good?"

Marge: *"I will smile and say, 'Thank you and I feel good too.' Then I'll let myself enjoy the moment."*

Laura: "Fantastic! Now I want you to call me the next few days and let me know how you are doing. Is that OK?"

Marge: *"That's fine. I feel much better."*

The next day when Marge called, she said, *"The crisis has passed and I had a great day. I ate normally, and I told people some simple answer when they said I looked good."* The following day Marge said, *"I ate well again today. I'm not hungry. I feel good about me, and I walked each morning the last two days."*

In addition to these skills, strategies such as learning how to develop a support system and continued therapist contact also encourage the maintenance of change. Family, friends, and the dietitian can support the client through the maze of maintenance. Change can be stressful and difficult, and the problems clients encounter are numerous and varied. Knowing the type of support needed and how to ask for it will help clients in the toughest times and provide the needed encouragement. Post-treatment contact that specifically targets maintenance skills has been found to be helpful. (9)

Our Responsibility

When beginning to counsel a new client, it is our responsibility to accurately assess which stage of change the client is in, and not present strategies for change that the client is not prepared to take. This will only discourage the client more, and set him or her up for repeat failure. Far too often counselors focus on the action stage without adequately exploring clients' motivation and commitment. (6)

Developing treatment plans for clients, addresses only half of the behavior change issue. Without a formal post-treatment program, the chances for maintenance of any dietary change will be slim. In the author's opinion, dietitians have an ethical responsibility to include a specific maintenance program that may last one year or longer.

Maintenance programs should be tailored to meet each client's needs; however, general guidelines exist which can increase the effectiveness of any plan you devise. The program should include an assessment of situations the client finds most difficult (10), skills training to equip clients to cope with post-treatment challenges, strategies for helping clients develop support, and continued professional guidance through formal contact, e-mails and phone calls. (9)

Learning Activities

1. Using the case study "What do you do when a client calls at 10pm?"
   Identify external situational variables that hampered the client's efforts to be successful.
   Describe maintenance skills that were used in assisting the client refocus her efforts.

2. Identify one personal lifestyle issue you would like to change to enhance your own health.
   What motivational processes can you identify for yourself?
   What barriers (external forces) limit your success?
   What maintenance skills have/can you use to enhance your change process?
   How will you measure success?

References
1. Danish SJ, Galambos NL, Laquatra I. Life development intervention: skill training for personal competence. In: Felner RD, Jason LA, Moritsugu JN, Farber SS, eds. *Preventive Psychology.* New York: Pergamon Press; 1983:49-61.
2. Kelman HC. Compliance, identification and internalization: three processes of opinion change. *Journal of Conflict Resolution.* 1958;2:51-60.
3. Brownell KD. Relapse and the treatment of obesity. In: Wadden TA, Van Ittallie TB, eds. *Treatment of the Seriously Obese Patient.* New York: The Guilford Press; 1992:437-455.
4. Marlatt GA, Gordon J, eds. *Relapse prevention: maintenance strategies in the treatment of addictive behaviors.* New York: The Guilford Press; 1985.
5. Bandura A. Self-efficacy: toward a unifying theory of behavioral change. *Psychosoc Rev.* 1977; 84: 191-215.
6. Shattuck, DK. Mindfulness and metaphor in relapse prevention: an interview with G. Alan Marlatt. *J Am Diet Assoc.* 1994;94:846-848.
7. Danish S. *"Advanced counseling skills."* Presentation at American Dietetic Association Annual Meeting, Orlando, FL, October 1994.
8. Kayman S, Bruvold W, Stern JS. Maintenance and relapse after weight loss in women: behavioral aspects. *Am J Clin Nutr.* 1990;52:800-807.
9. Perri MG. Improving maintenance of weight loss following treatment by diet and lifestyle modification. In: Wadden TA, Van Ittallie TB, eds. *Treatment of the Seriously Obese Patient.* New York: The Guilford Press; 1992:456-477.
10. Schlundt DG, Rea MR, Kline SS, Pichert JW. Situational obstacles to dietary adherence for adults with diabetes. *J Am Diet Assoc.* 1994;94:874-879.

Section III

Dealing with Weight and Chronic Disease

Chapter 15

Weight Management:
Counseling Challenges in Lifestyle Management

Bridget Klawitter, Ph.D., RD, FADA

After reading this chapter, the reader will be able to:
- ♦ Describe the prevalence of overweight and obesity.
- ♦ Identify medical conditions and diseases associated with obesity.
- ♦ Assess body mass index (BMI) and waist circumference along with other risk factors.
- ♦ Identify supportive counseling approaches for surgical treatment options.
- ♦ Describe and apply counseling strategies important to successful weight management.
- ♦ Assess diet, activity, cultural, and age-related factors that may impact counseling.

Obesity, both adult and pediatric, is on the rise not only in the United States but worldwide. In a study published in January 2003 (1), the Centers for Disease Prevention reported that obesity increased from 19.8% of American adults to 20.9% of American adults between 2000 and 2001. Currently, more than 44 million Americans are considered obese by body mass index (BMI), reflecting an increase of 74% since 1991. (2) Obesity increases the risk for developing chronic illnesses such as diabetes, hypertension, heart disease, hypercholesterolemia, stroke, some cancers, and arthritis. Addressing the underlying causes of obesity and developing effective lifestyle change interventions remains an unanswered challenge.

The statistics on pediatric obesity are even more sobering. Today's generation of children are predicted to become the most obese generation in U.S. history. (3) Children and adolescents with a Body Mass Index (BMI) greater than or equal to the 95th percentile have a significant risk of remaining obese as an adult. (4) In 1999, 13% of children aged 6 to 11 years and 14% of adolescents aged 12-19 years in the United States were overweight. (5) This prevalence has nearly tripled for adolescents in the past two decades.

There is significant research documenting that the traditional medical approach to preventing and treating obesity has failed. (6,7) In addition, the $117 billion dollars Americans spend annually on weight reduction products and services, including diet foods, products, and programs, has been equally ineffective. (8) Therefore, dietetic practitioners skilled in the newer approaches and counseling strategies for weight management have ample opportunities for intervention and outcome management.

CLINICAL ASSESSMENT

Obesity, as a chronic medical disease, has often been referred to as obesity syndrome. (9) Common co-morbidities include: hypertension, dyslipidemia, glucose intolerance, insulin resistance, and significant correlations with coronary heart disease. The initial clinical assessment of the obese patient should be comprehensive, covering several key areas.

Current Weight and Weight History
Standard anthropometric measurements (height, weight, and Body Mass Index [BMI]) should be done. In addition, waist circumference, weight patterns, highest and lowest adult body weight, and critical periods of weight gain over time are useful pieces of information. The NIH Clinical Guideline for BMI (10) (Table 15.1) can be used to determine degree of obesity.

Table 15.1	NIH Clinical Guidelines for BMI	
Classification	**BMI (kg/m^2)**
Underweight	<18.5
Normal weight	19 – 24.2
Overweight	25 – 29.9
Class I Obesity (Mild)	30 – 34.9
Class II Obesity (Moderate)	35 – 39.9
Class III Obesity (Extreme)	>40

Waist-to-Hip (WHR) ratio is an anthropometric measure commonly used to assess body fat distribution. (11) See Table 15.2. However, waist circumference has been positively correlated with abdominal fat content. Sex-specific cutoffs have been used to identify increased relative risk for the development of obesity-related risk factors in adults with BMI of 25 to 34.9. (12)

Table 15.2	Waist Circumference	High Risk
Men	>102 cm	>40 inches
Women	>88 cm	>35 inches

Health Status and Medical Risks
Assessment of risk requires identification of disease conditions and other obesity-related health problems. Common medical risks include cardiovascular disease, diabetes, or impaired glucose intolerance, sleep apnea, polycystic ovarian syndrome, osteoarthritis, depression, acid reflux disease, and stress incontinence. It is important to educate patients about the hazards of obesity and the overall health benefits of modest weight loss (5-10% of body weight). See table 15.3 for a list of common obesity-related diseases and conditions.

Table 15.3   Obesity-Related Diseases and Conditions

Hypertension
Coronary heart disease
Ischemic stroke
Hyperlipidemia
Impaired glucose tolerance
Impaired Fasting Glucose
Insulin resistance
Type 2 diabetes mellitus
Sleep apnea
Restrictive pulmonary dysfunction
Obesity-hypoventilation syndrome
Gallstones
Nonalcoholic steatohepatitis
Musculoskeletal disease:
- Osteoarthritis
- Hyperuricemia
- Gout

Malignancy:
- Cancer of the colon
- Endometrial cancer
- Postmenopausal breast cancer

Reproductive function:
- Menstrual irregularity
- Infertility
- Gestational diabetes

Other health conditions:
- Carpal tunnel syndrome
- Venous insufficiency
- Deep vein thrombosis
- Poor wound healing

Lifestyle and Cultural Factors

An assessment of work life, including type of work, physical exertion at work, work hours, sleep patterns, and meal times can be helpful in identifying barriers to regular meal planning and exercise. Special attention should be given to shift workers and unusual work patterns such as over-the-road truck drivers. The nutrition counselor may need to be creative with meal and activity suggestions feasible in these unique work settings.

The role of ethnicity and culture should not be overlooked. In some cultures, excess weight is desirable, especially for women. It is then important to understand the reasons an individual may desire a body image contrary to the culture in which they are surrounded. This may also impact weight management support systems available to the individual. In relation to foods, understanding the meaning of food, types of foods, and preparation methods are important as you work to develop meal plans and appropriate macronutrient intake to facilitate weight loss.

Behavioral and Psychological Barriers

The most difficult challenge to dietetic practitioners is to motivate patients to make significant lifestyle changes including diet and physical activity. Key areas to explore with the patient to assess motivation to lose weight include:

- patient understanding of obesity and health risks
- previous attempts at weight management (successful and unsuccessful)
- reasons for attempting weight loss now
- attitude towards physical activity/exercise and plans on increasing level as indicated
- perceived sources of support for weight management efforts
- perceived barriers to success and/or challenges to weight loss efforts

---

Certificate of Training in Childhood and Adolescent Weight Management

The country's leading health researchers call obesity the top nutrition problem in the United States. More than half of all adults are overweight and a third are obese, according to the National Institutes of Health, and as many as 20 percent of children are obese. Meanwhile, the Surgeon General's "Report on Physical Activity and Health" found exercise and physical activity among everyone from school-age children to adults to be at an all-time low. Childhood and adolescent obesity is an increasingly important predictor of adult obesity. This program is designed to produce providers of comprehensive weight management care for children and adolescents who also know when and how to refer patients to other specialists. It is open to ADA members, RDs, and DTRs.

The Certificate of Training Offers:

- Cutting edge information and skills shared by leading practitioners in the field
- Cases and exercises to allow hands-on experience
- Valuable resource materials and tools for immediate use and future reference
- An opportunity to showcase your expertise by earning a Certificate of Training
- 27 hours of continuing professional education units

What's Involved?

There are three components to the training program: a self-study module (9 hours of readings, activities, and a pre-test), a 2 ½ day live workshop, and a post test. Participants must pass the pre-test to attend the workshop. After successful completion of the course and take-home post-test, participants will be awarded a Certificate of Training in Childhood and Adolescent Weight Management.

What's Covered?

Fundamental Research and Current Practice Guidelines... Nutrition Assessment, Treatment, and Case Management... Medical Assessment and Management...Environmental and Genetic Influences on Pediatric Overweight... Prevention of Pediatric Overweight and Obesity...Physical Activity as Treatment...Behavioral Management: Assessment and Interventions...Motivational Interviewing...Pediatric Weight Management Programs.

For more information, please contact CDR by e-mail at **weightmgmt@eatright.org** or call 1-800/877-1600, ext. 5500.

One area this author has found helpful is to explore with patients the importance of food and the role food has played in their lives. Often this is the first insight patients have on how childhood experiences shape their adult food choices and behaviors. At times, it may also enlighten individuals about food behaviors (not always desirable) they are instilling in their own children.

Often patients will complain of cravings or feeling deprived. It is important to stress regular, scheduled meals, and no fasting or skipping meals. They should also learn there are no "forbidden" foods. All foods are allowed in moderation, and self-control over food behaviors is the ultimate long-term goal.

Lack of time is another barrier clients often encounter when considering lifestyle changes. Stress the overall benefits of a healthy lifestyle, including diet and exercise, and the importance of making time for themselves. Patients often find themselves caught up in the "hamster wheel of life" and need support in breaking the pace. (See Appendix 16-A on losing weight from a patient's perspective.)

Family and Social Support Networks

Involvement of the family may be helpful in reducing the progression of obesity in children, but the impact of this approach on adults is not clear. Obese adults report that family resistance to changes in lifestyle can often be barriers to weight loss. Dietetic professionals can assist in problem solving with the patient about family barriers that can disrupt even the most motivated patient.

It is also important to help patients identify who outside their family circle functions as support or barrier. For others, it helps to identify group support opportunities for social affiliations that facilitate weight loss success. Interesting research shows that patients' obesity significantly affected how their own physicians viewed and treated them. (13) Studies such as this suggest that physicians continue to play an influential role in the physical and psychological care of obese patients.

Often patients believe they must "eat different" from family members to be successful at weight management. The key is helping them identify positive health benefits their family may enjoy if many of the changes are made together as a family unit. Introducing changes slowly and gradually is usually the most beneficial and can enhance long-term lifestyle changes.

Occasionally, the nutrition counselor may encounter a patient who perceives "sabotage" by a spouse or partner. For example, the spouse will find frequent excuses to eat out or the parent will use high-calorie foods to show love. The nutrition counselor may want to educate the significant other on the need to be supportive and ways that can be accomplished. If unsuccessful, professional counseling may be indicated.

Goals and State of Readiness

Establishing why the patient seeks weight management intervention at this particular time can provide insight into the level of motivation and compliance. Asking patients if they are currently involved in any weight loss efforts (or considering trying to lose weight) can provide clues to readiness to change. To assess whether patients understand the changes required to achieve weight loss, ask how they will handle emotional eating, eating out of boredom, and social or family situations if they start or resume a weight loss program. Ask probing questions about what exercise options they plan to pursue. Establishing patient "readiness" is an important step to assure the time is right for successful weight management. (14) Several tools are also available to assist with this evaluation. (15-17)

Discussing patient goals should include both short-term (3-6 months) and long-term (>12 months) timeframes. Assisting with determining realistic goals, not just pounds lost but quality of life goals, can assist the patient in making small successful steps towards long-term lifestyle changes. For patients ready to make changes, emphasize gradual behavior changes over time and to avoid the short-term "diet mentality" or "quick fixes." When setting goals, it is important to acknowledge to the patient that lifestyle changes are possible, but difficult.

Energy Balance Requirements

Methods for estimating energy requirements in the obese remain controversial because bodies are so unique. Several predictive formulas have been suggested (18) and include simple ratios (such as calories per kilogram actual or adjusted body weight), common formulas not originally designed for use in the obese such as Harris Benedict (19), and predictive equations formulated specifically for the obese such as Ireton-Jones (20). Based on limited evidence to date, no clear method for estimating energy requirements in the obese has distinguished itself. In the outpatient or private practice setting, selection of a formula to calculate baseline estimated needs and clinical evaluation/monitoring of outcomes might be the method of choice unless indirect calorimetry is available. (Another simple method I have used successfully with athletes and people wanting to lose weight is estimating present caloric intake from food records. We start from where they are and reduce calories from there. King)

COUNSELING SURGICAL WEIGHT LOSS CANDIDATES

Although bariatric surgery has been around for about 50 years, the recent enthusiasm and media attention surrounding surgical weight loss has produced many new counseling challenges for dietetic practitioners. Between 1990 and 1997, the annual rate of bariatric surgery in the United States more than doubled without substantial changes in perioperative morbidity and mortality. (21) This trend was primarily impacted by the increased use of the gastric bypass procedure we are seeing so commonly today.

According to the National Institutes of Health (NIH) recommendations, weight loss surgery is an option for carefully selected patients with clinically severe obesity (BMI $\geq$ 40 or $\geq$ 35 with comorbid conditions) when less invasive weight loss methods have failed and obesity poses increased morbidity and mortality risks. (22) When counseling potential surgical weight loss patients, it is important to help them understand the relationship between BMI and health risk factors in relation to the impact of significant weight loss that usually occurs after such surgeries.

For most obese and morbidly obese patients, their diet history is a litany of unsuccessful fad diets, pills, fasting, prescription medications, and commercial or medically supervised diets. When counseling patients contemplating bariatric surgery it is important to review what has been tried in the past, amount of weight loss with each method, and the reasons for discontinuing those approaches. It is important for patients contemplating the surgical weight loss approach to realize surgery is only a tool, not a quick fix, and they will have to work on diet, exercise, and lifestyle changes to be successful long-term. Post-operatively, it is hard work, not a quick fix, and patients should clearly understand their role and responsibility after surgery. In this author's experience as a bariatric dietitian, many patients need to clearly understand the permanence of several of the surgical interventions, and the importance of making an informed decision on such surgery. Helping patients who have never known what it is like to be of normal size can be a psychological and nutrition counseling challenge. One must be prepared to counsel on both aspects both pre- and post-operatively to be a successful nutrition counselor.

Surgical weight loss procedures are designed to limit nutrient intake or restrict volume of food ingested or both. (23) The most popular procedure currently, open or laparascopic Roux-en-Y gastric bypass, actually is a combination of diminished volume capacity and nutrient malabsorption. The gastric bypass partitions the stomach into a small proximal pouch (usually about 15-30 ml capacity) and the remaining larger stomach fundus and antrum. The pouch is attached directly to the jejunum through a narrow anastamosis (often the size of a dime). Weight loss is accomplished by the limited pouch capacity and delayed pouch emptying, resulting in prolonged satiety and fullness. Potential and common acute and long-term complications the nutrition counselor may encounter include: vitamin-mineral deficiencies, protein-calorie malnutrition, dumping syndrome, anemia, dehydration, nausea/vomiting, constipation, gallstones, and ulcers. The use of surgical weight loss interventions in extremely obese pediatric patients is controversial in some circles. Physical growth and development status and emotional maturity to adjust to major lifestyle changes must be evaluated.

Counseling Considerations for Surgical Weight Loss
A multidisciplinary team should screen candidates before surgical weight loss procedures, assessing:
- extent of past weight loss efforts;
- anticipated compliance with necessary diet, exercise, and lifestyle changes;
- psychosocial history and anticipated support systems; and
- understanding of procedure and potential post-operative complications.

In many settings, patients are required to lose 5-10% of their weight pre-operatively to decrease hepatic steatosis and intra-abdominal adiposity. The role of the dietetic practitioner can be critical in accomplishing this pre-operative weight loss.

Despite a positive surgical outcome, successful weight loss is not guaranteed. Potential surgical candidates must be prepared to make lifelong diet and exercise changes. The dietetic practitioner must be prepared to provide long-term guidance and support as the patient develops and adjusts to a new body image. For patients who have not known what it is like to be of normal weight, they often struggle with how to respond to positive compliments or questions about their weight loss accomplishments. Despite significant weight loss, some patients may still possess a distorted body image of themselves and need assistance in adjusting to the "new me."

Besides individual nutritional counseling one-on-one post-operatively, it has been this author's observation that surgical weight loss patients often benefit greatly from a support group focused on their unique needs and situation. Pre-operatively, patients considering the surgical intervention can hear the challenges and successes of those who have been through the surgery. Key factors are skilled facilitators and the involvement of the interdisciplinary team in these support groups to ensure factual, unbiased, and supportive information is the focus.

PEDIATRIC OBESITY COUNSELING

Historically, intensive, behavior-based weight loss programs for pediatric obesity were successful in structured clinical settings. The exploding rates of obesity in the young have expanded the focus to include primary care interventions in the office setting. Recent recommendations for the primary care setting involve both health care provision and advocacy efforts. (24) Key points include:

- Identify and track patients at risk by virtue of family history, birth weight, socioeconomic, ethnic, cultural, or environmental factors.
- Calculate and plot BMI once a year in all children and adolescents.
- Use changes in BMI to identify rate of excessive weight gain relative to linear growth.
- Encourage, support, and protect breastfeeding.
- Encourage parents and caregivers to promote healthy eating patterns by offering nutritious snacks, such as vegetables and fruits, low-fat dairy foods, and whole grains. They should encourage children's autonomy in self-regulation of food intake, set appropriate limits on choices, and model healthy food choices.
- Routinely promote physical activity, including unstructured play at home, in school, in childcare settings, and throughout the community.
- Recommend limitation of television and video time to a maximum of two hours per day.
- Recognize and monitor changes in obesity-associated risk factors for adult chronic disease, such as hypertension, dyslipidemia, hyperinsulinemia, impaired glucose tolerance, and symptoms of obstructive sleep apnea syndrome.
- Help parents, teachers, coaches, and others who influence youth to discuss health habits, not body habitus (body build or propensity for disease), as part of their efforts to control overweight and obesity.
- Enlist policy makers from local, state, and national organizations, and schools to support a healthful lifestyle for all children, including proper diet and adequate opportunity for regular physical activity.
- Encourage organizations that are responsible for health care and health care financing to provide coverage for effective obesity prevention and treatment strategies.
- Encourage public and private sources to direct funding toward research into effective strategies to prevent overweight and obesity, and to maximize limited family and community resources to achieve healthful outcomes for youth.

As with most approaches, what works for adults does not always work for children and adolescents. Long-term weight management strategies allowing a child to grow in height while slowing weight gains can facilitate a gradual decline in BMI. For many children and adolescents, the psychosocial effects of obesity can be overwhelming, and include poor self-esteem, lack of peer relationships and friends, and the inability to participate in many activities with children their own age.

One key area for assessment of obesity in pediatric populations is physical activity level. Significant relationships have been found between childhood obesity and computer usage, television watching, and total hours in sedentary behavior. (25,26) Exercise is essential to build and maintain healthy bones, muscles, and joints. The lack of regular physical activity in children and adolescents can be addressed with caregivers, and often with the children themselves. The focus should be on creating an active environment in which the entire family participates in regular physical activity. Often, simply limiting television or computer time can open up time for more physical activity. In general, a minimum of 30-60 minutes per day spent in moderate physical activity is recommended for most children.

The focus of a pediatric obesity program should be healthy eating and activity. Steps recommended for families to help their overweight child have been suggested, and include: (27)

- Develop an awareness of current eating habits, activity, and parenting behavior.
- Identify problem behaviors.
- Modify current behaviors.
- Continue awareness of behavior and problems that may change as the child grows and matures.

CHRONIC CARE MODEL AND OBESITY MANAGEMENT

An application of the Chronic Care Model (see Chapter 18) has been developed (28) and provides a general framework for the management of overweight and obese adults.

Clinical information systems

- Automated screening reminders and tracking systems for weight, body mass index, and waist circumference
- Population based registry of overweight and obese patients
- Computer generated patient calls and provider reports

Delivery system design

- Weight management team (with nutrition, exercise, behavior change, pharmacy, and surgical expertise)
- Planned, proactive follow-up

Decision support

- Clinical practice guideline
- Online tools available through Internet
- Provider or team training and feedback

Self-management support

- Printed and web-based self-help materials
- Individual or group education or skills training
- Maintenance support

Weight Management DPG #26

The Weight Management DPG supports the highest level of professional practice in the prevention and treatment of overweight and obesity throughout the life cycle.

DPG Purpose

The purpose of the Weight Management DPG is to pursue professional excellence in comprehensive weight management by providing professional development and networking opportunities to its members. The group also strives to promote its members within and outside of ADA as a resource in the management of the chronic disease of obesity. This group will focus exclusively in the science and application of weight management prevention and treatment. This group will be a link between the public, organizations, and industry to dietetic professionals with an expertise in weight management.

DPG Benefits

- Newsletter
- Electronic Mailing List (EML)
- Advisory Board of Renown Obesity Experts
- Research Updates
- Resource Lists
- Mentoring Program

Community resources and partnerships
- Referral for additional resources (i.e., self-help and support groups)
- Liaisons with community based programs (i.e., work, school, church)
- Organizational leadership in the community for action or policy development

THE STATE OF OBESITY RESEARCH

Several studies or initiatives are being sponsored by the National Institutes of Health (NIH) and the National Institute of Diabetes, Digestive, and Kidney Disease (NIDDK), and focus on the prevention of obesity. NIH-sponsored workshops have brought together leading researchers who have initiated work on obesity prevention and facilitated the sharing of research information on intervention approaches, outcomes, successes, and challenges to obesity management. (29) The latest workshop report provides recommendations for future efforts in obesity prevention research initiatives including future clinical trials.

A bariatric surgery research consortium was created through NIH funding to provide the infrastructure for bariatric surgical research and coordination of outcomes data. (30) This consortium will provide a resource for clinical research involving the mechanisms by which surgical weight loss interventions affect obesity-related co-morbid conditions, energy expenditure, mechanisms of appetite and nutrient absorption, and psychosocial factors.

Ghrelin, a recently identified hormone, usually plays a role in increasing hunger and food intake. However, researchers have found that individuals who undergo gastric bypass surgery for obesity are significantly lower in the hormone than lean, obese pre-gastric bypass surgical or obese non-surgical subjects. (31) This research may provide clues to the fullness, early satiety, and decreased appetite so common in post-gastric bypass patients. Common questions/concerns this author has encountered pre-operatively from patients include, "I'm afraid I'll be hungry and overeat after the surgery," or "How will I ever be full on such a tiny amount of food!" Explaining this research on ghrelin often assists patients pre-operatively deal with fears of excess uncontrolled food consumption and hunger post-operatively.

The National Weight Control Registry (NWCR) was established in 1994 to study factors associated with successful weight loss maintenance. (32) The NWCR is a longitudinal prospective study of individuals 18 years of age and older, who have successfully maintained a 30-pound or more weight loss for a minimum of one year. As of August 2003, approximately 3000 individuals are enrolled in the registry.

SUMMARY

Weight management presents a dynamic and challenging arena for today's dietetic practitioners. Historically, weight loss approaches have met with variable success. Motivating patients to make permanent long-term lifestyle changes requires nutrition counseling approaches that can empower individuals to self-manage food and physical activity. The booming increase in surgical interventions to diminish meal capacity and, in some cases, cause malabsorption, provides yet another layer of counseling challenges.

Learning Activities

1. Locate demographic statistics on obesity rates for your state and/or local community. What conclusions can you draw? What programs/resources are available for weight management in your local community?

2. Compare and contrast adult and pediatric obesity. What are the key similarities and differences that would impact counseling strategies?

3. Observe three different counseling sessions:
   - Pediatric (child or adolescent)
   - Adult pursuing non-surgical management of obesity
   - Adult pursuing surgical management of obesity

   What components of the clinical assessment did you observe? What components would you have focused on? Describe patient/significant other role in each case.

4. Compare and contrast at least three different types of surgical intervention for obesity management. What are the short- and long-term nutritional implications of each? What key counseling points should be included for each procedure?

References

1. Mokdad AH, Ford ES, Bouman BA, Dietz WH, Vinicor F, Bales VS, Marks JS. Prevalence of obesity, diabetes, and obesity-related health risk factors. *J Am Med Assoc.* 2003; 289 (1): 76-79.
2. *Centers for Disease Control and Prevention. New state data show obesity and diabetes still on the rise.* Department of Health and Human Services Press Release December 31, 2002.
3. Hill JO, Trowbridge FL. Childhood obesity: future directions and research priorities. *Pediatrics.* 1998; 101: 570-574.
4. Guo SS, Roche AF, Chumlea WC, Gardner JD, Siervogel RM. The predictive value of childhood body mass index values for overweight at age 35. *Am J Clin Nutr.* 1994; 59(4): 810-819.
5. *Overweight in children and adolescents: fact sheet.* http://www.surgeongeneral.gov/topics/obesity/calltoaction/fact_adolescents.htm
6. Grodstein F, Levine R, Tray L, Spencer T, Colditz GA, Stampfer MJ. Three-year follow-up of participants in a commerical weight loss program: can you keep it off? *Arch Intern Med.*
7. Foster GD, Wadden TA, Kendall PC, Stunkard AJ, Vogt RA. Psychological effects of weight loss and regain: a prospective evaluation. *J Consult Clin Psychol.* 1996: 64(4): 752-757.
8. http://www.trendsetters.com/health-trend/9001,1,obesity.html Accessed August 4, 2003.
9. Blackburn GL, Miller D, Chan S. Pharmaceutical treatment of obesity. *Nurs Clin North Am.* 1997; 32(4): 831-848.
10. NHLBI Obesity Education Initiative. *Clinical guidelines on the identification, evaluation, and treatment of overweight and obesity in adults: the evidence report.* Washington: National Institutes of Health, 1998.
11. Seidell JC, Bakx JC, DeBoer E, Deurenberg P, Hautvast J. Fat distribution of overweight persons in relation to morbidity and subjective health. *Int J Obesity.* 1985; 9(5): 363-374.
12. Bray GA. *Contemporary diagnosis and management of obesity.* Newtown PA: Handbooks in Health, 1998: pp 140.
13. Hebl MR, Xu J. Weighing the care: physicians' reaction to the size of a patient. *Int J Obes Relat Metab Disord.* 2001; 25(8): 1246-1252.
14. Fontaine KR, Wiersema L. Dieting readiness test fails to predict enrollment in a weight loss program. *J Am Diet Assoc.* 1999; 99(6):664.
15. Pendleton VR, Poston WS, Goodrick GK, Willems EP, Swank PR, Kimball KT, Foreyt JP. The predictive validity of the Diet Readiness Test in a clinical population. *Int J Eat Disord.* 1998; 24(4): 363-369.
16. Brownell KD. Dieting readiness. *Weight Con Digest.* 1990; 1: 5-10.
17. Carlson S, Sonnenberg LM, Cumming S. Dieting readiness test predicts completion in a short-term weight loss program. *J Am Diet Assoc.* 1994; 94(5):552-554.
18. Salzman E, Shah A, Shikora SA. Obesity. In: Gottschlich MM, ed. *The science and practice of nutrition support: a case-based core curriculum.* Dubuque IA: Kendall/Hunt Publishing Company; 2001: pp 677-699.
19. Glynn CC, Greene GW, Winkler MF. Predictive versus measured energy expenditure using limits of agreement analysis in hospitalized, obese patients. *JPEN.* 1999; 23(3): 147-154.
20. Ireton-Jones CS, Francis S. Obesity: nutrition support practice and application to critical care. *Nutr Clin Pract.* 1995; 10(4): 144-149.
21. Pope GD, Birkmeyer JD, Finlayson SR. National trends in utilization and in-hospital outcomes of bariatric surgery. *J Gastrointest Surg.* 2002; 6(6): 855-861.
22. Gastrointestinal surgery for severe obesity. National Institutes of Health Concensus Development Conference Statement. *Am J Clin Nutr.* 1992; 55(2 Suppl.): 615S-619S.
23. http://www.weightlosssurgeryinfo.com/pages/wls/surgery-options.jsp#cr-mp
24. Committee on Nutrition. Prevention of pediatric overweight and obesity. *Pediatrics.* 2003; 112(2): 424-430.

25. Arluk SL, Branch JD, Swain DP, Dowling FA. Childhood obesity's relationship to time spent in sedentary behavior. *Mil Med.* 2003; 168(7): 583-586.
26. Proctor MH, Moore LL, Gao D, Cupples LA, Bradlee ML, Hood MY, Ellison RC. Television viewing and change in body fat from preschool to early adolescence: the Framingham Children's study. *Int J Obes Relat Metab Disord.* 2003; 27(7): 827-833.
27. Meerschaerr CM. Treating obesity: what works? *Today's Dietitian.* 2003; 5(5): 38-40.
28. Glasgow RE, Orleans CT, Wagner EH. Does the chronic care model serve also as a template for improving prevention? *Milbank Q.* 2001; 79: 579-612.
29. National Institutes of Health. *2nd Investigators Workshop on Innovative Approaches to the prevention of Obesity: Workshop Report.* Washington, DC: August 12-13, 2002.
30. *Working Group on Bariatric Surgery: Executive Summary.* May 8-9, 2002 National Institutes of Health, National Institute of Diabetes and Digestive and Kidney Diseases (NIDDK). Accessed at http://www.niddk.nih.gov/fund/crfo/Bariatric-Surgery-final.pdf
31. Tritos NA, Mun E, Bertkau A, Grayson R, Maratos-Flier E, Goldfine A. Erum ghrelin levels in response to glucose load in obese subjets post-gastric bypass surgery. *Obes Res.* 2003; 168(7): 583-586.
32. *National Weight Control Registry* http://www.uchsc.edu/nutrition/WyattJartberg/nwcr.htm

ADDITIONAL READING AND RESOURCES:

Nutrition in Clinical Practice Vol 18 No 2, April 2003 (Entire issue devoted to obesity treatment.)

The National Heart, Lung, and Blood Institute Expert Panel on the Identification, Evaluation, and Treatment of Overweight and Obesity in Adults. Executive Summary of the clinical guidelines on the identification, evaluation, and treatment of overweight and obesity in adults. *J Am Diet Assoc.* 1998; 98(10):1178-1191.

Institute of Medicine. Weighing the options: criteria for evaluating weight-management programs. Washington DC: National Academy Press; 1995.

Rippe JM, ed. The Obesity Epidemic: A mandate for a multidisciplinary approach. October 1998 (a supplement to the Journal of the American Dietetic Association).

Bessesen DH, Kushner R. Evaluation and Management of obesity. Orlando FL: Hanley and Belfus; 2002.

Pediatrics Specific:

Barlow SE, Dietz WH. Obesity evaluation and treatment: expert committee recommendations. *Pediatrics.* 1998; 102(3): e29.

P Bundred, D Kitchiner, I Buchan. Prevalence of overweight and obese children between 1989 and 1998: population based series of cross sectional studies. *BMJ*, February 10, 2001; 322(7282): 326 - 326.

Barlow SE, Dietz WH. Management of child and adolescent obesity: summary and recommendations based on reports from pediatricians, pediatric nurse practitioners, and registered dietitians. *Pediatrics.* 2002 Jul;110(1 Pt 2):236-8. Review.

Ikeda J. Dietary approaches to the treatment of overweight pediatric patients: childhood and adolescent obesity. *Pediatric Clinics of North America* 2001;18(1): 966-968.

Nichols MR, Livingston D. Preventing pediatric obesity: assessment and management in the primary care setting. *J Am Acad Nurse Pract.* 2002 Feb;14(2):55-62; quiz 63-5. Review.

Prevalence of overweight among children and adolescents: United States, 1999-2000; http://www.cdc.gov/nchs/products/pubs/pubd/hestats/overwght99.htm

Story MT, Neumark-Stzainer DR, Sherwood NE, Holt K, Sofka D, Trowbridge FL, Barlow SE. Management of child and adolescent obesity: attitudes, barriers, skills, and training needs among health care professionals. *Pediatrics*. 2002 Jul;110(1 Pt 2):210.

Wray S, Levy-Milne R. Weight management in childhood: Canadian dietitians' practices. *Can J Diet Pract Res*. 2002 Fall;63(3):130-3.

WEBSITES: GENERAL REFERENCE

Centers for Disease Control: Obesity Trends
www.cdc.gov/nccdphp/dnpa/obesity/trend/index.htm
View online or download Obesity Trends slides to see the spread of the U.S. waistline.

Clinical Guidelines on the Identification, Evaluation, and Treatment of Overweight and Obesity in Adults
www.nhlbi.nih.gov/guidelines/obesity/ob_home.htm
Publications available in full-text online or downloadable versions in PDF and for Palm OS users, includes interactive BMI calculator.

NHLBI Obesity Education Initiative
www.nhlbi.nih.gov/about/oei/index.htm
OEI was developed to reduce the occurrence of obesity and physical inactivity associated with cardiovascular disease. Consumer and professional publications and programs are available, along with an online menu planner.

NIDDK National Taskforce on Prevention and Treatment of Obesity
www.niddk.nih.gov/fund/divisions/DDN/obesitytaskforce.htm
Access practitioner reports/statements based on synthesis and critical analysis of current scientific finding for the treatment and prevention of obesity.

Weight Control Information Network
www.niddk.nih.gov/health/nutrit/win.htm
Science based information on obesity, weight control, and nutrition. The site includes publications (including fact sheets and brochures), a quarterly newsletter for health professionals, information on ordering audiovisual and educational materials, and a listing of weight loss and control organizations and resources.

Certificate of Training in Adult Weight Management Program
Over half of American adults are overweight or obese. A dietetics professional, trained to have a comprehensive knowledge of the field and management options, can enable long-term patient compliance and sustained success. This program is designed to produce providers of comprehensive weight management care who also know when and how to refer patients to other specialists. It is open to ADA members, RDs, and DTRs.

The Certificate of Training Offers:
- cutting edge information and skills shared by leading practitioners in the field
- cases and exercises to allow hands-on experience
- valuable resource materials and tools for immediate use and future reference
- an opportunity to showcase your expertise by earning a Certificate of Training.
- 27 continuing professional education units

What's Involved?
There are three components to the training program: a self-study module (6-8 hours of readings, activities, and a pre-test), a 2 1/2 day live workshop, and a post test. You must pass the pre-test to attend the workshop. After successful completion of the course and take-home post-test, a Certificate of Training in Adult Weight Management suitable for framing is awarded.

What's Covered?
Current Research and Future Possibilities... Clinical Management of Overweight and Obesity... OTC Dietary Supplements... Behavior Modification... Application of Popular Diets and Weight Loss Programs... Formulas for Weight Loss... Medical Complications of Weight Loss... Role of Exercise... Pharmacotherapy... Bariatric Surgery as a Treatment Option...Case Studies

For more information, please contact CDR by e-mail at **weightmgmt@eatright.org** or call 1-800-877-1600, ext. 5500.

American Obesity Association
www.obesity.org

Websites: Pediatric Obesity
www.hugs.com A non-diet program with a component for teens designed to instill confidence for personal decisions on health, energy, and emotional needs.

www.committed-to-kids.com Tools and resources for an individualized approach to weight management conducted in an outpatient, group setting.

www.trimkids.com Unique twelve-week plan that gives parents and children a positive, safe initial approach to lifetime weight management.

www.waytogokids.com Nutrition and fitness program for kids designed specifically for registered dietitians to teach overweight and under-active kids ages 8 to 13 years.

www.shapedown.com Involves families in creating an active lifestyle and a healthy diet using age-appropriate materials for children, adolescents, and parents.

www.fns.usda.gov/tn/default.htm USDA's Team Nutrition site where the goal is to improve children's lifelong eating and physical activity habits by using the principles of the Dietary Guidelines for Americans and the Food Guide Pyramid.

www.walktoschool.org Walk to School Initiative; links and resources for anyone interested in creating a more walkable community for children and parents.

www.actionforhealthykids.org Action for Healthy Kids Initiative; information, tools, and resources to help improve kids' health and educational performance through better nutrition and physical activity in schools.

www.healthykidschallenge.com Nationally recognized program offering a multi-level approach of assistance to schools and communities for making a healthy difference for kids.

www.kidnetic.com Interactive site for kids with a focus on increased activity and healthy diet; tells kids about how their body works, how eating right helps them play better and feel good and how staying active is lots of fun!

www.brightfutures.org/nutrition/index.html Emphasizes prevention and early recognition of nutrition concerns for infancy through adolescence; nutrition guidelines and tools for healthy child nutrition practices.

http://www.mchlibrary.info/KnowledgePaths/kp_childnutr.html Child and adolescent nutrition resources and tools for health professionals, educators, researchers, and parents.

Chapter 16

Empowerment and Nondiet:
Using the Feminist Therapy Perspective

Monica A. Dixon, PhD, RD
Author, Love The Body You Were Born With!

After reading this chapter, the reader will be able to:

♦ Identify two major assumptions in counseling women using feminist theory.

♦ Describe counseling issues related to external pressures that may affect the nutrition habits of women.

♦ Identify "stuckness" in counseling a client and describe appropriate methods to address the issue.

In private practice, nutrition therapists counsel more women clients than men, more women with eating disorders, and a disproportionate number of clients with obesity as a primary or secondary diagnosis. As mentioned earlier in this book, white men of Northern European heritage developed the major counseling therapies commonly used in the U.S. Because of the limitations of their orientations, new types of therapy have emerged to better accommodate and match the needs of other segments of the population. Multicultural and Feminist therapies are two of the more recent therapies to evolve.

Feminist therapy is typified by three basic tenets: 1) a close counselor-advocate to client relationship, 2) bolstering a person's self-image, and 3) empowerment. As counseling in general becomes more relationship-oriented, this therapy does not seem so novel as it once did. Now that traditional gender roles are less well defined and men face many of the same social pressures as women like weight biases, this type of therapy has broader application.

WOMEN AND WEIGHT ISSUES

Few Americans eat simply in response to hunger. We eat because the clock deems it is time, dinner is ready, we really SHOULD have that glass of milk, our friend offers us a "bite" of a new dessert, the special included "all you could eat," or the hot cookies just came from the oven.

Quietly lurking beneath our "land of plenty" hide many complicated and emotional issues involving food, dieting, and feelings about one's body. The prescription of a 1400-calorie diet to an overweight person is seldom a sufficient or effective method in attaining weight loss goals. Adherence to the dietary regimen becomes difficult if not impossible for many clients in light of other more pressing needs that may not be getting resolved. The exploration of these needs in the nutrition counseling session can help increase the chances of success for the client, yet will demand the keenest of counseling skills.

Dietitians may feel uncomfortable or unqualified to encounter issues besides food with a client, even though these issues may be deeply woven and inextricable parts of their clients' eating behaviors. Although there are areas that dietitians are not qualified to enter into in the counseling session, all can assist in empowering the client for greater success. Dietitians should have insight into the tenets of feminist psychology, enhancement of counseling skills and increased confidence in one's intuitive nature to determine acceptable counseling limits.

The first step in separating complicated weight issues with women is the perspective gained when viewing clients through a feminist view of psychology that praises the feminine in all women and does not stereotype them under the male model of psychological thought. Women have an entirely different set of life experiences from men, therefore, adopting a feminist perspective in counseling is an essential first step in empowering female clients. Feminist therapy (1) may be characterized as allowing clients to determine their own destinies without the construction of culturally prescribed sex-role stereotypes based upon assumed biological differences. This approach attempts to work toward equality in personal power between females and males. It allows women the space and skills to design a personal vision for their lives that is grounded in their unique and individual needs.

> **A feminist perspective of women's weight issues is essential if we are to move away from the ineffective "blaming-the-victim" approach, the endless behavioral modification treatments, or the "deep-rooted psychological problems of the obese" perspective.**

The feminist viewpoint insists that those painful personal experiences arise from the social setting into which females are born, and within which they develop to become adult women. The fact that compulsive eating and eating disorders are overwhelmingly a woman's problem suggests that it has less to do with individual experiences and more to do with the social context in which women live their lives.

TWO GUIDING ASSUMPTIONS OF FEMINIST THERAPY

First Assumption: Look to the Environment

There are two guiding assumptions offered by feminist therapy that closely relate to women's weight issues. The first of these is that *the primary source of women's pathology is social, not personal; and external, not internal.* (2) This does not discount the woman's role and responsibility in the choices she makes as an adult in relationships, career, and so on. In your counseling, seek to be constantly aware of external forces that have brought the client to you. How has this woman's life been influenced by the social context she lives in? What external forces are influencing the decisions she has made? How independent, codependent, or dependent is this woman in the context of her daily life? How connected is this woman to those passions that drive her life, offer her purpose and reason for living, and provide the foundations of her existence?

External pressures to conform to the cultural model. The cultural worship of thinness in America is a significant external force on women and can hold enormous power for many. Although this value is external, it has been internalized by many American women, as is evidenced by the skyrocketing of eating disorders and obsessive dieting. (3) How many of us have seen clients who come for weight loss, yet are not considered obese by medical standards? Or clients who want to lose ten pounds only for their class reunion or a big party coming up? Recognition and discussion of this power in the counseling session is an important first step in setting the stage for further growth for the client. There are several methods of doing this:

1. Ask the client to go back to previous stages in her life and describe the feelings she had about her body. How did she feel as a child? What types of messages did she receive about her growing body? What types of comments does she remember hearing about her body during puberty? What were the feelings she had about food and her relationship with it? How did her feelings about her body and food affect her social relationships as she grew into adulthood?

2. Help her to identify where she received the messages about how much she should weigh. Was it her parents? Her physician? Her boyfriend or husband? Her girlfriends? Or was the magical number one she pulled from a hat? Have different individuals had varying effects on her weight goals throughout the years? Identifying where her weight goals have come from can aid her in beginning to see how external goals have been determined for her by others.

3. Gather a weight history from the client during the initial assessment. Find out her weight at high school graduation, during college or her early years and before and after childbirth if she has children. Search for a specific picture of how the natural female life cycle has altered both her weight and her perceptions of it.

4. Have her identify a time in her life when she was most pleased with her weight, felt comfortable, happy and relatively healthy. Is this weight realistic for her now? What types of things did she have to do to maintain that weight and is she willing to do them again?

5. Ask her for specific reasons she is pursuing nutrition counseling at this time. Have her identify why she feels the time is right for her, especially if prior attempts at lifestyle change have not been remarkably successful. What factors in her life have changed that will make it work for her now? This helps to begin to put the responsibility on the client for the changes she will make in future sessions with you.

These questions and explorations can help the client to identify an internal goal that she may be happier with than an external goal that may have been influenced by someone else. She can also separate the "shoulds" regarding weight from a healthy and individual weight goal. They can also help you assess her readiness at this point to make lifestyle changes. Too often, dietitians feel obligated to continue with the counseling process, even when they have a "gut feeling" or sometimes even obvious evidence that the client is not ready to adopt the changes being recommended. Perhaps the client is initiating counseling for reasons related to external pressures to change their weight without having thought through her own preferences first. Gathering this information during the initial session can help both the counselor and client save valuable time, money, and effort by assessing direction or desires clearly at the outset.

External forces want women to conform to cultural stereotypes. Social forces play other important roles in women's lives besides their view of how they should look and weigh. It is difficult, if not impossible, to get a woman to begin an exercise program if she is the prime provider of care for four young children or if she bears the burden of all the housework. It becomes important for success in the weight management process to help the woman construct a view of her present reality that will help her in defining and working toward her goals. In addition to acquiring the requisite dietary history/assessment, gather information from the woman so you can "mentally" draw a picture of her life.

1. **Ask her to describe a typical day.** What does she do? What responsibilities does she have? How does she spend her time?
2. **Ask her about additional responsibilities.** What committees does she serve on, groups she volunteers with or other situations in her life that occupy her time. This will help you begin to view her life as a complete picture and aid her in designing realistic goals that will be successful within her own framework.
3. **What type of things is she doing she doesn't necessarily enjoy?** Are there responsibilities she may give up in favor of completing her lifestyle and health goals?

Gathering this information will help you determine how realistic her weight change and personal goals are. You will also gain a sense of her readiness to alter her life with the guidance you have to offer.

External forces and "stuckness" cause havoc in women's lives. For many women, being caught in the trap of "today" and the stress of everyday life does not afford the opportunity to look to the future and envision where the treadmill of life is taking them. The term "stuckness" is a highly descriptive term coined by Fritz Perls (4) to describe the opposite of "intentionality," or purpose and direction in life. Other words used to describe "stuckness" are immobility, inability to achieve goals, or limited life script. The nutrition counselor using advanced level skills will be able to help the client recognize "stuckness" and enable her to take the steps necessary to move on. Often, clients will come to the nutrition counselor because they are stuck with old eating habits and old ways of seeing their body, or they have grown tiresome of "yo-yo" dieting and seek intentionality in their lifestyle habits.

Begin by asking the woman to draw you a mental picture of where she would like to be in five years. What will she look like? Who will she socialize with? Where will she live? How will she spend her days? What will she do for leisure? What type of work will she do? Allow her to tap into her creative powers to draw this vision. Let her relax and her thoughts flow. Do not interrupt her nor judge her. Seldom are we allowed the safety of being able to "dream." You are there to listen.

Some clients will have a very difficult time with this exercise. They may respond, "Well, gee, I never really thought about it" or "I have absolutely no idea!" Clients such as these are clearly manifesting their "stuckness" in life and are perfect candidates for help in broadening their vision of the future. Urge her on. Encourage her to begin to identify thoughts she may only have remotely sketched out for her future, such as, "I often think about returning to night school to finish my degree," or, "I would love to take a dance class and be involved in a dance group." The main goal is to allow her "mind wander" to what could be in her future. The external pressures felt by many women in our society do not always allow their thought processes to think about the bigger picture.

This exercise can be used in a variety of ways. I have often found it extremely helpful when working with an eating disordered client who may be amenorrheic or so caught up in binge/purge or dieting cycles that she can't find her way out. "How will you get from not menstruating to birthing the children you dream about?" or "How might you graduate from college if you can't go to your classes because of your laxative use?" It is also helpful in allowing your client to begin to free herself from what her external circumstances may have dictated she follow, such as family and friends' expectations, which may not necessarily mesh with the goals your client has dreamed of pursuing.

It is important to pay serious consideration to the incredible amount of energy continued dieting demands from a woman. Constantly thinking about what to eat or not eat, when and how much to exercise, counting calories and fat grams, reading diet books and beating themselves up over their failure to have the perfect body all combine to drain a woman's soul. With weight loss maintenance recidivism rates nearing 98%, the majority of women are squandering valuable internal resources on unattainable externally defined goals. Attention to this in the nutrition counseling session can help women invest their personal resources to work toward a healthy balance of mind, body and spirit.

Counseling Skills Necessary in Changing The Paradigms
Helping a client draw a road map to their future goals requires some advanced level counseling skills. These include:

1. Observe your client's nonverbal behavior. Watch for indicators of discomfort, as you may be treading on areas that are very sensitive to the client. Is the client crossing her arms in front of her to fend you off, or leaning toward you indicating excitement about the ideas? What kinds of expressions are on her face? Use the client's comments to provide cues for the direction of your future questioning.

2. Note the client's verbal behavior. Does the client sound angry and resentful when discussing her plans for the future, or excited and determined? Does she express anger at others in her life? Regrets? Happiness? The counseling skill of active listening is one of the most important. Hear what your client has to say, not just what you want her to say. Our world would be a better place if more people really listened to others.

3. Your most important skill will be determining client discrepancies. Watch for incongruities, mixed messages, contradiction, and conflict throughout the interview. An effective counselor will be able to identify these discrepancies, to name them appropriately, and when appropriate, to feed them back to the client. These discrepancies may be between nonverbal behaviors (client is laughing while describing the total sense of powerlessness she feels about dieting), between two statements (client says she really wants to be thinner but cannot give up any type of high-fat foods), between what clients say and what they do (client says she wants to lose weight but continually misses appointments), or between statements and nonverbal behavior (client says she loves low-calorie foods, but hangs her head and looks at the floor while she talks about them). They may also represent a conflict between people or between a client and a situation (client says her family has attempted to enforce a diet on her since she was ten).

As these examples demonstrate, incongruity is common in the nutrition counseling process. Using confrontational skills appropriately can help move your client toward intentionality. While all counseling skills are concerned with development, it is the confrontation of these discrepancies that acts as the lever for the activation of human potential. It is actually a combination of skills such as open-ended questioning, confrontation, and feedback that often results in a client's examination of core issues. With some clients, it may be adequate simply to identify and label the incongruity with the client. *Focus on the elements of the incongruity, and not the person. Often the simple question, "How do you put these two together?" will lead a client to begin thinking about her inconsistency and possible resolution.*

If this is not effective, you may need to move to summarizing the incongruity for the client. "Mrs. Jones, on the one hand you say that you really wish to lose weight, but on the other hand you say you will not eat low-fat foods," or " Jennifer, you say that you really want to start changing your diet, but each week you come without having done your food records." Follow this with, "How does that fit for you?" Many clients are unaware of their incongruities and mixed messages; pointing them out gently but firmly can be extremely beneficial to them. For some clients, even your summarization will be inadequate to help them recognize their inconsistencies, and only your repeated disclosure of the discrepancy over time will help them move away from denial of the problem and accept responsibility.

The Road Map to Change

Now that you have gathered your data regarding your client's perceptions of her weight, her feelings toward her goals and identified any discrepancies she may have, it is time to move her from here to there. The next step in this process is to help the client identify her resources, both external and internal. Resources can be defined as anything that will be helpful to the client in attempting to work toward her goals. It is also important to identify those forces that will hold her back or act as barriers to her goals.

Suppose that the vision your client has created involves having a healthy body one year from now that she feels proud of, buys nice clothes for, and treats with respect. What type of resources will help her get there? Does she need money to join her local exercise club? Does she need to buy a set of running shoes? Does she need to go to the library and check books out about exercise programs or meet with an exercise physiologist? Does she have friends who will exercise with her? Is she the tenacious type, who will be determined to follow her goal? Does she need someone to watch the children while she is gone? Each resource that the two of you can help her identify will move her closer to her goals. Many women aren't accustomed to thinking about what they have going for them in their personal inventory.

Your client will face obstacles to her success. What types of forces will work against her? Does her best friend offer her donuts every time she attempts to begin exercising? Will her partner support her or sabotage her efforts? Does she procrastinate when given a difficult task? Is her employer accommodating to a schedule change? Is there money available to buy the things she might need to get started? If not, how will she find the money?

Helping your client identify her resources and assets will demand creativity on both your parts. Helping her to change the paradigms of thinking that have restricted her ability to see things from a variety of different perspectives will surely stretch your imagination. The more well thought out the barriers and assets are that she will meet in her endeavors, the greater her chances for success, as she will meet few obstacles she has not already thought out in her session with you.

In the goal setting and resource inventory stages with the client, it is important to allow the client to develop her own ideas. She MUST own the solutions to her problems. Some dietitians I have worked with often become frustrated and upset because the course of action for a client is so obviously clear, and why don't they "just do it"? **Your position is to empower their process, not design it. The road map must be drawn and owned by the client.** If not, chances for success are slim. Solving her concerns and giving her solutions only makes you guilty of exactly that which you are attempting to disassemble—pressure to conform to an external model she must live under.

Following are key concepts for an empowerment-based practice, no matter the diagnosis or gender of the client: (5)

- Emphasis on the whole person
- Setting negotiated goals
- Transference of decision-making and leadership
- Promotion of the person's inherent drive towards health and wellness
- Education for informed choices about treatment options
- Patient selection of learning needs
- Self-generation of problems and solutions
- Treatment plans viewed as ongoing experiments

Case Study

The following is a scenario that may help you in visualizing this process at work:

Audrey is a 19-year-old client who presents with symptoms of Anorexia Nervosa. She is referred by her physician referral, due to recent weight loss and onset of amenorrhea, but has not yet been given the DSM diagnosis of Anorexia Nervosa. Audrey insists that she is eating well and is getting plenty of food. The diet history you gather reflects otherwise. Her protein and calorie intake are exceedingly low for her height and weight. Throughout your first and second session with Audrey, she continues to insist that she is eating adequate calories and does not need to eat anymore. As you develop a rapport with her, you sense that there are incongruities in her message, and in fact, she is experiencing significant hunger pains, dizziness, and apathy.

Audrey: *I'm really feeling better than I ever have in my life. I really don't understand why everyone is making such a fuss.* (Client states denial.)

Counselor: You say you are feeling quite good, yet last week you complained about feeling tired and unable to get through your workday. How does that fit for you?
(Counselor points out discrepancy in information.)

Audrey: *Well, that is just sometimes. I usually feel almost euphoric and in control of my life.*
(Client again denies a problem.)

Counselor: Tell me how you feel in control of your life.
(Counselor uses open-ended question to gather more information.)

Audrey: *I am strong and I can make my own decisions about the food I eat. No one else can tell me what to do. My mom used to always try to make me eat certain foods and now I can do what I want to.* (Client seeking identity through resistance.)

Counselor: What other kinds of things do you want to do? (Counselor works toward moving client out of current paradigm of "stuckness" and looking at future.)

Audrey: *I'd like to get into college eventually when I save enough money and I would like to get married and I suppose have some kids.*
(Client identifies some disconnected, not clearly defined goals.)

Counselor: How will you save enough money to get into college if you are missing so much work because you are weak and tired now?
(Counselor identifies discrepancy between verbal statement and actions.)

Audrey: *Well, I suppose sometimes I don't feel I have the energy I used to, but that really has more to do with my heavy schedule, don't you think?*
(Client is beginning to internalize the discrepancies and seek counselor's approval.)

Counselor: It has more to do with the lack of calories your body is getting to do the things you need to do today. What you eat today and tomorrow and the next day not only fuels your body to have the energy to do your daily activities, but it also affects your attitude and the way your body will perform in the future. Your menstrual cycle will not return until you provide your body enough calories for the rest of its activities, and you will probably not have children until your menstrual cycle returns. You will not have the strength to complete your studies until you eat enough calories. Only you can make the changes in your diet that will result in a healthy future for you. (Counselor confronts client with reality of her actions and behaviors and focuses responsibility on client.)

Audrey: *I guess I never really thought about those things. But I am pretty afraid. And what kind of food can I eat that will not make me "blimp out"?*
(Client identifies fear of change, but ability to begin the process.)

At this point, the counselor has confronted Audrey with her inconsistencies in her statements, helped her identify a vision for her future that is incongruent with her activities today, and helped increase Audrey's awareness that the responsibility rests on her to change. Obviously, a client of this background would be much more complicated to work with, and results would never be this quick, but the confrontation and movement toward intentionality process has begun.

The Second Guiding Assumption: Each Individual Must Still Take Responsibility

Feminist therapy includes viewing a woman in the social context within which she lives her life, and using that information to help her move towards creating her own vision of the future void of the "stuckness" she may have exhibited. The second assumption of feminist therapy important for the nutrition counselor is that the focus on environmental stress as a major source of pathology is *not* used as an avenue of escape from individual responsibility. (2) Each individual, regardless of her social condition, is responsible for making the changes necessary within her own life. No one else, including the counselor, can maintain that responsibility. Feminist therapy believes that women must be free to make their own decisions. In many cases this may require therapy work that is beyond the scope of the nutrition counselor, yet there are appropriate nutrition counseling strategies that can begin the process to help women regain power and control over their own lives.

Since women are expected to devote enormous energy to the lives of others, often the boundaries between their own lives and the lives of those close to them become blurred. Molding their lives to others' concerns, feeding others, or not knowing how to make time in their lives for themselves are frequent issues for women. A mother is constantly at the beck and call of others; everyone else's needs become more important. This becomes important in weight counseling sessions as the woman returns week after week never having found the time to complete the tasks you have jointly agreed upon. She may be having difficulty defining her needs as important in the greater family picture.

Although this may be an appropriate time for the use of the confrontation skills discussed earlier, it is also an appropriate time for aiding her in learning to set her own boundaries. For some women, they are treading into unfamiliar territory. She must begin by first determining what exactly is hers in terms of time, goals, and resources. Assist her in defining limits. What block of time during the day can she save only for herself? What must she give up in order to find the time? What benefits would she gain? Who else can she delegate responsibility to? Where does she begin and others end? In my many years of counseling women, I have found this is by far the most difficult task, primarily because of societal expectations about what the "ideal" woman should be and also lack of learning in the early years that our identities and needs are separate and unique from others.

Help the woman explore her uniqueness and individuality. Ask her what traits she has that make her different from others in her life. How can she use those traits as assets to alter her lifestyle and pursue her own goals? Give her homework where she establishes her needs with significant others in her life and discusses how they can help with her new lifestyle changes. Clients have had great success with a small assignment I have them do each morning. Answer on a sheet of paper the questions, "Today I want..." and "Today I feel..." Many of your clients will say, "I want....WHAT??? I don't understand what you mean." You will need to teach them how to identify their wants in life. Do they *want* to go out to lunch with their nagging friend? Do they *want* to take a short nap today to catch up on lost sleep? Do they *want* to clean the house, or would a walk in the woods be more desirable? The same happens with "Today I feel..." Help them learn to pinpoint their feelings each day. A wonderful quote I use from Alice Koller's book, *An Unknown Woman* (6) is *"Is this thing I'm doing worth being alive for?"*

Most importantly, how much better could she meet the needs of others in her life if she allotted time for her own needs first? A garden left unattended in the hot sun proffers no fruit. Women, much like gardens, need frequent water, healthy, nourishing food, fresh air, and adequate rest. Nurturing our own needs first and taking great care of our powerful bodies puts us far ahead when needing to nurture others.

Change Does Not Come Without Risk

"And the trouble is, if you don't risk anything, you risk even MORE." Erica Jong

Risks to the Counselor. Empowering women to accept responsibility for their own lives, establish decisive boundaries, determine their own goals, and create a vision for their future does not come without risk. There is risk involved for both the counselor and the client. Awareness of these risks will help you determine ahead of time how far you feel comfortable pushing the limits.

The risks to the counselor are that you may broach significant emotional issues the woman has had hidden for some time. Ironically, using your advanced level counseling skills to establish a unique rapport with the client can put you in the position of being the first person that really *ever* sat and listened to her at length. You must be prepared for numerous types of latent concerns that can provoke great emotion in your client. Remembering life goals that have been waylaid, prior sexual trauma, verbal or physical abuse, and current domestic violence at home or within the family can all come to the forefront in your sessions. You must be prepared to deal with these issues. Think through your own feelings. Many advanced counselors can benefit from seeking counseling themselves to understand where they stand on important life issues. Be sure you have resolved your own troubles with these emotional traumas before you attempt to help someone else discuss them. In addition, learn to pay attention to your senses and intuition. I believe that far too much emphasis has been put on "proper" ethical counseling behavior, and not enough on the human side. For many of your female clients who become upset over emotional wounds, a hug and a shoulder to cry on may be the best immediate response you can give them. Trust your own intuition and the knowledge you gather from the client, both verbal and nonverbal, to determine when a hug might be necessary or when a referral to a specialized therapist is necessary.

I remember a client early in my career that came to me with little in her charts except notes by a frustrated physician unable to get information from her. She appeared to be significantly underweight, pale and with poor affect. She never responded verbally to me once during our entire first session. I reluctantly set an appointment for a second session with her. The entire week following her visit I spent trying to determine what the problem was and how I might help her nearly catatonic state. At her second appointment, I walked to her and held her. Again, she never uttered a word, but cried in my arms for her entire second session. Finally, on her third visit she began to slowly speak to me about the Anorexia Nervosa that was rampaging her body. Only through connecting with her on a basic human level was I able to get from her information that she did not disclose to her physician and school counselors.

Risks to the Client. The risk to the client who is learning to empower her life can be great as well. A woman who decisively makes lifestyle changes, pursues her goals, and with determination follows her dreams can be an intimidating force to a partner who is unaccustomed to seeing his mate behave this way. Her newfound self, sense of boundaries, and freedom to choose her destiny may be setting her up for abusive situations with her partner if he is a batterer. This is one of the many risks of being in the counseling business, yet another responsibility the client must own. You cannot take responsibility of this magnitude upon yourself. Refer women who are at risk to the local Women's Shelter, found in the phone book, or refer them to the National Domestic Abuse Hotline at 1-800-333-7233. All women's shelters maintain advocates who can help your client get help and protection. The call must be the responsibility of your client. The social support networks can do nothing until the battered woman herself takes the first step. Even well trained domestic abuse counselors experience the frustration of being unable to intervene. This number can be helpful to you as well in gaining information on how to identify potential battering, determining the level of danger a woman may be in, or learning of other resources available in your area. Although the risk of this situation happening may be slim, it is important information for the counselor who concerns herself with the greater picture of her clients' lives.

Where Does Nondiet Fit?

The Nondiet approach to weight counseling originated from the 1970's women's movement when people started recognizing that women were treated differently than men regarding weight and health issues. (7) Over the past thirty years this movement has grown in popularity and developed into what is referred to as Health At Every Size (HAES). (7,8,9,10) The basic conceptual framework includes acceptance of: (7)

- The natural diversity in body shape and size
- The ineffectiveness and dangers of dieting
- The importance of relaxed eating in response to internal body cues
- The critical contribution of social, emotional, and spiritual, as well as physical, factors to health and happiness

See Table 16.1 for a comparison of the traditional approach to weight and health enhancement. HAES philosophies can be found in the books: *Moving Away From Diets*, 2nd edition by Kratina, King, and Hayes, *Big Fat Lies* by Gaesser, and *Intuitive Eating* by Tribole and Reisch. (See Suggested Additional Reading.)

For the practitioner using the HAES approach, assessment and treatment of a client's health status proceeds in the same manner regardless of the person's weight: address the present health problem, do not make size-related assumptions (thin clients may be sedentary and have poor habits), provide reasons not to diet, and focus on other well-being parameters. (7)

Figure 16.1

Comparing Traditional and Health at Every Size (HAES) Approaches to Health Enhancement

	Traditional Approach	**HAES Approach**
Ideology	Excessive fatness, as defined by standardized tables, is unhealthy. Goal is weight loss or weight maintenance.	Healthy weight is highly individualized and cannot be determined by a standardized table. The healthiest weight is a natural weight one can maintain without dieting, Goal is to enhance health and treat medical problems if present.
Weight	Counsel clients to reach and maintain the defined weight even if it means permanent food restriction.	Teach clients that the body will seek its natural weight as one eats in response to bodily cues and is physically active. This weight may be higher than society advocates.
Hunger	Assist clients to suppress or ignore hunger in order to be able to follow meal plan. Hunger and satiety typically irrelevant in eating patterns.	Assist clients to relearn to eat in response to internal cues of hunger and satiety. Explain that doing so (most of the time) will aid the body in returning to and maintaining natural weight and reinforce need to trust these cues.
Food	Externally regulated eating. Counsel clients to follow meal plan, teach avoidance of "bad," "illegal," or "unhealthy" foods and to use cognitive behavioral methods to restrict caloric intake. If clients relapse, counsel to return to food plan.	Internally regulated eating. Explain to clients food is not the problem, but *restricting* certain foods is (making food forbidden and more desirable); therefore, no foods are forbidden. Assist clients with a gentle openness that allows them to listen to their bodies' feedback without judgment. They will begin to desire healthier food when they have nonjudgmental free access to all foods.
Self/Size Accept-ance	Assist with weight loss because clients will feel better about themselves at closer to an ideal weight. Clients typically feel more powerful when starting diet but lose self-esteem if they are one of the 95% of those who fail to lose and maintain weight loss.	Work with clients to increase self-esteem and personal power from self-determined eating style and movement. Help clients realize that healthy bodies come in all shapes and sizes; cultural norms can be dangerous, and pursuit of them can interfere with quality of life. Refer clients to support for reinforcement required to make these changes.
Trust/ Distrust of Self and Body	Clients' trust is put in the health care provider. Clients often come to distrust their own body and sense of judgment, especially when there is a history of failure with dieting.	Teach clients to trust themselves and their bodies. Trust in other areas builds as clients learn they can eat when hungry, stop when satisfied, and enjoy movement. Ensure clients are learning to live without judgment or criticism of own or others' weight and eating.

Rethinking the Nutrition Counseling Paradigm

Feminist therapy differs from traditional therapies in that it views women's problems as being external in origin and influenced by the social setting in which women live. It encompasses a broader and more descriptive view of the specific world women exist in and the lifespan issues that women face that are unique to being a woman in our society. The social stresses that women live under are not viewed as an exemption from personal and individual responsibility. Every woman is entitled to learn to establish her own boundaries, create her own vision for her life plan, determine her future goals, and choose healthy lifestyle choices to empower her body to seek her goals. Nutrition counselors will find that adapting a feminist perspective to counseling women can enhance their chances for success. The nutrition counselor is the woman's ally in her unique and individual process, gently challenging, prompting, prodding, and supporting her growth in changing her current paradigms.

To see how this theory can be adapted to counseling by a man to men and women clients with disordered eating and gross obesity, read the personal story by Bob Wilson, DTR in Appendix 16-A. Today, Bob is going a step further by bringing spirituality, self-nurturing, and placing self-love before trying to care-take and nurture others in order to recover and live a more balanced life.

> *"The symptoms people come to me with are really their deep emotional process work and they are asking me to shut it off so they can continue to live their busy, rushing lives, and avoid their process. "*
> *Anonymous Physician*

Learning Activities

1. Attend a group weight management session of your choice where the majority of participants are women. Listen closely to conversations/discussions regarding weight issues. What do you learn? Can you identify external pressures related to culture? "Stuckness"?

2. Observe a counseling session for a woman with weight management issues, preferably with a therapist trained in counseling. How does the therapist address cultural issues? What strategies are used to identify weight issues?

3. Analyze one popular woman's magazine *from the feminist therapy perspective*. What issues do you identify? What impact do you suspect this has on women? How would you change the publication?

Suggested Additional Reading

Bordo S. *Unbearable weight: feminism, western culture and the body.* Berkeley: Univ. of Calif. Press; 1995.

In this provocative book Bordo untangles the myths, ideologies, and pathologies of the modern female body. Likening the womanly form to the image of a voracious animal of "unbearable weight," Bordo explores our tortured fascination with food, hunger, desire, and control and its effects on women's lives. A fascinating read for anyone involved in counseling women with weight issues.

Dixon M. *Love the body you were born with!* New York: Putnam; 1996.

An interactive workbook to use with clients that can change the way they think and treat their bodies. By working through the entertaining, thought-provoking steps, women will gain the knowledge and the strength they need to get off the diet roller coaster, stop abusing their body, and begin appreciating themselves for the powerful and wonderful person they are! A MUST for every woman who has ever squandered her resources by dieting or beaten herself up for not being thin enough.

Kratina K, King N, Hayes D. *Moving Away From Diets: Healing Eating Problems and Exercise Resistance,* 2nd edition. Lake Dallas, TX: Helm Publishing; 2003.

This classic book is for counselors who want to learn about and embrace the nondiet/ Health At Every Size tenets. It covers the nondiet research, philosophies, and therapy to re-teach clients about healthy eating and movement for fun. Best selling self-study courses for dietitians and nurses with camera-ready handouts.

Omichinski L. ***You Count, Calories Don't.*** Winnipeg, Canada: Hugs International;1992.

    This was one of the first books published by a dietitian on the nondiet approach to weight counseling. Linda provides a wealth of thoughtful ideas and strategies.

Orbach S. ***Fat is a feminist issue.*** New York: Berkley Group; 1978.

    Orbach's book pioneered the field of compulsive overeating and its relationship to the cultural stereotypes and roadblocks' women find themselves trapped in. Orbach's classic book details many methods of implementing feminist psychology into therapy with women suffering with compulsive overeating or eating disorders.

Pinkola Estes C. ***Women who run with the wolves: myths and stories of the wild woman archetype***. New York: Ballantine Books; 1997.

    Within every woman there is a wild and natural creature, a powerful force, filled with good instincts, passionate creativity, and ageless knowing. Her name is Wild Woman, but she is an endangered species. Though the gifts of wildish nature come to us at birth, society's attempt to "civilize" us into rigid roles has plundered this treasure, and muffled the deep, life-giving messages of our own souls. This book stretches the current paradigms of thinking about being a woman in our society; not only a useful tool for counselors of women, but also a thought provocative book for every woman who seeks to understand her own individuality and uniqueness.

References
1. Rawlings E, Carter D. *Feminist and nonsexist psychotherapy.* Springfield, IL: Charles C. Thomas; 1977.
2. Brodsky A, Hare-Mustin R, eds. *Feminist therapy.* New York: Guilford; 1980.
3. Fontaine KL. The conspiracy of culture: women's issues in body size. *Nursing Clinics of North America.* 1991; 26: 669-676.
4. Perls *FS. Gestalt Therapy Verbatim.* Moab, UT: Real People Press; 1969.
5. Funnell MM, Anderson RM, Arnold MS. Empowerment: A winning model for diabetes care. *Practical Diabetology.* 1991: May-June: 15-18.
6. Koller A. *An Unknown Woman: a journey to self-discovery.* New York: Bantam; 1983.
7. Robison J, Kratina K. An Alternative: Health at Every Size, Health for Every Body. In: Kratina K, King N, Hayes D. *Moving Away From Diets,* 2nd ed. Lake Dallas, TX: Helm Publishing; 2003.
8. Satter EM. Internal Regulation and the Evolution of Normal Growth as the Basis for Prevention of Obesity in Children. *J Amer Diet Assoc.* 1996:9:860-64.
9. Berg FM. Nondiet Movement Gains Strength. *Obesity and Health.* 1992; 6:5: 85-90.
10. Omichinski L. *You Count, Calories Don't.* Winnipeg: Hugs International;1992.

Chapter 17

Counseling Clients with Eating Disorders

Eileen Stellefson Meyer, MPH, RD
Adapted from *Winning the War Within: Nutrition Therapy for Anorexia and Bulimia Nervosa*

After reading this chapter, the reader will be able to:
♦ Identify at least three special considerations when working with someone with an eating disorder.
♦ Explain why the language might need to be altered when working with this population.
♦ List five biochemical abnormalities that must be watched.
♦ Calculate a refeeding program for a client.

The role of the Nutrition Therapist is to assist with the normalization of the client's weight and eating behavior. It is useful to break these tasks down into eight basic principles: (1)
1. Recognize the client's symptoms and DSM-IV criteria for diagnosing an eating disorder.
2. Evaluate the client's current food intake patterns.
3. Estimate and determine the client's appropriate weight goal.
4. Support the client as she tries new eating behaviors.
5. Help the client normalize her eating pattern.
6. Assist the client in understanding the connection between emotions and behaviors.
7. Teach the client how to maintain a healthy body weight.
8. Work together with other professionals providing treatment to the client.

Continuum of Counseling
Figure 17.1 schematically outlines the counseling process when working with a client with eating disorders. Initially, rapport is built as the client and Nutrition Therapist learn about each other. Goals are discussed and established for therapy. The motivated client moves forward with guidelines to improve her intake, while the unmotivated client continues to work on reasons for wanting to change. The motivated client, having a blueprint for a healthy eating plan, works through the Cognitive Behavioral Therapy (CBT) exercises that help her challenge her irrational thoughts and beliefs. She sometimes gets scared and retreats to unmotivated behavior at which time there is a break in the CBT sessions as you help her become re-motivated by reviewing costs and benefits to change. Assisting a client with an eating disorder takes years rather than months. With assistance, approximately 2/3 of the clients improve. (2,3)

STEPS OF COUNSELING

Establishing Trust
No counseling strategy is effective without first establishing rapport with your client. Do not move forward with the exercises in this book until you have established a good relationship with your client. Typically, the client with an eating disorder only trusts her own gut feelings. It is important for her to see you as a knowledgeable and experienced counselor. She may want to check your credentials or speak with some of your clients. If you are just starting to work with clients with eating disorders, emphasize that you are already a competent Nutrition Therapist.

Continue your education on eating disorders and become proficient in advance counseling skills through books and supervision. The more you understand and empathize with your clients, the greater likelihood of establishing trust and bonding with them.

Figure 17.1 CONTINUUM OF COUNSELING

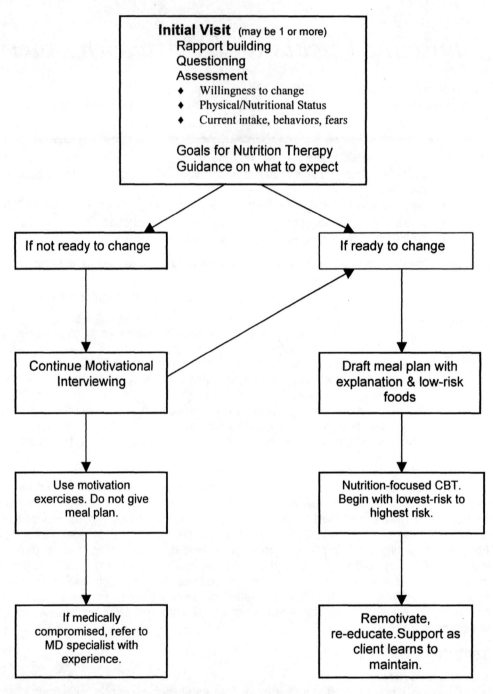

Language, Meanings, and Thoughts

Do not assume the meanings of your client's words mirror your own. Conversely, your words may not be interpreted literally. The person with an eating disorder may distort the meaning of language as much as she distorts body image. Following are some typical comments and their common misinterpretations:

"You are looking much healthier."	I must be getting too fat.
"You seem to be eating better."	I am no longer special.
"You gained a pound this week. Great job."	I must be getting fat. I am losing control.
"You're just 5 pounds from your goal weight."	I must be getting fat. My life is over.

Remind your client before leaving your office, she may hear these comments from friends and family members. Rehearse with her some appropriate responses to these situations.

This chapter will help you develop strategies to challenge your clients' distorted thoughts (including those related to food). Intellectually, the person with an eating disorder is often a big challenge, but she may know that her thoughts about food and weight are irrational. The challenge for her will be to learn to identify and dispute these irrational thoughts, and then learn how to consider more rational alternatives and take action to improve her life. You will play a major role in helping her make that transition.

Assessment

Assessment is a dynamic, comprehensive, and organized system of gathering information relevant to the nutritional care of your client. It should identify, along with using good interviewing skills, contributing factors to the eating disorder, starting points for therapy, and whether goals are met along the way. (4,5) See Appendix 17-A for Expected Outcomes; Appendix 17-B Outcomes Report; Appendix 17-C Medical Nutrition Therapy Protocols for Anorexia and Bulimia; and Appendix 17-D for Drug-Nutrient Interactions.

Assessment should be part of each session, not just an activity for the first session. Good, unbiased interviewing skills are essential to gathering an accurate picture of the client. A thorough assessment should include an evaluation and understanding of the client's:

- Present nutritional status
- Present lifestyle and health risk status
- Present biochemical and anthropometric values
- Psychosocial, cultural, ethnic, literacy, developmental skills, physical limitations, and economic factors
- Family dynamics
- Understanding
- Motivation and readiness to change

Interviewing

Although you may want to see only motivated clients, one of your goals will be to help clients with eating disorders become motivated to make changes. The very first session often is crucial in setting the stage for long-term outcome. It is important to utilize good interviewing skills from the start and to avoid the common traps that can hinder progress: (5)

- At the beginning of a counseling session, it is easy but inappropriate to begin asking only simple, basic yes or no questions. This can set the stage for your client feeling that it is better to give short, concise answers rather than more in-depth, thoughtful ones that give you much more needed information. If yes/no questions need to be asked, do so on a written questionnaire before the first session, or only briefly as necessary.
- Another common counseling mistake is moving too quickly. This can happen when you tell the client what her problem is before asking if she thinks there is a problem. Often this leads to more denial. For example, after asking a new client questions on her eating and weight history, don't say, "You know, this meets the criteria for anorexia nervosa." If the client was already ambivalent about seeing you, she may be put on the defensive. Just using a label, especially one with such negative "baggage," can make a person more defensive, so try to avoid using one or helping the client use one. Consider instead the following conversation:

  Client: *Do you think I have anorexia nervosa?*
  Counselor: Let me ask you first if you think you struggle with eating a healthy diet?

Client: *I know I don't eat right, and that's why I came for help.*
Counselor: Then, let's start by finding out about your eating struggles, and how I can be helpful to you. We will look at the diagnosis criteria and symptoms.

From your training in dietetics you know the basics of interviewing:
- Ask open-ended questions (ones that allow the client to "explore").
- Listen reflectively (repeat or rephrase what you hear the client say to see if your interpretation is correct, see Table 9.1 Basic Listening Skills).
- Affirm and support your client (let her know when you agree; support her right to feel as she does).
- Summarize periodically in order to reinforce it and let the client know you have heard what she said.
- Facilitate the client's expression of her self-motivational statements. Self-motivational statements fall into four general categories: (5)
  1. The first is problem recognition where the client expresses, "I guess there is more of a problem here than I thought."
  2. The second is the expression of concern about perceived problems. A good example would be the client saying, "I'm really worried about this."
  3. The third is a direct or implicit intention to change where the client may say, "I'm sick of this eating disorder. I need to do something about it."
  4. The fourth category is optimism about change such as when the client says, "No matter what it takes, I'm going to lick this thing."

Assessment questions should be presented in a motivational fashion. For the client who doesn't really think there is a problem, you can begin by saying, "Maybe you are right. Is it okay to ask you some questions so we'll have a better idea of what is going on?" For the motivated person, you can say, "I'd like to ask you some questions so we can determine the best place to begin."

Table 17.1 lists Physical Assessment Concerns. Table 17.2 gives guidance on how to normalize her weight. Table 17.3 lists specific questions about eating disorder behaviors to explore with the client. Complete details of dietary assessment are beyond the scope of this manual but need to be addressed.

Biochemical Assessment

Be aware of the biochemical markers that are indicative of nutritional concerns when an eating disorder is suspected. It has been suggested that low serum albumin concentration is an indicator of increased risk of B6 and Riboflavin deficiencies. (8) Hypercarotenemia is present in 30-60 percent of clients because of the excessive intake of vegetables such as carrots (conversion of provitamin A to Vitamin A is regulated by the body, and hypercarotenemia neither promotes nor increases risk for hypervitaminosis A). (9) Hypercholesterolemia may be seen with anorexia nervosa. This should not be interpreted as a concern requiring a reduction of dietary fat, but instead as a biochemical indicator of malnutrition. (10)

Calcium nutriture is important to assess in eating disorders because anorexia nervosa is associated with an increased risk of low bone density. Several physiological features of anorexia nervosa contribute to bone loss regardless of dietary calcium intake, such as low estradiol and hypercortisolemia. Calcium intake seems to play more of a permissive, rather than primary, etiological role in bone loss in these patients. (11)

Electrolyte abnormalities, especially hypokalemia and hypochloremia can occur as a result of the purging behavior. It is important that biochemical markers in clients with eating disorders be interpreted within the context of the neuroendocrine and physiological abnormalities that are present. (12-17)

It may take several sessions for you to gather the information you want. It may be difficult for your client to open up with specifics about her eating disorder behavior, due to embarrassment, until you have established rapport with her.

Table 17.1 PHYSICAL ASSESSMENT CONCERNS

- **What is the client's biochemical status?**
- **What is the client's average body weight for her height, age, and body frame?**
- **What is the client's percent of average body weight (needed as part of the diagnosis for anorexia nervosa)?**
- **What is the client's heaviest weight? What is her lowest weight as an adult (if an adult)?**
- **At what weight did her menstrual cycle become irregular? At what weight did she become amenorrheic?**
- **What is the client's desired weight and why?**
- **What are the caloric requirements of the client?** Some studies suggest differences in energy requirement among the subtypes of anorexia nervosa with restricting-type anorexia nervosa patients having a relatively higher energy requirement (36 kcal/kg) when compared with anorexia nervosa patients of the binge-purge type or compared to patients with bulimia nervosa (28 kcal/kg). See Table 17.2 below.
- **What is the client's percent body fat?** Body fat is best measured using skinfold calipers rather than bioelectrical impedance methods since bioelectrical impedance relies on body water that is more varied in the client with an eating disorder (overhydrated or dehydrated).
- **What is the client's current food intake?** It is often difficult to assess portion size and assess behaviors such as hiding food. Food models are helpful. The client can rationalize or defend choices on the basis of taste preferences when in actuality foods are chosen to maintain a reduced energy intake.
- **What is the client's eating pattern?** Check out idiosyncratic patterns such as avoidance of or excessive intake of sweets. The client is most likely to have foods categorized into good and bad foods. Find out which foods are in which lists. Check for eating unusually seasoned foods or combinations of foods, prolonged meal time, eating alone, constantly thinking about food, preparing foods for other people and then not eating anything herself. These behaviors are present as a general response to semi-starvation and have even been observed in semi-starved people without eating disorders.

Table 17.2 NORMALIZATION of WEIGHT (6,7)

Initial Phase
- 30 kcal/kg
- No less than 1200 calories
- Adjusted formula for obesity: wt (kg) – ABW (kg) x 0.25 + ABW (kg)

Weight Gain
- Partial program (increase 300-500 kcal every 3-7 days) until goal weight or client gains over 3 pounds per week
- Outpatient
    Begin with meal plan for weight gain at least 1 lb / week
    Discuss contract with team with consequences for not achieving

Sustaining Calories
    Anorexia nervosa   ~34 kcal / kg
    Bulimia nervosa   ~28 kcal / kg
    Preference is to ingest commonly available foods 3 meals / day

---

Table 17.3 ASSESSMENT QUESTIONS ON EATING DISORDER BEHAVIORS
Have you ever or do you currently:

- Binge eat? What does binge eating mean to you? (See criteria to assess for bulimia or binge eating disorder). How often do you binge? For what reason do you binge?
- Use laxatives? How many at a time? How many times a day/week/month? What reason?
- Use diuretics?
- Use diet pills?
- Vomit? How many times per episode? Do you use ipecac?
- Exercise? (This should include walking, cleaning, yard work, sit ups, etc) How much? How often? How intense? For what reason?
- Weigh yourself more than once a day? How many times? For what reason? What might you do if it goes up during the day? If it goes down during the day?
- Drink alcoholic beverages? How often? How much? For what reason?
- Use drugs (list some such as marijuana, cocaine)? How often? How much? For what reason? Some studies show that especially women choose to use cocaine for its appetite suppressing effects.
- How often do you have a bowel movement? After how long of a time period would you feel that there would be a problem if you did not have a bowel movement?
- Have any rituals that you do before, during and after eating? (Such as washing hands, cutting all foods into bite-sized pieces, exercise every day, drink water before eating; not drink water during eating; mix food; don't let different foods on the plate touch; chew 20 times before swallowing?) This not only provides a better picture of the eating behavior, but also may bring out other tendencies such as obsessive-compulsive behavior. Breaking rituals may be as much of a struggle for the client as eating healthier foods.

Diet Assessment

When gathering a diet history, make sure the client realizes your goal is not to judge but to have a better understanding of her food choices. In order to obtain the most accurate assessment of dietary intake, use of the 24-hour recall, a food frequency questionnaire, and a three- to seven-day food record are helpful tools. The 24-hour recall is a quick way to get an example of the client's daily intake, however, it may not be representative of a typical intake. The food frequency questionnaire helps to identify how often specific foods or food groups are consumed by the client.

Food records can provide meaningful information, not only on types and quantities of food eaten, but also patterns of intake. You may see that the client doesn't start eating each day until 5:00 p.m. or only eats when no one else is home. Once the client is introduced to CBT, ask her to complete the record in Appendix K that also includes thoughts and feelings accompanying each eating episode. Food records are invaluable throughout the counseling process in providing data on actual changes being made. Records must be checked for accuracy of content and amounts. For example, if the client recorded she ate a turkey sandwich:

Counselor: You have written that you ate a turkey sandwich. How much of it did you eat?
Client: *I ate about half.*
Counselor: You actually ate the equivalent of one slice of regular bread and how much turkey?
Client: *Well, there was one slice of turkey on the whole sandwich.*
Counselor: This slice (showing food model)?
Client: *Yes.*
Counselor: And were there any condiments on the sandwich?
Client: *There was a little mustard.*
Counselor: Anything else?
Client: *No.*
Counselor: One more thing. That bread was regular or diet bread?
Client: *Actually it was diet bread.*

You see that although the food record listed one turkey sandwich, the actual intake was the equivalent of a 40-calorie slice of bread and ½ ounce of turkey. This is smaller than an "average" turkey sandwich. The bottom line is to fill in the details of the food record.

In gauging the client's willingness to improve her nutritional intake, it may be most helpful to ask her to describe her concept of healthy eating with her reasons for why she considers it healthy. You might ask the client to list ten or more examples of "healthy foods," and ten or more examples of "not so healthy foods." These exercises will help you both design meaningful changes that your client may be willing to make. Without obtaining the client's input and reading her nonverbal behavior, you may rush into suggestions she is unwilling to try, and she may never return for a follow-up appointment.

Dietary Treatment

Refeeding. For the client with anorexia nervosa, the greatest barrier to gaining weight is her own fear. Often the client will say, "I want to get better. I just don't want to gain weight." Additional obstacles for this client are physiological changes, which may make gaining weight difficult. "Refeeding" is a term often used in eating disorder literature when discussing the weight-gaining phase of treatment. The refeeding process can be divided into four phases as described in Table 17.4.

Krahn and colleagues measured the resting metabolic rates and percent body fat in ten adult patients during the four phases of treatment. (16) During the initial Phase, all subjects were fed 1200 calories. In Phase two, they were fed 1500 calories per day, and in Phase three, patients were fed 3600 calories per day. Phase four consisted of maintenance calories once the subjects achieved their goal weight. Six subjects completed the study. Resting energy expenditure varied from 30 calories per kilogram at initial feeding to a high of 37.3 calories per kilogram at 3600 calories per day, to a maintenance level of 34.5 calories per kilogram. In summary, it took greater than 30 calories per kilogram of body weight to maintain the body weight of someone with anorexia nervosa. In other studies of resting energy expenditure in people with bulimia nervosa, 28 calories per kilogram of body weight seemed sufficient for maintenance. An explanation for this difference has yet to be determined. (6,7,18-21) A table showing the results of the Krahn study is shown in Appendix 17-E; share it with your clients. Help them see the evidence that metabolism does increase with refeeding.

The parameters may shift when considering children. These calculations must take growth into account. To achieve weight gain for clients with anorexia nervosa, it is necessary to raise calorie levels to a greater extent than when working with a non-eating disordered underweight client. Table 17.5 provides information on the energy, protein, and fluid needs of pediatric patients of different ages. Table 17.6 lists the energy needs of pediatric patients based on height. (22)

Determining Goal Weight

Goal weight refers to the weight that will restore normal physiological functioning. There is no exact method for predetermining the specific number at which goal weight is achieved. One method averages the client's premorbid weight, the midpoint of the 1979 Build Study height-weight table, and the 50th percentile of the Frisch table (www.valueoptions.com/provider/Eating Disorders.pdf). Goal weight should approximate the individual's "set point." Set Point refers to a weight range that the client can maintain without needing to restrict her intake or overexercise; a weight where she is no longer preoccupied with food.

Nutrition Education

Changing food attitudes and behaviors in clients with eating disorders requires education as well as therapy. Before proceeding with the exercises in this manual, it is important that you explain to the client what she might expect as her eating habits change:
1. Discuss the medical and physical consequences of weight-related behaviors (Tables 17.7 and 17.8).
2. Discuss the side effects that occur with improved nutrition, "refeeding" (Table 17.4).
3. Discuss the evidence which suggests that vomiting and laxative use are ineffective for weight control. (24-26)
4. Discuss basic principles of nutrition.
5. Reinforce for your client that *food is medicine*.

Table 17.4   REFEEDING PHASES AND SIDE EFFECTS

Phase 1: Initial increase in caloric intake Difficulties with weight gain occur because of an increase in resting energy expenditure (REE). This is due to improved nutrition, an increase in body temperature, and an increased T3 level.

- **Fluid Weight Gain or Edema:** (Occurs with anorexia and bulimia.) *Rebound edema*: It is not that the client is getting fat; it is that the body is holding on to more fluid than it needs. This fluid retention is temporary and will resolve as long as the client continues to normalize her eating behaviors. It may be significant with as much as 10-15 pound weight gain occurring during the first week. Results from muscle and vascular rehydration, intestinal hyperosmolality, and delayed gastric emptying. Edema is most commonly seen with bulimia nervosa. Refeeding too quickly can cause edema. *Shortness of breath*: from the increase in fluid volume. (Occurs with anorexia and laxative abuse in bulimia.) *Remedy:* Caloric content should begin at 30 Kcals/kg of current body weight. Encourage the client to include protein sources with carbohydrates, which should lessen fluid weight gain. There is no need to restrict sodium.

- **Constipation**: (Occurs with anorexia or withdrawal from laxatives.) Caused by lack of gastrointestinal muscle tone, the consequence of fluid abnormalities, or insufficient nutrient intake to keep the bowels functioning properly. *Remedy:* The problem should resolve itself by consuming higher fiber foods and drinking more fluids. May need to add nonaddictive stool softener if problem does not resolve easily.

- **Delayed Gastric Emptying**: (Occurs in anorexia.) May be a consequence of a reduction in enzyme activity and GI muscular atrophy. *Abdominal pain may result* from the delayed gastric emptying; food empties more slowly causing client to feel very full for hours after the meal has ended. *Remedy:* During the first week of improved intake, keep meal plan low-fat and low-lactose (milk products have been known to cause bloating, gas, and pain). Limit intake of gas-producing foods because of generalized gas production occurring from improved intake.

Phase 2 and 3

Post-meal and nighttime sweating: from the increased metabolic rate and production of heat. (15-18) This is an indicator that the client has significantly increased her caloric intake. Caused by increase in T3 and heat dissipation with increased ATP production. *Heat intolerance:* from increased body temperature and new sensation of heat production. *Remedy:* Layered clothing.

Phase 4

Maintenance of weight: Requires individualized caloric adjustment and frequent monitoring.

Adapted from: Anderson A. *Practical Comprehensive Treatment of Anorexia Nervosa and Bulimia.* Baltimore, MD: John Hopkins University Press; 1985.

Table 17.5 Nutritional Needs of Children   Adapted from Dietary Allowance Committee, Food & Nutrition Board. Washington, DC; National Academy Press.

Age (years)	Energy (kcal/kg)	Protein (g/kg)	Fluid (ml/kg)
0.0-0.5	108	2.2	120-150
0.5-1.0	98	1.6	125-145
1-3	102	1.2	114-115
4-6	90	1.1	90-110
7-10	70	1.0	70-85
11-14 Boys	55	1.0	70-85
Girls	47	1.0	70-85
15-18 Boys	45	.9	50-60
Girls	40	.8	50-60

Table 17.6 Height Related Energy Needs of Children (14,22)

Male:	11-14 years:	15.9 kcal/cm
	15-18 years:	17.0 kcal/cm
Female:	11-14 years:	14.0 kcal/cm
	15-18 years:	13.5 kcal/cm

Skill is needed in interviewing the client to prevent her from feeling judged, thus making her uncomfortable and defensive. Time spent educating the client on what to expect with refeeding often increases the therapist's credibility when the client begins to experience the changes.

CLASSIFICATION OF DISORDERED THOUGHTS

"How are you today, Ann?"
"Fine."
"And how was your eating this week?"
"Fine."
"And how was your exercise?"
"Fine."
"And how did you do with staying off the scale?"
"Fine."

From the above set of questions, you can see that the Nutrition Therapist did not get much useful information from her client. Although she might have asked better questions to elicit a "better" answer, the point is that the word "fine" is a common one-word response you will hear from clients with eating disorders. This may be related to the client's insensitivity to her own thoughts or feelings, an indication of her resistance to treatment, or a response she gives to please the therapist.

Styles of Distorted Thinking
It is helpful to understand some of the dysfunctional/distorted thinking which is typical of the person with an eating disorder. Here are some illustrations of frequently made "cognitive errors." (4, 27-30)

Filtering. This distortion is characterized by tunnel vision. It is focusing on one element of a situation to the exclusion of everything else. A person with an eating disorder might be told that she is, "too thin, except her thighs are big, like a runner." The client only hears that her thighs are big and never hears, "she is too thin." She leaves the situation depressed about her big thighs. Filtering exaggerates all her fears, losses, and irritations.

Dichotomous thinking (also referred to as black and white thinking). With this type of distortion, there is no middle ground. If you aren't perfect, then you are a failure. In behaviors, "if you eat one cookie, then you might as well eat the whole box," or "you better not eat anything else for the rest of the day."

Overgeneralization. With this distortion, the person reaches a generalized conclusion from one single incident. One slip with eating means, for example, "I'll never be able to control my eating." Some nutritional overgeneralizations are, "I can't eat butter because it will make me fat," or "I can't eat after 6:00 pm because people who eat after 6:00 pm are fat."

Mind reading. Mind reading involves "jumping to conclusions" about what others are supposedly thinking. Although there may be no evidence for what she believes, the client feels she "really knows." These assumptions are mostly untested, basically hunches or intuition, and often incorrect. A person with an eating disorder may believe that people who see her eat think she is eating too much and is gluttonous. She also may believe that people are thinking she is fat, even though she is obviously thin. Mind reading sometimes involves projection, which is a process of expecting other people to think, feel, or act the same way you do.

Catastrophizing. This error involves accepting the worst possible outcome as the most likely. It typically involves a major distortion of probability like "If I gain weight, I'll become obese and totally unattractive." Some people see the glass half empty instead of half full.

Personalization. With this type of thinking, the person is always comparing herself to others or perceiving she is the center/cause of others' actions, "My parents divorced because I couldn't keep them together." Or, "My friend is the same height I am, but I can't afford to eat as much as she does."

Discounting. With this disordered way of thinking, an individual cannot give herself credit or accept positive feedback. "I only ate my meal plan today because my mother was around." She has not learned to say, "Thank you for saying that. I've been working on it."

Self-fulfilling Prophecy. A typical statement of a person with an eating disorder is, "I can't." By generating the outcome before it occurs, the biased negative expectation can be made more likely to occur. Also, it's easier *not* to expect something to happen; it takes less work. She might say, "If I feel too full, I'm so uncomfortable I have to vomit."

"Shoulds." With this distortion, the person acts from a set of inflexible rules. For the person who overexercises, "I should go to Karate because I'm way behind and I need to test for a belt next week." Other common *shoulds* include, "I should be able to get an A," or "I should stay in this relationship because no one in my family divorces," or "I should go see my mother even though she always talks about dieting."

Once the client has learned to identify her distorted thinking, she then can begin to see how this way of thinking affects her emotions and behavior. Often, you must clarify the difference between what she thinks and what she feels. In American culture we have been taught to say, "I feel," at times when describing our thoughts, not emotions. For example, "I don't like to eat meat because it makes me feel disgusting." Exercises in this manual will help your client better understand her thoughts, as distorted as they might be, and examine this self-talk. "When I eat red meat, I think all grizzle and fat will stick to my body. I think it will never get digested and it will be with me forever." In this example, the person's thoughts are distorted, and they become emotional issues.

214

Underlying Assumptions

Underlying assumptions are the personal rules or beliefs that govern a person's thinking and the way she sees herself, the world, and the future. (31) It doesn't take traumatic events to influence beliefs. Beliefs can be influenced by our gender, neighborhoods, family beliefs, cultural and ethnic backgrounds, and religion. It is easy to provide an example of a cultural belief in western society. A girl could conclude from her environment that being pretty is the key to being well liked. A boy could conclude being tall, strong, and athletic are the keys to being well liked. Our culture teaches us to make these connections.

It may be important to know how the client developed her ideas or cognitions about reality, how she chooses and decides from the many possibilities, and how she acts and behaves in relationship to reality.

In disputing thoughts, it is helpful to have the client recognize the specific rule that governs her thinking. It may be helpful, at times, to ask the client for an example of a nonfood assumption. For example, "If you want to be rich, you have to work hard." Some examples of underlying assumptions that are related to food and eating follow:

"No one will like me if I'm fat."
"I will not be happy or successful if I am fat."
"My mother and father divorced because she was fat."

Helping your client change maladaptive assumptions can reduce the number of negative, distorted, automatic thoughts she may have. Developing new assumptions can lower her anxiety and make it easier for her to change her behavior. Techniques found useful in treating eating disorder thoughts include the following:

Decatastrophizing helps the client evaluate her belief system. (4) It involves first evaluating the client's fear of an identified situation and what she considers a horrible negative outcome. Then help the client to acknowledge that this belief and resulting emotion are unfounded. For example:

Nutrition Therapist: You say, no one will like you if you gain weight. Help me understand that.
Client: *No one likes people who are fat.*
Nutrition Therapist: Well, I'd like to bring up two issues here. Do you really think that no one likes people who are fat? And the second issue is how will eating the food on your meal plan make you fat?
Client: *You know how fat people are treated in this society. They just don't get respect. And I know that I don't like people who are fat, so why should anyone like me if I was fat?*
Nutrition Therapist: I must agree with you that society is tough on those who are overweight, but I know many people who are overweight who are very well liked, very successful, and they like themselves. What makes you not like people who are fat?
Client: *My mother always said fat people were lazy, unreliable, and unpopular. I'd rather have friends who are popular, smart, and nice. That's also why I would never let myself get fat.*
Nutrition Therapist: Okay. But, back to my second point. How would following your meal plan make you fat? It is calculated to keep you in your goal weight range. So, help me understand how you will be fat and disliked, if you follow your meal plan.
Client: *I'm just afraid that I will be fat following the meal plan.*
Nutrition Therapist: The calculations are based on research that was done to determine how many calories it takes to maintain various weights. The exercises we will go through in the sessions will help you better understand this, but can I ask you to trust that your meal plan will not make you fat?
Client: *I will try to trust you but it's hard to believe it.*
Nutrition Therapist: I know. I will help you see the evidence about food intake and weight as we progress.

Challenging the "shoulds" is essential to break down the irrational belief system. (4) Without the dichotomous thinking inherent in these self-imposed rules, irrational thinking would not occur. Since no one can be perfect, any break from what the client feels she should do leaves her feeling inadequate. As the Nutrition Therapist, you will develop an awareness of these beliefs and work to dispel the myth of the "shoulds."

Reattribution is used to help the client perceive an attribute of her self, differently. (4) You question the validity of the perception and create an atmosphere of ambiguity in order to get the client to see that her thinking may be irrational. For example, "You have said that you think Mary is thin. Mary actually is the same height as you, but weighs 20 pounds more than you do. How can she be so thin and you be so fat if you weigh less than her?"

Decentering is useful when helping the client see issues from other people's perspectives (reality) versus her own (distortion). (4) For example:

Client: *I almost didn't come in today because I knew my weight was up and I didn't want anyone to see me.*

Nutrition Therapist: How did you know your weight was up?

Client: *I actually followed my meal plan so I know it's up.*

Nutrition Therapist: Would you mind getting on the scale to check it out?

Client: *OK. I know it's up. I am so fat.*

Nutrition Therapist: Your weight is up one pound. That is just what we hoped to accomplish. I know you feel bad about this right now, but this weight gain means you are closer to getting better. Now, let's spend a few minutes talking about you feeling so much fatter with only one pound weight gain. Do you feel it is noticeable?

Client: *Of course it is. I can really feel it.*

Nutrition Therapist: Can you tell when your friends gain one pound, or even two or three pounds?

Client: *No, I guess not.*

Nutrition Therapist: I would guess that through normal fluid fluctuations that my weight is up or down within three pounds every time you come in. Do you notice?

Client: *No, I can't tell.*

Nutrition Therapist: Do you think someone can tell your one pound gain?

Client: *I guess not.*

Nutrition Therapist: That's right. No one can tell. I want to stress that I do understand you think people can tell, but let me reinforce that neither of us can tell. Let's discuss how we can continue to move forward this week and progress toward reaching your goal.

SUMMARY

The identification of automatic thoughts forms the basis of cognitive-behavioral therapy. It is necessary to help your client understand her thought processes and how cognitive errors in thinking occur. You can then proceed to challenge both the errors in thinking and the underlying assumptions that may have contributed to them. When the automatic thought of the client is identified, her mood and behavior makes sense. When she recognizes that her thought stems from cognitive error, it makes change more likely to occur.

References

1. Reif D, Reif K. *Eating Disorders: Nutrition Therapy in the Recovery Process.* Mercer Island, Washington: Life Enterprise Publication; 1997.
2. Fichter MM, Quadflieg N. Six-Year Course of Bulimia Nervosa. *International Journal of Eating Disorders.* 1997; 22: 361-384.
3. Strober M, Freeman R, Morrell W. The Long-Term Course of Severe Anorexia Nervosa in Adolescents: Survival Analysis of Recovery, Relapse, and Outcome: Predictors over 10-15 years in a Prospective Study. *International Journal of Eating Disorders.* 1997; 22: 339-360.
4. King K, Klawitter B, eds. *Nutrition Therapy: Advanced Counseling Skills,* 2nd ed. Lake Dallas, Texas: Helm Publishing; 2003.
5. Miller WR, Rollnick S. *Motivational Interviewing: Preparing People to Change Addictive Behavior.* New York: Guilford Press; 1991
6. Ebert M, George T, Gwirtsman H, Jimmerson D, Kaye W, Obarzanek E. Calorie Intake Necessary for Weight Maintenance in Anorexia Nervosa: Nonbulimics Require Greater Caloric Intake than Bulimics. *Am J Clin Nutr.* 1986; 44: 435-443.
7. Weltzin TE, Fernstrom MH, Hansen D, McConaha C, Kaye WH. Abnormal Caloric Requirements for Weight Maintenance in Patients with Anorexia Nervosa and Bulimia Nervosa. *American Journal of Psychiatry.* 1991; 148: 1675-1682.

8. Rock CL, Vasantharajan S. Vitamin Status of Eating Disorder Patients: Relationship to clinical indices an effect of treatment. *International Journal of Eating Disorders*. 1995; 18:227-262.
9. Rock CL, Jacob RA, Bowen PE. Update on the Characteristics of the Antioxidant Micronutrients: Vitamin C, Vitamin E, and the Carotenoids. *J Amer Diet Assoc.* 1996a; 96:693-702.
10. Banji S, Mattingly D. Anorexia Nervosa: Some Observations on "dieters" and "vomiters," Cholesterol and Carotenes. *British Journal of Psychology.* 1981; 139: 238-241.
11. Rigotti NA, Neer RM, Skates SJ. The Clinical Course of Osteoporosis in Anorexia Nervosa: a longitudinal study of cortical bone mass. *Am J Clin Nutr.* 1991; 265: 1133-1138.
12. Mordasini R, Klose G, Greter H. Secondary Type II Hyperlipoproteinemia in Patients with Anorexia Nervosa. *Metabolism.* 1978; 27: 71-79.
13. Biller BK, SaxV, Herzog DB, Rosenthal DI, Holzman S, Kilbanski A. Mechanisms of Osteoporosis in Adult and Adolescent Women with Anorexia Nervosa. *Journal of Clinical Endocrinology and Metabolism.* 1989; 68: 548-554.
14. The American Dietetic Association. Nutritional Assessment. In: *Handbook of Clinical Dietetics.* 2nd ed. New Haven, Connecticut: Yale University; 1992: 5-39.
15. Rock C, Yager J. Nutrition and Eating Disorders: A Primer for Clinicians. *International Journal for Eating Disorders.* 1987; 6(2): 267-280.
16. Krahn DD, Rock C, Dechert R, Nairn K, Hasse S. Changes in resting energy expenditure and body composition in anorexia nervosa patients during refeeding. *J Am Diet Assoc.* 1993; 93: 434-438.
17. Curran-Celentano J, Erdman JW, Nelson RA, Grater SJE. Alterations in Vitamin A and Thyroid Hormone Status in Anorexia Nervosa and Associated Disorders. *Am J Clin Nutr.* 1985; 42:1183-1191.
18. Kiyohara K, Tamai H, Takaichi Y, Nakagawa T, Kumagai LF. Decreased Thyroidal Triiodothyronine Secretion in Patients with Anorexia Nervosa: Influence of Weight Recovery. *Am J Clin Nutr.* 1989; 47:989-994.
19. Stordy BJ, Marks BS, Kalucy RS, Crisp AH. Weight Gain, Thermic Effect of Glucose, and Resting Metabolic Rate during Recovery from Anorexia Nervosa. *Am J Clin Nutr.* 1977; 30:138-146.
20. Vaisman N, Rossi MF, Corey M, Clarke R, Goldberg E, Pencharz PB. Effect of Refeeding on the Energy Metabolism of Adolescent Girls who have Anorexia Nervosa. *European Journal of Clinical Nutrition.* 1991; 45: 527-537.
21. Gwirtsman H, Kaye W, Obarzanek K, et al. Decrease caloric intake in normal-weight patients with bulimia: comparison with female volunteers. *Am J Clin Nutr.* 1989; 49:86-9
22. Samour PM, King K, eds. *Handbook of Pediatric Nutrition.* Gaithersburg, MD: Aspen Publishers; 1999.
23. Anderson A. *Practical Comprehensive Treatment of Anorexia Nervosa and Bulimia.* Baltimore, MD: John Hopkins University Press; 1985.
24. Bo-Linn GW, Morawski SG, Fordtran JS. Purging and Caloric Absorption in Bulimic Patients and Normal Women. *Annals of Internal Medicine.* 1983; 99:14-17.
25. Kaye WH, Weltzin TE. Neurochemistry of Bulimia Nervosa. *Journal of Clinical Psychiatry.* 1991; 52S: 21-28.
26. Lacey JH, Gibson E. Does Laxative Abuse Control Body Weight? A comparative study of purging and vomiting bulimics. *Human Nutrition:Applied Nutrition.* 1985; 39:36-42.
27. Dobson KS, ed. *Handbook of Cognitive-Behavioral Therapies.* New York: The Guilford Press; 1988.
28. Beck AT, Rush AJ, Shaw BF, Emery G. *Cognitive Therapy of Depression.* New York: The Guilford Press; 1979.
29. Beck AT. *Cognitive Therapy and the Emotional Disorders.* New York: New America Library; 1979.
30. Schuyler D. *A practical Guide to Cognitive Therapy.* New York: W.W. Norton and Company; 1991.
31. Greenberger D, Padesky C. *Mind Over Mood.* New York: The Guilford Press; 1995.

For more complete nutrition therapy counseling strategies for people with anorexia and bulimia, see *Winning the War Within,* a Cognitive Behavioral Instructor's Manual with Camera-Ready Handouts by Eileen Stellefson Meyer, MPH, RD, FADA. Published by Helm Publishing (www.helmpublishing.com).

Chapter 18

Counseling People with Chronic Disease

Bridget Klawitter, PhD, RD, FADA

After reading this chapter, the reader will be able to:
- ♦ List the major U.S. chronic diseases.
- ♦ Identify six essential components of the Chronic Care Model.
- ♦ Tell the difference between self-management and other forms of communication.
- ♦ Discuss the positive aspects of evidence-based practice.

U.S. HEALTH CARE

Providing care for individuals with chronic illness in the current healthcare environment of cost containment and outcomes management has led to a focused effort to move toward disease case management. Chronic disease is defined as a disease that persists over a long period as compared with the course of an acute disease. The symptoms of chronic disease are sometimes less severe than those of the acute phase of the same disease. Chronic disease may be progressive, result in complete or partial disability, or even lead to death. (1)

The myriad of diseases that contribute to morbidity and mortality in America have changed significantly over the last 100 years. Chronic diseases such as cardiovascular disease, cancer, and diabetes are among the most common, costly, and preventable of all health problems. (2) Seven out of every ten Americans who die each year, or more than 1.7 million people, die of a chronic disease. The chronic nature of many of these diseases also contributes to the extended periods of disability and declining quality of life often reported by individuals. Since more than 90 million Americans live with chronic illnesses, and chronic, disabling conditions cause major limitations in activity for more than 25 million Americans, it only appears to be increasing yearly.

A major contributing factor to the rising incidence of chronic disease is the aging American population. The elderly are the most rapidly growing group in the United States. By the year 2030, one in five Americans will be over age 65, and the population of individuals over age 85 will double. (3) Hospital use, measured in days per 1000, for older adults is triple that of younger age groups. Visits to health care providers' offices are more frequent as age increases.

It is a well-known fact that the incidence of chronic disease in the United States is increasing. Such diseases as type 2 diabetes, obesity, asthma, and osteoporosis continue to increase. Coronary arterial atherosclerosis remains the primary cause of death in the United States. It was estimated that in the year 2000, 125 million Americans (45 percent) lived with chronic conditions. Of those with chronic conditions, 44 percent (or 55 million) are living with two or more different chronic conditions. (4)

The degree to which individuals maintain their physical health and functional independence can be correlated with lifestyle factors including nutrition and physical activity. Although the leading causes of death in the United States are usually the result of over-nutrition, epidemiological studies have indicated that adults age 65 and older are at a disproportionate risk for under-nutrition. (5) The role of the dietetic practitioner in addressing physical, as well as social and environmental factors, which can contribute to over- and under-nutrition are invaluable.

The costs of chronic diseases are staggering. It is impossible to effectively address escalating health care costs without addressing the problem of chronic disease (2):

- The medical care yearly expenses of individuals with chronic diseases account for more than 75 percent of the nation's medical care costs.
- Chronic diseases account for more than one-third of the years-of-potential-life lost before age 65.
- Direct and indirect costs of diabetes care alone are currently near $100 billion per year.
- In 2001, approximately $300 billion was spent on all cardiovascular diseases.
- Direct medical costs associated with a sedentary lifestyle were nearly $76 billion in 2000.

The increase in chronic disease means more complex patients. Physicians, in a limited-time office visit, are ill equipped to provide the scope of services needed by the medically complex patient. This affords dietetic practitioners the opportunity to target such needs as counseling on lifestyle changes, reinforcement of positive health behaviors, modifying or negotiating nutrition plans of care, and linking patients to other needed services.

Overview of Chronic Disease Care
Usual chronic illness care in the United States has emphasized episodic and reactive treatment of acute illness. Multiple, short hospitalizations to resolve acute symptoms focus on physician treatment with little or no emphasis on the patients' role in self-management of their conditions. Recognition that chronic disease care is very different from acute illness care has contributed to a more collaborative, multidisciplinary approach to patient-centered, self-management models.

The health care team should be proactive and integrated across time, place, and condition, when developing a chronic illness care plan. The medical literature suggests interventions, such as the use of protocols and practice guidelines, improved patient education, improved access to expertise, and greater availability of clinical information, can improve outcomes for these patients. (6)

Benefits of Nutrition in Chronic Disease Care
In 1997, the Nutrition Screening Initiative (NSI) developed a nutrition care manual specific to chronic disease care. (7) The NSI is a multidisciplinary coalition led by The American Dietetic Association, the American Academy of Family Physicians, and the National Council on Aging in collaboration with more than 25 national health- and aging-related organizations. See Chapter 10 for more information on the NSI.

Patient–Centered Care
Patient-centered care emphasizes long-term, continuous, healing relationships. Patients want to be partners in their care and receive more responsive care from healthcare providers. Care is individualized based on the patient's needs and values, and emphasizes patient control in the health care process. Empowering patients through the provision of information is at the heart of patient-centered care. In a chronic disease model of care, patients partner with healthcare providers to determine the approach to care.

Overview of the Chronic Care Model
Dr. Edward Wagner and the Improving Chronic Illness Care program developed the Chronic Care Model (8) using available literature and addressing strategies for chronic illness management. See Figures 18.1 and 18.2. The model identifies the essential elements for chronic disease management:

- Community
- Health system
- Self-management support
- Delivery system design
- Decision support
- Clinical information systems

Figure 18.1   Overview of the Chronic Care Model
(Source: Wagner EH. Chronic disease management: What will it take to improve care for chronic illness? Effective Clinical Practice. 1998;1:2-4.)

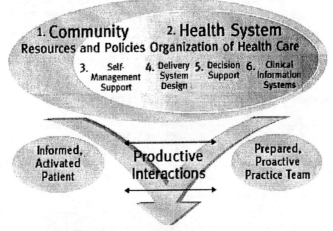

Functional and Clinical Outcomes

Changes in the health system will only improve chronic illness care if active, informed patients work together with provider teams.

Figure 18.2   CHRONIC CARE MODEL by Dr. Edward Wagner
Source: http://www.improvingchroniccare.org/change/model/components.html

The Chronic Care Model is based on the premise that functional and clinical outcomes can be improved through collaborative efforts among various providers of healthcare. Dietetic practitioners, whether engaged in private practice or employed in structured healthcare delivery systems, can benefit from an understanding of the elements and their implications on chronic care this model addresses.

1. **Community**—Community programs can support care for the individual with chronic illness. Unfortunately, national and state health policies and legislation can affect the provision of services available. National organizations such as the American Diabetes Association may have free resources to promote self-care. Local linkages with programs and facilities can enhance community-based resources for individuals to self-manage their disease. Community resources may include adult day care, congregate meal sites, food assistance programs, home care services, and assisted living facilities.

2. **Health Systems**—In the organizations providing healthcare services on a local level, they must re-evaluate their approach to chronic disease management. Care must be convenient and affordable for patients to promote early intervention for symptoms and illness. Case management has become more common in health systems, especially those who have evolved into integrated systems. Outreach clinics, free community education programs, speaking to community groups and media can be areas hospital-based dietetic practitioners can tap into to promote nutrition and lifestyle changes and encourage individuals to seek nutrition counseling. Collaboration and/or linkages with health systems may also be an avenue those in private practice may consider.

3. **Self-Management Support**—Herzlinger (9) has provided significant insight into developing healthcare movement where patients are starting to "call the shots". A disease management program empowers individuals to care for their disease themselves, hence self-management. Self-management support is an integral part of chronic disease care. Self-management of chronic illness requires patients to recognize, treat and manage their condition(s) on an ongoing, often daily basis. Multiple studies (10-14) have demonstrated that self-management can improve health status, reduce healthcare resource utilization, and improve self-care skills.

221

Living with a chronic disease has often been compared to having a second full-time job. In order to keep chronic illnesses under control, patients must be empowered to take better care of themselves. This requires counseling on ways to minimize symptoms, complications, and long-term disability. For example, the individual with diabetes must learn how to achieve glycemic control. Effective nutrition counseling gives individuals primary responsibility to determine their care. The counselor works collaboratively with the patient to define problems and barriers, set priorities, establish goals, create treatment plans, and solve problems along the way. (15)

Self Management [4]	
What it isn't	What it is
Didactic patient education	Emphasis on patient role
You should….	Self-care skills
Finger pointing	Self-assessment
Lecturing	Problem-solving
Waiting for patients to ask for help	Care planning
One-time effort	Ongoing
Commercial websites	Empowering
Remote monitoring	

4. **Delivery System Design**—Process evaluation and improvement to ensure patients with chronic diseases obtain timely, consistent care, is key to a proactive approach. Frequent follow-up procedures should be standard practice to assure patients receive long-term monitoring of outcomes. For dietetic practitioners, this may mean evaluating counseling skills and the ability to form relationships that enhance return visits and longer-term follow-up. This becomes key as we, as a profession, struggle to demonstrate our positive impact on patient outcomes and costs to legislators, the payers, and the public at large.

5. **Decision Support**—Treatment decisions and counseling approaches need to be based on explicit, proven guidelines. In dietetic practice, this approach is often referred to as evidence-based practice.

Evidence-Based Practice
The goal of evidence-based practice is to improve care using sound research. Treatment decisions should be based on explicit, proven guidelines supported by at least one scientific study. Evidence-based practice (EBP) is the reliance on scientific data and the results of scientific studies as the basis for practice decisions. (16) It is important for dietetic practitioners to have a systematic method for applying new knowledge and research data, regardless of practice setting, in order to achieve quality outcomes. The strength of the evidence supporting a practice decision, or used in developing a guideline or protocol, determines:
- the strength of the approach
- the strength of any recommendations
- the likelihood of achieving desired outcomes
- the likelihood of reimbursement, and
- the likelihood of legislative recognition supporting MNT coverage

With evidence-based practice, nutrition care is pre-planned according to the patient's diagnosis, condition, or procedure. Pre-planned nutrition care incorporates the best practices, according to existing evidence, but allows for individualization of care when indicated. Examples of pre-planned nutrition care resources include the MNT Protocols and Nutrition Practice guidelines for diabetes (17,18), hyperlipidemia (19), pre-renal disease (20), as well as other chronic conditions (21,22). See Chapter 22 for a more detailed look at outcomes management and its importance for reimbursement efforts. The American Diabetes Association (23) has issued a position statement reiterating the need for evidence-based nutrition principles and recommendations for the treatment and prevention of diabetes and related complications. See Chapter 19 for a more specific application of counseling approaches for individuals with diabetes.

6. **Clinical Information Systems**—Effective chronic disease care requires systems to track individual patients as well as populations of patients. (24) In larger systems, a data registry or data repository may be put in place to compare treatment to recommended guidelines, measure outcomes, and offer reminders for follow-up care. For dietetic practitioners, data collection sheets, simple spreadsheets, or data entry programs on an office computer, can be designed to track patient outcomes and create summary reports on effectiveness of interventions. This information can be invaluable when attempting to become a payer-provider, negotiate reimbursement rates, and/or justify staffing for outpatient counseling programs. For dietetic practitioners initiating an outcomes project, it is important that the outcomes measured are clinically relevant, and have a significant impact on the quality and cost of care or the service being provided. (25)

SUMMARY

Providing disease prevention and health promotion nutrition counseling to older adults and those younger with chronic diseases presents a growing challenge to dietetic practice. A focus on health promotion to young and old alike can improve functional ability as well as health conditions. Nutrition therapy interventions can often address such simple problems as loss of appetite or lack of understanding a prescribed diet using a relatively low cost approach. This can contribute not only to positive health outcomes, but also save significant healthcare dollars in the future.

Chronic disease self-management has been shown to be effective in reducing healthcare utilization and costs. Intensive programs with frequent follow-up can improve the patient's functional status, mood, and satisfaction with care. Dietetic practitioners should emphasize the patient's central role in managing their illness. At each visit, assess the patient's self-management knowledge, behaviors, self-confidence, and perceived barriers. Collaborative care planning and problem-solving with other members of the healthcare team is vital to provide effective behavior change interventions and ongoing support. In the long run, utilization of a chronic disease model approach can improve patient outcomes.

Learning Activities:

1. Discuss the role of nutrition in aging and the implications/considerations for nutrition counseling.

2. What characteristics can be contributing factors to malnutrition in those individuals with chronic illness? Discuss implications/considerations for nutrition counseling.

3. How do the principles of patient-centered care support the concept of nutrition counseling and adult learning theory?

4. Using the Chronic Care Model, discuss applications and considerations for dietetic practitioners in the following settings:
   - Hospital-based inpatient
   - Hospital-based outpatient
   - Public health
   - Private practice
   - Work site wellness programs

References
1. Anderson DM. *Mosby's Medical, Nursing and Allied Health Dictionary*, 6th ed. St. Louis: Mosby; 2002.
2. *National Center for Chronic Disease Prevention and Health Promotion.* August 30, 2002. http://www.cdc.gov/nccdphp/overview.htm
3. US Bureau of the Census. *Statistical Abstract of the United States: 1996*, 116th ed. Washington DC; 1996.
4. Hyatt JD. *The weakest link: self-management of chronic disease.* Presentation at the 27th annual National Wellness Conference; July 17, 2002.
5. Marwick C. NHANES III health data relevant for an aging population. *J Am Med Assoc.* 1997; 277:100-102.
6. Wagner EH, Austin BT, Vonforff M. Improving outcomes in chronic illness. *Managed Care Qtrly.* 1996; 4 (2): 12-25.
7. White JV, ed. *The role of nutrition in chronic disease care.* Washington DC: The Nutrition Screening Initiative; 1997.
8. Source: http://www.improvingchroniccare.org/change/model/components.html
9. Herzlinger R. *Market-driven healthcare: who wins, who loses in the transformation of America's largest service industry.* Boulder, CO: Perseus Books Group; 1999.
10. Gibson PG, Coughlan J, Wilson AJ. Self-management education and regular practitioner review for adults with asthma. *The Cochrane Database of Systemic Reviews.* 2001;1.
11. Norris S, Engelgau MM, Narayan KM. Effectiveness of self-management training in Type 2 diabetes. *Diabetes Care.* 2001; 24 (3): 561-587.
12. Linden W. Psychosocial interventions for patients with coronary artery disease: a meta-analysis. *Archives of Internal Medicine.* 1996; 156 (7): 745-752.
13. Philben E. Comprehensive multidisciplinary programs for the management of patients with congestive heart failure. *J General Int Med.* 1999; 14 (2): 130-135.
14. Lorig KR. Effect of self-management program on patients with chronic disease. *Effective Clinical Practice.* 2001; 4(6): 256-262.
15. VonKorff M, Gruman J, Schaefer JK, Curry SJ, Wagner EH. Collaborative management of chronic illness. *Ann Int Med.* 1997; 127: 1097-1102.
16. Splett PL. *Developing and Validating Evidence-based Guides for Practice: A tool kit for dietetic professionals.* Chicago IL: The American Dietetic Association; 1999.
17. *The American Dietetic Association: Nutrition Practice Guidelines for Type 1 and Type 2 Diabetes Mellitus.* Chicago IL: The American Dietetic Association; 2001.
18. *The American Dietetic Association: Nutrition Practice Guidelines for Gestational Diabetes Mellitus.* Chicago IL: The American Dietetic Association; 2001.
19. *The American Dietetic Association: Hyperlipidemia Medical Nutrition Therapy Protocol.* Chicago IL: The American Dietetic Association; 2001.
20. *The American Dietetic Association: Chronic Kidney Disease (non-dialysis) Medical Nutrition Therapy Protocol.* Chicago IL: The American Dietetic Association; 2002.
21. The American Dietetic Association and Morrison Health Care. *Medical Nutrition Therapy Across the Continuum of Care (MNTACC).* Chicago IL: American Dietetic Association; 1998.
22. The American Dietetic Association and Morrison Health Care. *Medical Nutrition Therapy Across the Continuum of Care (MNTACC).* 2nd ed. Supplement 1. Chicago IL: American Dietetic Association; 1998.
23. American Diabetes Association. Position Statement: Evidence-based nutrition principles and recommendations for the treatment and prevention of diabetes and related complications. *J Amer Diet Assoc.* 2002;102(1): 109-118.
24. Wagner EH. Population-based management of diabetes care. *Pat Educ Couns.* 1995; 16: 225-230.
25. Niedert KC, ed. *Nutrition care of the older adult: a handbook for dietetic professionals working throughout the continuum of care.* Chicago: American Dietetic Association; 1998: p. 37.

Chapter 19

Motivational Interviewing and Diabetes Education: Fostering Commitment To Change

Jeffrey J. VanWormer, MS and Jackie L. Boucher, MS, RD, LD, BC-ADM, CDE
HealthPartners Center for Health Promotion, Minneapolis, MN

After reading this chapter, the reader will be able to:
- ♦ Define motivational interviewing.
- ♦ Identify four general principles of motivational interviewing.
- ♦ Discuss applications of motivational interviewing to nutrition counseling.

BACKGROUND

Lifestyle modification is the cornerstone of successful diabetes prevention and management. (1) Consistent carbohydrate intake, regular physical activity, and blood-glucose monitoring are some of the key recommendations that call for behavior changes. Unfortunately, convincing others to modify unhealthy habits can be a challenging endeavor, especially when it involves clients who are not ready to change. Clinicians can easily become frustrated by an inability to foster commitment within this group. Motivational interviewing (MI) is a counseling style that focuses on using a nonconfrontational and client-centered approach. (2) It is designed specifically to help resolve ambivalence, reduce resistance, and foster commitment-three critical components to intentional behavior change.

MI was originally developed for use in the treatment of alcohol abuse and drug addiction. (3) More recently, however, MI has been successfully applied to other areas of health promotion and disease management, even during brief clinical encounters. (4) The purpose of this article is to provide an overview of MI and to review the literature regarding its efficacy for modifying eating behavior. Conclusions and practice recommendations for diabetes educators will also be discussed.

MOTIVATIONAL INTERVIEWING OVERVIEW

MI is formally defined as a client-centered, directive method for enhancing intrinsic motivation to change by exploring and resolving ambivalence. (2) It is particularly recommended for use with clients in the pre-action stages (i.e., pre-contemplation, contemplation, and preparation) of change. (5) The primary role of the counselor or clinician is to help clients explore self-generated arguments for change versus having those arguments presented to them. Four general principles guide MI and include: 1) Express empathy, 2) Develop discrepancies, 3) Roll with resistance, and 4) Support self-efficacy (see Table 19.1).

Expressing empathy is best accomplished via skillful reflective listening that avoids judging, criticizing, or blaming the client for his/her problems. (2) To express empathy, clinicians strive to provide an atmosphere of respect, understanding, and acceptance, even if they don't agree with the client's position.

Table 19.1	General Principles of Motivational Interviewing	
Principle	**Purpose**	**Example**
1. Express empathy	To respect, understand, and accept the client's position	"Sounds like checking your blood glucose every day is demanding. Many people struggle with it from time to time. Tell me more about what it's like for you."
2. Develop discrepancies	To amplify the "gap" between the client's current status and long-term goals/values	"So on the one hand you are not checking your blood glucose every day, but on the other hand you think keeping your blood glucose within normal limits is very important. How do you think this situation may affect your diabetes?"
3. Roll with resistance	To avoid confrontation, identify barriers, and emphasize autonomy	"It can be very frustrating to make all these changes. May I tell you about some different options that have worked well for others? I would be glad to help you problem-solve around some of the barriers, but you ultimately decide what is best for you."
4. Support self-efficacy	To increase self-confidence under difficult circumstances	"I see your recent A1c is substantially lower than the previous one. What worked so well for you?"

Developing discrepancies is a way to cultivate motivation for change. When the client can see the "gap" between his/her current behavior and long-term goals, change is more likely to occur. This is chiefly accomplished by exploring and focusing on the client's important life values. Clients are then encouraged to discover the discrepancy between their current behavior(s) and their desired behavior(s).

Rolling with resistance is related to expressing empathy. To roll with resistance means clinicians may invite new perspectives but try to avoid arguments and confrontation. They acknowledge resistance and ambivalence as normal components of the behavior-change process and as signals for them to respond differently to their clients.

Finally, clinicians support self-efficacy throughout the counseling process. The idea is to enhance and foster the client's self-confidence for changing lifestyle behaviors, even under difficult circumstances. This can be accomplished by affirming past success (i.e., reinforcement), presenting related success stories of others (i.e., modeling), and verbal encouragement.

Some MI skills, such as reflective listening and exploring life values, can be complicated and time-consuming to use in a demanding medical setting. Extensive training may also be required to teach clinicians such in-depth techniques. (4,6,7) Rollnick and Miller (8), however, have argued that adhering to the "spirit" of MI, rather than just using a few techniques, is the most important aspect of fostering behavior change. Sticking to the general principles and applying basic MI techniques such as agenda setting and scaling questions are recommended for brief clinical encounters. (9,10)

Agenda setting involves letting clients choose the topic(s) of interest. (11) Clinicians may present a series of lifestyle changes they feel are important (based on objective test results, epidemiological research, clinical experience, etc.), but clients are encouraged to become active decision-makers in identifying areas they would like to work on changing. Scaling questions are quick, directed queries designed to get clients talking about the personal and/or environmental factors that influence their behavior. (10) Clients are asked to rate their level of motivation and confidence for making a particular lifestyle change. This is followed up with a couple of probes that ask why they did not choose a lower rating and what it would take to get them to a higher rating. Such questions help to generate statements related to motivation and barriers.

ELIGIBILITY REQUIREMENTS – CERTIFIED DIABETES EDUCATOR (CDE)

Definition of Diabetes Self-Management Education

Diabetes self-management education is performed by health care professionals who have appropriate education and experience consistent with their profession's scope of practice. The process of diabetes self-management education is defined by:

- Performance of an individualized biopsychosocial and cognitive assessment of the individual with diabetes and/or the caregivers.
- Formulation of an education plan including collaboratively identified goals and objectives based on a core body of knowledge in diabetes content topics and self-care behaviors.
- Implementation of the education plan based on established principles of teaching-learning theory and lifestyle counseling.
- Evaluation(s) to assess the individual's understanding and utilization of diabetes management skills and knowledge, including reassessment of needs.
- Proper documentation of all education encounters.

Eligibility Requirements for Initial Certification

To qualify for the Certification Examination for Diabetes Educators, the following requirements must be met:

1. Professional Education

A. An active, unrestricted license from the United States or its territories as a registered nurse, occupational therapist, optometrist, pharmacist, physical therapist, physician (M.D. or D.O.), physician assistant, podiatrist, or registration as a dietitian by the Commission on Dietetic Registration.

OR

B. A minimum of a master's degree, from a United States college or university accredited by a nationally recognized regional accrediting body, in one of the following areas: nutrition, social work, clinical psychology, exercise physiology, health education, or specified areas of study in public health.*

NOTE: Individuals who meet both A. and B. (above) **must apply** under A., current license or registration
*Advanced degrees in public health must be in an area of concentration specific to health education, health promotion, health and social behavior, or health communication.

2. Professional Practice Experience

After meeting the education requirement and before applying for the Certification Examination, all *(A through C)* of the following requirements must be met:

A. A minimum of two years (to the day) of professional practice experience in diabetes self-management education in health care settings within the United States or its territories.*

- Only experience occurring AFTER completing the education requirement may be counted toward this requirement.

AND

B. A minimum of 1,000 hours of diabetes self-management education experience within the past five years.*

- Work experience is defined as employment in diabetes education for compensation.
- All experience must be in health care settings within the United States or its territories.

AND

C. Current employment in a primary role as a diabetes educator a minimum of four hours per week, or its equivalent, at the time of application.

For more information contact: National Certification Board for Diabetes Educators
330 East Algonquin Road, Suite 4 Arlington Heights, Illinois 60005
Voice 847 228-9795 Fax 847 228-8469
Email info@ncbde.org

MI AND EATING BEHAVIOR

Modifying eating habits (e.g., carbohydrate distribution, meal timing, fat intake) is perhaps the most common behavior change recommended in diabetes education. (12) A literature search using MEDLINE and PSYCINFO online databases was performed to identify studies that employed an MI-based, dietary counseling intervention. Key words included motivational interviewing, diet, nutrition, and diabetes. Six studies were identified and are summarized in Table 19.2 available at www.dce.org.

Intervention trials were evenly split between primary and secondary prevention. Most studies used only two or three MI counseling sessions within the context of a broader nutrition education program. Primary outcomes varied somewhat depending on the population of interest, but typically included nutritional intake and weight loss.

Generally speaking, MI was effective in improving diet. Two studies noted significant reductions in fat intake (13, 14), one study observed significant reductions in sodium intake (15), and another study found significant increases in fruit/vegetable consumption. (16) The effects of MI on weight loss were mixed. One study (15) noted an advantage for MI participants relative to controls, while two others found no advantage of MI beyond standard care. (17, 18) Nearly all studies reported significant improvement in some facet of program adherence (e.g., session attendance, self-monitoring, use of materials) as a result of MI. (13,14,16,17)

Despite the importance of dietary recommendations, few studies have specifically investigated MI with diabetes patients. Smith and colleagues (17) randomized obese adults diagnosed with type 2 diabetes to either a standard weight-loss program or the same program with the addition of three MI counseling sessions. While nutrient intake was not directly assessed, participants in the MI condition showed superior glycemic control, session attendance, and food diary completion compared to the standard group. In addition, MI participants were more likely to self-monitor their daily blood-glucose levels. Both groups lost weight relative to baseline, but did not differ from each other significantly.

CLINICAL APPLICATION

Education alone does not address the complex factors that influence eating behavior, especially among clients who are not ready to change. Fortunately, MI appears to offer much promise as an effective adjunct to nutrition education. Participants with and without chronic diseases have demonstrated improvements in fat reduction, fruit/vegetable consumption, and program adherence as a result of MI counseling.

How effective MI is in the context of diabetes education is less clear. Despite the general success of MI in modifying various health-related behaviors (4), MI-based counseling techniques are not widespread among diabetes educators. (19) In addition, few studies to date have included participants with diabetes. One trial found that MI helped to improve glycemic control, but not weight loss, relative to standard care. (17) Only one other MI-diabetes study was identified (20), but it was excluded from the review because of poor procedural reliability. (Only 19 percent of clinicians adhered to the MI-based intervention throughout the experiment.) Fortunately, at least two other randomized trials are currently under way to assess how MI can affect fruit/vegetable intake and physical activity. (21,22) One is specifically geared toward patients with diabetes. (22) Results of these investigations will help researchers draw more firm conclusions on the overall effectiveness of MI.

Notwithstanding, several MI-based counseling protocols have already been promoted for use in diabetes education. (11, 23, 24) One emerging tool that may be particularly attractive to clinicians is computer-aided assessments. Such tools help to streamline the counseling process by providing key psychosocial information before clients are even seen for an office visit.

The Accu-Chek Interview is a MI-based, computer-aided assessment that is specifically designed to help people with diabetes identify important lifestyle areas (along with barriers and motivational readiness) they would like to change. (25) Such technology offers a promising avenue for future research aimed at improving the scalability of MI for diabetes educators and other healthcare professionals.

For more information on MI, readers are encouraged to review the latest edition of Miller and Rollnick's book (2) and explore the MI homepage at www.motivationalinterview.org.

Table 19.2 Motivational Interviewing and Dietary Behavior Change - Intervention Studies

Study	Participants	Intervention	Measures	Results
Woollard J, Beilin L, Lord T, Puddey I, MacAdam D, Rouse I. (1995)	166 adults diagnosed with hypertension	*Treatment Length = 18 weeks* 1) Control – Usual general practitioner care 2) Low Intervention – One face-to-face appointment and 5 MI phone counseling sessions (15 min) with a nurse counselor 3) High Intervention – Six face-to-face MI counseling sessions (45 min) with a nurse counselor	1) Weight 2) Dietary intake (alcohol, salt, & fat) 3) Leisure-time physical activity 4) Smoking status 5) Blood pressure (systolic & diastolic)	Both intervention groups significantly lowered their systolic and diastolic blood pressure compared to controls. The low intervention group significantly reduced their salt and alcohol intake compared to controls. The high intervention group significantly reduced their weight compared to controls.
Smith DE, Kratt PP, Heckemeyer CM, Mason DA (1997)	22 older obese adult women diagnosed with type 2 diabetes	*Treatment Length = 16 weeks* 1) Standard Weight Control Program – 16 group sessions covering nutrition, exercise, and behavior modification 2) MI – Identical to standard group with the addition of 3 individual MI sessions	1) Weight 2) GHb 3) Treatment adherence (attendance, food diaries, & glucose monitoring)	Both groups lost a significant amount of weight during treatment but did not differ significantly. The MI group achieved significantly better glucose control, session attendance, food diary completion, and glucose self-monitoring compared to the standard group.
Mhurchu CN, Margetts BM, Speller V. (1998)	121 adults diagnosed with hyperlipidemia	*Treatment Length = 3 months* 1) Standard Dietary Intervention – 3 sessions of lipid-lowering dietary advice from a clinical dietitian 2) MI Intervention – Identical to standard group with the addition of MI techniques during counseling sessions	1) Lipid profile (total cholesterol, HDL, Total/HDL ratio, & triglycerides) 2) Nutrient intake (energy, fat, protein, carbohydrates, fiber, alcohol, & cholesterol) 3) BMI	Both groups improved their BMI and lipid profile relative to baseline, but did not differ significantly. Both groups significantly reduced their energy, fat, carbohydrate, and cholesterol intake, but did not differ from each other significantly.
Berg-Smith SM, Stevens VJ, Brown KM, Van Horn L, Gernhofer N, Peters E, Greenberg R, Snetselaar L, Ahrens L, Smith K. (1999)	127 adolescents with elevated LDL-cholesterol	*Treatment Length = 3 months* Participants received one face-to-face MI session with a second follow-up MI session 1-3 months later. MI treatment was done after receiving three years of dietary counseling in the Dietary Intervention Study in Children (no control group)	1) Dietary intake (total fat, saturated fat, & cholesterol) 2) Adherence to dietary guidelines 3) Readiness-to-change (dietary behavior)	Participants significantly decreased their calories from fat and dietary cholesterol compared to baseline. Dietary adherence and readiness-to-change significantly increased from baseline levels.
Resnicow K, Jackson A, Wang T, De AK, McCarty F, Dudley WN, Baranowski T. (2001)	1,011 African-American adults (14 churches cluster-randomized to conditions)	*Treatment Length = 1 year* 1) Self-help – diet video, cookbook, quarterly newsletter, dietary cues, and 1 phone call prompting the use of materials 2) Self-help plus MI – same as self-help group with the addition of 3 MI phone calls (4 total) 3) Comparison – standard nutritional education materials	1) Mean fruit and vegetable intake 2) Outcome expectations 3) Self-efficacy 4) Low-fat and high-fat vegetable preparation practices 5) Portion size knowledge	The MI group significantly increased their fruit and vegetable consumption compared to the self-help and comparison group. Also, MI participants significantly increased their use of the cookbook and low-fat vegetable preparation practices compared to the comparison group.
Bowen D, Ehret C, Pedersen M, Snetselaar L, Johnson M, Tinker L, Hollinger D, Lichty I, Bland K, Siversten D, Ocken D, Staats L, Beedoe JW. (2002)	175 adult women participating in the Women's Health Initiative Diet Modification Trial (WHIDMT)	*Treatment Length = 5 months* 1) Intensive Intervention Program (IIP) – 3 MI sessions with a dietitian in addition to regular WHIDMT activities 2) Control – Regular WHIDMT group sessions	1) Fat intake 2) Attendance at WHIDMT groups sessions 3) Self-monitoring of fat consumption	IIP participants significantly reduced their fat consumption compared to controls. IIP participants also tended to show better attendance and self-monitoring compared to controls, but differences were not significant.

BOARD CERTIFIED - ADVANCED DIABETES MANAGEMENT (BC-ADM)
A Certification for Advanced Clinical Practitioners Specializing in Diabetes Management

Jointly Sponsored by:
American Nurses Credentialing Center and American Association of Diabetes Educators
Collaborators Include:
American Dietetic Association
Diabetes Care and Education Practice Group
American Pharmaceutical Association
American Diabetes Association
In Consultation with: National Certification Board for Diabetes Educators

The Advanced Practitioner in Diabetes Management has an advanced degree and is able to:
- perform complete and or focused assessment,
- recognize and prioritize complex data in order to identify needs of patients with diabetes across the life span; and
- provide therapeutic problem solving, counseling and regimen adjustment.

The scope of advanced clinical practice includes management skills such as medication adjustment, medical nutrition therapy, exercise planning, counseling for behavior management and psychosocial issues. Attaining optimal metabolic control may include treatment and monitoring of acute and chronic complications. The depth of knowledge and competence in advanced clinical practice and diabetes skills affords an increased complexity of decision-making, which expands the traditional discipline specific practice. Research, publications, mentoring and continuing professional development are expected skill sets.

Eligibility:
This certification and credential is offered for Registered Dietitians (RD's), Registered Nurses (RN's), and Registered Pharmacists (RPh's).

License: Registration by Commission on Dietetic Registration (RD), active, unrestricted Licensed Registered Nurse (RN) or Licensed Pharmacist (RPh)

Education: Advanced Degree
RN: Masters in Nursing preferred. Minimum of BSN with Masters in a clinically relevant area, such Masters in Health Care Administration, Public Health, MEd, Counseling, Gerontology, etc.*
    * State board requirements differ from state to state. If a state requires a specific type of advanced degree for prescriptive privileges, this certification does not supersede the state statue.

RD: Masters in a clinically relevant area. Such as MS in nutrition, Masters in Public Health, MEd, Exercise, Sports Nutrition, Counseling, Gerontology
RPh: Masters or Doctorate degree in Pharmacy or currently practicing in a state recognized collaborative diabetes clinical practice.
Experience: 500 hours of clinical diabetes experience (after discipline licensure) within 48 months prior to application

Applications are accepted and processed continuously. After acceptance and receipt of admission ticket, an exam time may schedule any time within 90 days of receiving the admission ticket at any of the designated testing centers nationwide.
Application: http://www.nursecredentialing.org/certification/catalogs/ADMcat.pdf
Paper applications can be requested from the American Nurses Credentialing Center - www.Nursingworld.org, 600 Maryland Ave SW Ste 100 West, Washington, DC 20024-2571

Learning Activities

1. For each of the following principles of motivational interviewing, develop three example statements for use in counseling a person with diabetes:
   - Expressing empathy
   - Developing discrepancies
   - Roll with resistance
   - Support self-efficacy

2. Locate at least one of the motivational interviewing-based counseling protocols (references 11, 23, 24). Critique the protocol and its application to diabetes nutrition counseling practice.

3. Observe an individual, 1:1 counseling session. Was motivational interviewing observed during the session? How would you incorporate motivational interviewing principles into what you observed?

Additional Readings and Resources

On the Cutting Edge: A Peer Reviewed Publication of the Diabetes Care and Education DPG. Summer 2003; 24(1). (Entire issue devoted to behavioral science applications in diabetes counseling.)

Sawyer-Morse MK. The mechanics of motivational interviewing. *Today's Dietitian.* 2002; 7: 16-17.

Scales R, Miller JH. Motivational techniques for improving compliance with an exercise program: skills for primary care clinicians. *Curr Sports Med Rep.* 2003 Jun;2(3):166-72.

Thorpe M. Motivational interviewing and dietary behavior change. *J Am Diet Assoc.* 2003;103(2):150-151.

Burke B L, Arkowitz H, Dunn C. The efficacy of motivational interviewing. In: Miller WR, Rollnick S. *Motivational interviewing: Preparing people for change,* 2nd ed. New York: Guilford Press; 2002.

DiClemente CC, Velasquez MW. Motivational Interviewing and the Stages of Change. In: Miller WR, Rollnick S. *Motivational interviewing: Preparing people for change,* 2nd ed. New York: Guilford Press; 2002.

Wen DB, Ehret C, Pedersen M, Snetselaar L, Johnson M, Tinker L, Hollinger D, Ilona L, Bland K, Sivertsen D, Ocke D, Staats L, Beedoe JW. Abstract Results of an adjunct dietary intervention program in the Women's Health Initiative. *J Am Diet Assoc.* 2002 Nov;102(11):1631-7.

DiClemente CC, Marinilli AS, Singh M, Bellino LE.The role of feedback in the process of health behavior change. *Am J Health Behav.* 2001 May-Jun;25(3):217-27.

Konkle-Parker DJ. A motivational intervention to improve adherence to treatment of chronic disease. *J Am Acad Nurse Pract.* 2001 Feb;13(2):61-8

Shinitzky HE, Kub J. The art of motivating behavior change: the use of motivational interviewing to promote health. *Public Health Nurs.* 2001 May-Jun;18(3):178-85.

Selected Diabetes Resources

American Diabetes Association. Clinical Practice Recommendations. *Diabetes Care.* 2003; 26(Supp 1).
   Entire issue every January provides an update of current recommendations for diabetes care.

Mensing C, et al. National standards for diabetes self-management education. Diabetes Care 2000; 23(5).
   History of National Standards: The National Standards for Diabetes Patient Education Programs were developed and tested under the auspices of the National Diabetes Advisory Board (NDAB) and first published in *Diabetes Care* in 1984. Designed to promote quality education nationwide for every person with diabetes, the Standards were developed, tested, and distributed by a steering committee of the NDAB made up of many diabetes organizations. The American Diabetes Association (ADA) endorsed the Standards in 1983 and participated in the nationwide pilot testing of the Standards and review criteria in 1984. In 1986 the ADA developed an application and review process to determine whether an education program met the Standards. The first programs to meet the Standards were recognized by the ADA in 1987. The Standards were reviewed and revised in 1995 and most recently in 2000. A task force of representatives from the diabetes community completed a review of the 1995 Standards in January 2000. The task force reviewed the Standards for their appropriateness, relevancy, scientific basis, specificity and ability to be implemented in multiple settings. The revised Standards are now called the National Standards for Diabetes Self-Management Education and have been endorsed by the organizations involved in their development. The Standards are designed to be flexible enough to be applicable in any health care setting, from physicians' offices and HMOs to clinics and hospitals.

Nutrition Practice Guidelines for Type 1 and Type 2 Diabetes Mellitus CD-ROM (2002) ADA

Nutrition Practice Guidelines for Gestational Diabetes Mellitus CD-ROM (2002)

- The Nutrition Practice Guidelines for Type 1 and Type 2 Diabetes Mellitus and Gestational Diabetes are to be used with Medicare beneficiaries when providing the Medicare Part B benefit for MNT diabetes services effective January 1, 2002.
- A feature you will find in the ADA *Medical Nutrition Therapy Evidence-Based Guides for Practice* is the research, which is the foundation for the guides, organized in evidence worksheets showing the quality and strength of recommendations.
- For additional questions, send an email to: mntguides@eatright.org.

The American Diabetes Association (ADA) bookstore www.diabetes.org The bookstore offers a variety of books and other educational and professional materials to assist you in counseling persons with diabetes. Discover new cookbooks, meal planners, self-care guides and more.

The American Association of Diabetes Educators (AADE) www.diabeteseducator.org AADE offers a number of publications and products to help today's health professionals keep pace with the ever-changing field of diabetes education. Members of AADE can enjoy discounts on many products and receive notices whenever an update or new products are released.

REFERENCES

1. Behavior change is centerpiece of new DM approach for diabetics. *Dis Manag Advis.* 2001;7:118-121.
2. Miller WR, Rollnick S. *Motivational interviewing: Preparing people for change,* 2nd ed. New York: Guilford Press; 2002.
3. Miller WR. Motivational interviewing with problem drinkers. *Behav Psychother.* 1983;11:147-172.
4. Resnicow K, DiIorio C, Soet JE, et al. Motivational interviewing in health promotion: It sounds like something is changing. *Health Psychol.* 2002;21:444-451.
5. Prochaska JO, Velicer WF. The transtheoretical model of health behavior change. *Am J Health Promot.* 1997;12:38-48.
6. Doherty Y, Hall D, James PT, et al. Change counselling in diabetes: The development of a training programme for the diabetes team. *Patient Educ Couns.* 2000;40:263-278.
7. Miller WR, Mount KA. A small study of training in motivational interviewing: Does one workshop change clinician and client behavior? *Behav Cognitive Psychother.* 2001;29:457-471.
8. Rollnick S, Miller W. What is motivational interviewing? *Behav Cognitive Psychother.* 1995;23:325-334.
9. Emmons KM, Rollnick S. Motivational interviewing in health care settings: Opportunities and limitations. *Am J Prev Med.* 2001;20:68-74.
10. Rollnick S, Mason P, Butler C. Health behavior change: A guide for practitioners, 11th ed. Edinburgh: Churchill Livingstone; 1999.
11. Stott NCH, Rollnick S, Rees MR, et al. Innovation in clinical method: Diabetes care and negotiating skills. *Fam Pract.* 1995;12:413-418.
12. Leggett-Frazier N, Swanson MS, Vincent PA, et al. Telephone communications between diabetes clients and nurse educators. *Diabetes Educ.* 1997;23:287-293.
13. Berg-Smith SM, Stevens VJ, Brown KM, et al. A brief motivational intervention to improve dietary adherence in adolescents. *Health Educ Res.* 1999;14:399-410.
14. Bowen D, Ehret C, Pedersen M, et al. Results of an adjunct dietary intervention program in the Women's Health Initiative. *J Am Diet Assoc.* 2002;102:1631-1637.
15. Woollard J, Beilin L, Lord T, et al. A controlled trial of nurse counseling on lifestyle change for hypertensives treated in general practice: Preliminary results. *Clin Exp Pharmacol Physiol.* 1995;22:466-468.
16. Resnicow K, Jackson A, Wang T, et al. A motivational interviewing intervention to increase fruit and vegetable intake through Black churches: Results of the Eat for Life Trial. *Am J Public Health.* 2001;91:1686-1693.
17. Smith DE, Kratt PP, Heckemeyer CM, et al. Motivational interviewing to improve adherence to a behavioral weight-control program for older obese women with NIDDM. *Diabetes Care.* 1997;20:52-54.
18. Mhurchu CN, Margetts BM, Speller V. Randomized clinical trial comparing the effectiveness of two dietary interventions for patients with hyperlipidaemia. *Clin Sci.* 1998;95:479-487.
19. Brown SL, Pope JF, Hunt AE, et al. Motivational strategies used by dietitians to counsel individuals with diabetes. *Diabetes Educ.* 1998;24:313-318.
20. Roisin P, Stott NCH, Rollnick SR, Rees M. A randomized controlled trial of an intervention designed to improve the care given in general practice to type II diabetic patients: Patient outcomes and professional ability to change behaviour. *Fam Pract.* 1998;15: 229-235.
21. Resnicow K, Jackson A, Braithwaite R, et al. Healthy Body/Health Spirit: A church-based nutrition and physical activity intervention. *Health Educ Res.* 2002;17:562-573.
22. Clark M, Hampson SE. Implementing a psychological intervention to improve lifestyle self-management in patients with type 2 diabetes. *Patient Educ Couns.* 2001;42:247-256.
23. Doherty Y, Roberts S. Motivational interviewing in diabetes practice. *Diabet Med.* 2002;19(suppl 3):1-6.
24. Heins JM, Delahanty L. Tools and techniques to facilitate eating behavior change. In: Coulston AM, Rock CL, Monsen ER, eds. *Nutrition in the prevention and treatment of disease.* San Diego: Academic Press; 2001:113-115.
25. Welch G, Guthrie DW. Supporting lifestyle change with a computerized psychosocial assessment tool. *Diabetes Spectrum.* 2002;15:S203-207.

Chapter 20

Counseling People with Renal Disease

Bridget Klawitter, PhD, RD, FADA

After reading this chapter, the reader will be able to:
- ♦ Discuss the incidence of renal disease in the U.S.
- ♦ Identify the major symptoms and risk factors of renal disease.
- ♦ List three important considerations when counseling people with renal disease.

Chronic kidney disease (CKD) is permanent kidney damage due to injury or disease. Caring for kidney disease involves controlling the person's diet, blood pressure, and medications to delay heart complications and the need for dialysis. Unfortunately, many patients do not know they have chronic kidney disease and do not get the early care they need to delay complications. More than 20 million Americans—one in nine adults—have chronic kidney disease, and more than 20 million others are at increased risk. (1) More detailed statistics related to the incidence of kidney disease can be accessed from data collected by the United States Renal Data System. (2)

Risk factors for kidney disease include older age, family history of kidney disease, African-American ethnic background, diabetes, and high blood pressure. Diabetes and high blood pressure are the two leading causes of ESRD, accounting for more than 60 percent of new cases. (2) Anyone can develop kidney disease; however, people over the age of 50 and certain minority populations, including African Americans, Native Americans, Hispanics, Asians, and Pacific Islanders are disproportionately affected by ESRD. (4) Approximately 360,000 Americans suffer from ESRD, and this number increases by about seven percent each year. Kidney disease can also develop from infection, inflammation of blood vessels in the kidneys, development of kidney stones, and cysts. Other possible causes include prolonged use of pain relievers and use of alcohol or other drugs (including prescription medications). The warning signs of kidney disease include:

- High blood pressure
- Swelling of the face and ankles
- Puffiness around the eyes
- Frequent urination (especially at night)
- Rusty or brown colored urine
- Back pain just below the rib cage

In 2002, the National Kidney Foundation developed recommendations for chronic kidney disease as part of an effort to improve quality of care. (5)

In a study done by the United States Renal Data System (USRDS), only 46 percent of patients with end stage renal disease starting dialysis had seen a dietitian as a chronic kidney disease failure patient. (2) This is indefensible, since Medical Nutrition Therapy (MNT) had been an accepted part of the comprehensive management of either chronic or end-stage renal disease since 1973. (6) In January 2002, the Centers for Medicare and Medicaid Services (CMS) added MNT as a benefit for Medicare beneficiaries who have chronic kidney disease (including post-transplantation) or diabetes. This was important legislation, as it sets precedent for the coverage of MNT for specific diagnoses by other payers. See Chapter 22 for the MNT codes and descriptions, as well as further guidance on reimbursement requirements.

Intensive nutrition counseling for chronic and end-stage renal disease has been recommended in the National Kidney Foundation's Kidney Disease Outcome Initiative (K-DOQI) clinical practice guidelines. (5) Healthy People 2010 (7) also has included chronic kidney disease as one of its 20 focus areas. The goal is to increase the number of chronic kidney disease patients receiving nutrition counseling prior to reaching end-stage renal disease.

GENERAL COUNSELING CONSIDERATIONS

The psychological consequences of living with a life-threatening disease can often be misinterpreted or missed by the dietetic practitioner. When faced with a chronic disease requiring major changes in food and fluid intake, individuals often feel deprived and powerless. They often will put off appointments or seek alternative cures in the hope things will change. At the first visit, it is important to set the stage by preparing the patient for their MNT counseling experience, not only during the initial visit, but also for subsequent follow-up encounters. (8)

Before counseling on the restrictions related to the renal diet, it is important to determine the patients' knowledge or perceptions about what dietary changes they will be expected to make. This provides an opportunity to clarify misperceptions and misinformation, and clear the way for new diet information. The "what" question technique can provide insight into what patients think is related to the subject at hand. (8) For example, "What do you think you need to know about your kidney disease to make it easier to follow the diet?" or "What do you think is the best way for you to decrease your protein intake?" When presenting complex diet information, such as in renal disease, it is easy for the inexperienced counselor to present extensive information (i.e., facts, lists, and information sheets) in an overwhelming way that prevents the patient from feeling in control. Simply providing the information will not guarantee comprehension or compliance!

Counseling Applications for Chronic Renal Failure

The individual diagnosed with chronic renal failure (CRF) may often feel overwhelmed and confused about MNT interventions. At the initial visit, a detailed assessment of current diet intake is critical to determine baseline intake of protein, calories, potassium, sodium, phosphorus, calcium, and magnesium. Asking the patient to keep a detailed food diary for at least 3-4 days prior to the appointment can provide insight into day-to-day variations. Several tools are available for obtaining diet histories. (9,10)

The goal of MNT counseling in CRF is to slow the decline in renal function, hence decreasing long-term cumulative healthcare cost and prolonging an independent quality of life. Due to the large and growing number of patients faced with long-term dependence on dialysis, ESRD is among the most expensive diseases to treat on a per capita basis. Fortunately, since 1972 the cost of dialysis and kidney transplantation for most Americans is covered through Medicare. In 2000, the total combined direct medical payments for ESRD by public and private sources was estimated at more than $19.35 billion (latest year for which figures are available). (1) As the population ages and as other at-risk populations increase, ESRD incidence is sharply on the rise. In fact, the U.S. incidence rate is the highest in the world—210 per million. While dialysis and improved treatments keep most ESRD patients alive far longer than we were able to just two decades ago, these developments also mean that more people are living with this debilitating and costly disease. (11)

Initial visits with newly referred CRF patients are usually quite complicated and require extra time by the dietetic practitioner. (12) Because many individuals have prior experience with calorie-controlled diets that limit fat and carbohydrate, the mind-shift required to adopt the pre-renal diet with emphasis on high-calorie, high-fat, high-carbohydrate components, is a difficult concept to grasp. The social aspects of eating quickly become restrictive and patients perceive they no longer "fit in."

The patient with CRF needs consistent, long-term monitoring to sustain renal function as long as possible. Studies have indicated that self-monitoring and dietitian-support were the most helpful components of diet intervention. (13) New information should be reviewed and reinforced often so it can become part of their existing knowledge. (8) Varying the reinforcement techniques helps achieve a better match with individual learning styles. For example, after reviewing general principles of the low-protein diet, allow the patient to plan a meal using food models and count the protein points together.

Counseling Applications for End-Stage Renal Disease
The most common symptoms experienced by the ESRD patient include:
- Weakness, fatigue, nausea
- Physical limitations and loss of function
- Loss/change in employment and income
- Changes in appearance

The most common psychological problem for such patients is depression. (14) Diabetes, coupled with ESRD, contributes to chronic complications such as impairment of vision and circulation.

Due to multiple diet components in the dialysis renal diet, staging or setting priorities for adjustment to the restrictions of the diet may be challenging but effective in facilitating compliance. This process allows the patient to focus on one diet restriction (i.e., phosphorus for an elevated serum level) while starting to modify diet behaviors for other restrictions (i.e., protein, fluid, and sodium). Snetselaar (11) has suggested three factors counselors should consider when staging:
- Identify problem that, if solved, will provide the most success.
- Identify barriers that may need to be dealt with first to allow patient to work on diet restrictions.
- Identify problem(s) that are moderately challenging and assist patient in ranking in order of priority.

Inadequate nutrient intake caused by such factors as anorexia, uremia, taste changes, limited income, mental health and addiction issues, co-morbid acute or chronic illnesses, chewing or swallowing difficulties, cultural preferences, and/or inadequate knowledge of dietary restrictions can result in chronic malnutrition. (15) The dietetic practitioner is then challenged to balance repletion with renal diet restrictions to restore nutritional status. Care must be taken to clearly explain to the patient the reasons why common diet restrictions are being relaxed and the amount of leeway given.

SUMMARY

Renal disease is just one specific example of the role dietetic practitioners can play in increasing self-management skills through effective nutrition counseling. Skilled nutrition counselors use sound counseling principles to assess learning needs, establish rapport, determine readiness to learn, and build knowledge and confidence in patients to self-manage their illness. With the multiple diet restrictions and medication schedules, it becomes important to provide encouragement and affirm the patient's hard work and persistence, as well as successes, however small. Active listening and collaborative decision-making can enhance the potential for compliance. Future research to provide a better understanding of the effects of nutrition counseling methods (including Quality of Life scales) is needed.

Additional Resources

Rollnick S, Mason P, Butler C. Health behavior change: a guide for practitioners. New York: Churchill Livingstone, 1999.
National Institute of Diabetes and Digestive and Kidney Disease, National Kidney Disease Education Program accessed at www.nkdep.nih.gov/
The National Kidney Foundation 1-800-622-9010 or access at www.kidney.org
The American Dietetic Association: Chronic Kidney Disease (nondialysis) Medical Nutrition Therapy Protocol. Chicago IL: The American Dietetic Association, 2002.

Board Certification as a Specialist in Dietetics Renal (CSR)

The Commission on Dietetic Registration currently offers Board Certification as a Specialist for registered dietitians in the area of renal nutrition. Board Certification is granted in recognition of an applicant's documented practice experience and successful completion of a clinical problem simulation examination in the specialty area. Renal nutrition practice experience that qualifies includes: Working directly with adults and/or children with acute or chronic renal dysfunction or failure, under treatment by kidney transplantation, dialysis, or other modalities in a variety of settings (home, hospitals, other treatment centers, etc.), or indirectly as documented by management, education, or research practice linked specifically to renal nutrition.

Dietetic Practice Group #21 Renal Practice Group of the American Dietetic Association is an organization of Registered Dietitians and other dietetic professionals who specialize in the care of patients with kidney disease. The Renal Dietitians Dietetic Practice Group (RPG) consists of Registered Dietitians and other dietetic professionals who provide renal nutrition counseling in dialysis facilities, clinics, hospitals, and private practice. RPG's purpose is to offer direction, leadership, and education to help members provide quality renal nutrition practice. RPG promotes continuing education programs for dietitians and other health professionals, and is an information resource for those who specialize in renal nutrition. The group includes renal dietitians working with pre- or end-stage renal (kidney) disease, acute renal failure, adult and pediatric dialysis, and kidney transplant patients. For more information, access the web site at www.renalnutrition.org

References
1. K/DOQI Clinical Practice Guidelines for Chronic Kidney Disease: Evaluation, Classification, and Stratification. *A J Kidney Dis.* 2002; 39(2, Suppl 1):S1-S266.
2. United States Renal Data System. *USRDS 2002 Annual Data Report. Bethesda, MD: National Institute of Diabetes and Digestive and Kidney Diseases, National Institutes of Health (NIH), DHHS; 2002.* Available at www.usrds.org.
3. National Kidney Foundation. *2002 Annual Report.* Available at www.kidney.org/general/annualreport02.pdf Accessed 9/4/03.
4. National Kidney Foundation. Diagnosis and evaluation of patients with chronic kidney disease: recommendations from NKF. *Ann Int Med.* 2003; 139(2): 1-36.
5. National Kidney Foundation. *K/DOQI clinical practice guidelines for chronic kidney disease: evaluation, classification and stratification.* Available at www.kidney.org/professionals/kdoqi/guidelines_ckd/toc.html Accessed 8/29/03.
6. Pavlinac J. Medical nutrition therapy (MNT): reimbursement for nutrition intervention in chronic kidney disease and its impact on the renal care community. *Dialysis & Transpl.* 2001; 30(9): 584-585, 614.
7. *Healthy People 2010.* Accessed at www.healthypeople.gov/
8. Doak CC, Doak LG, Root JH. *Teaching patients with low literacy skills,* 2nd ed. Philadelphia: JB Lippincott Company, 1996.
9. Snetselaar LG. Chapter 7: Nutrition counseling in treatment of renal disease. In: *Nutrition Counseling Skills for Medical Nutrition Therapy.* Gaithersburg MD: Aspen Publishers Inc. 1997: pp 271-309.
10. Wiggins K. *Guidelines for Nutritional Care of Renal Patients,* 3rd ed. Chicago: American Dietetic Association, 2002.
11. www.coloradohealthsite.org/dialysis/dialmain.html Accessed 8/25/03.
12. Dolecek TA, Olson MB, Caggiula AW, Dwyer JT, Milas C, Gillis BP, Hartman JA, DiChiro JT. Registered dietitian time requirements in the modification of diet in renal disease study. *J Am Diet Assoc.* 1995; 95(11): 1307-1312.
13. Gillis BP, Caggiula AW, Chiavacci AT, Coyne T, Doroshenko L, Milas NC, Nowalk MP, Scherch LK. Nutrition intervention program of the modification of diet in renal disease study: a self-management approach. *J Am Diet Assoc.* 1995: 95(11): 1288-1294.
14. Rosen LS. The trauma of life-threatening illness: end-stage renal disease. *Dialysis & Transpl.* 2002; 31(5): 295-300.
15. Dwyer JT, Cunniff PJ, Maroni BJ, Kopple JD, Burrows JD, Powers SN, Cockram DB, Chumlea WC, Kusek JW, Makoff R, Goldstein DJ, Paranandi L. The hemodialysis pilot study: nutrition program and participant characteristics at baseline. The HEMO study group. *J Ren Nutr.* 1998; 8(1): 11-20. Erratum in *J Ren Nutr.* 1998; 8(4): 230.

Chapter 21

Counseling a Person with HIV/AIDS
Jean E. Schreiner, MS, RD

After reading this chapter, the reader will be able to:
  ♦ Identify five nutritional concerns of particular importance to this patient population.
  ♦ List at least three counseling strategies that may improve patient compliance.

Counseling a person with AIDS (referred to as PWA in medical settings) about nutrition is an essential component for overall management of the disease. Also, early intervention allows time to establish a relationship and develop rapport with the patient.

By delaying the wasting and malnutrition commonly seen in AIDS patients, dietitians can presumably improve a patient's prognosis. The degree of body cell mass depletion may be a better predictor of survival than any analysis of any specific underlying infection or a CD4 count. (1) Supportive nutrition and dietary measures may significantly improve symptomatic relief and contribute to a higher quality of life. As early as 1994, the position of both the American Dietetic Association and the Canadian Dietetic Association was that nutrition intervention and medical nutrition therapy, along with education, should be components of the total healthcare provided to persons infected with the human immunodeficiency virus (HIV). (2)

PREPARING FOR THE COUNSELING SESSION

A nutrition therapist must be concerned about all the factors that affect the patient's current nutrition status and his or her ability to buy, prepare, and eat food as the disease progresses. Prepare for the counseling session by first evaluating the patient's current symptoms, individual abilities, and needs. Use all data available including any recent interview information, charts, nutritional assessments, and information from any others involved in his/her care. Consider psychosocial conditions, economic factors, and support systems to develop a workable and realistic plan. If friends, family, or funds are limited, enlist the aid of Social Services, local HIV/AIDS support groups, and meal delivery services. Check the patient's existing insurance coverage and such options as nutritional supplements to see if they are reimbursable. Develop a flexible plan with prioritized goals that will improve the patient's quality of life and nutritional status.

The following is a brief review of nutrition-related concerns, along with other possible complications to consider as you create the individualized plan. Detailed discussions of nutritional concerns and interventions can be found in the resources listed at the end of this article. See Appendix 20-A Nutritional Assessment Form, Appendix 20-B Nutritional Assessment Data Tracking Form, and Appendix 20-C Diet History Checklist.

Weight Status
If nutritional support is delayed until after significant weight loss, it may be more difficult to change the patient's malnutrition status. Deliberate weight gain may help improve his or her chances of surviving longer with HIV. (3,4) Check weight status and weight history. Use nutritional assessment data to determine which body compartments are depleted. Determine the energy, protein, and nutrient goals.

Anorexia
Determine the cause by checking for depression, mouth sores, dementia, anxiety, medications, and fear of increased diarrhea. Focus on a calorically dense diet and supplements.

237

Nausea/Vomiting
Identify cause(s) and counsel patients regarding appropriate food/liquid choices and timing of meals. If needed, recommend anti-nausea medications to physician.

Dyspnea/Fatigue/Pain
Check patient's ability to eat and evaluate actual intake. Make meal suggestions that include easy food preparation techniques, and possibly, meal delivery or helpers to assist at mealtimes. Consider alternative food routes to achieve adequate intake and counsel patient on these options.

Infection/Fever
Check for presence of fluid and nutrient losses, and assume increased tissue breakdown. Adjust patient's calorie/protein/nutrient goals, and counsel accordingly.

Mouth and Esophageal Sores
To avoid aggravating their mouth problems, counsel patients regarding food consistency, types of foods to avoid or comfort foods, and temperatures.

Diarrhea and Malabsorption
Discuss fluid and electrolyte replacement. Counsel patients to avoid caffeine and increase soluble fiber. Consider possible lactose and fat restriction. Add appropriate supplements specifically for PWAs.

Food Safety
PWAs have an increased vulnerability to food borne illness. They should be counseled concerning food safety at home and eating out, as well as safety of their water sources.

Nutritional Supplements
Check any supplements the patient is using. Counsel in a nonjudgmental way regarding potential harm or concerns about the unorthodox supplements. Prevent and correct any deficiencies in the person's diet (goal = approximately 200% RDI).

Enteral and Parenteral Feedings: Check into physical facilities and adequacy of feeding equipment. Counsel caregivers and patient (perhaps along with the home health nurse) on the formula and how to administer the feeding. (See Resource list for detailed information.)

Drug/Nutrient or Food Interactions: Note all medications used including over-the-counter ones and look for potential influence on nutrient needs, absorption, and side effects. Counsel and educate accordingly.

COUNSELING CONSIDERATIONS FOR THE PERSON WITH AIDS

After considering your client's needs and appropriate interventions, prioritize your recommendations. What is an essential intervention and what can be delayed?

Plan the session so that it will be in tune with the patient's condition. Is morning nausea the rule? Will talking during the meal distract the patient from eating a needed high-calorie intake? Make sure any home visit or outpatient appointments are planned in the best interest and convenience of the patient's and caregiver's schedules. Avoid conflicts with meal delivery times, visits from home health aids, or any other events related to management of the patient's care and well-being.

Depression can occur, and may be related to the stress of dealing with a life threatening illness, or from medications, or the underlying disease itself. Be aware and sympathetic. AIDS patients may at times feel too depressed to shop, plan meals, or eat nourishing foods. For this and other reasons, it is important to include any friends, family, or caregivers in any counseling sessions.

One study revealed the most prominent feelings of PWAs are uncertainty, anxiety, and anger over the treatment of their illness by caregivers. (5) Demonstrate your concern and willingness to listen. A positive and nonjudgmental attitude is important. It helps to encourage a patient to be involved in his or her care as much as possible. Making decisions regarding food choices and the diet plan can help promote feelings of self-control and esteem. One client once remarked he felt like he to his hospital room. An on-site tour of the nourishment area of the hospital kitchen complete with a "taste test" of various supplements got him involved in his care in a positive way.

Information for the client can be provided in an endless number of creative ways. Depending on the patient's needs, the following resources can be useful: verbal plans, written plans with grocery lists, menu ideas, shake recipes, resource lists, eating hints, and the address of the nearest food bank. Individual instruction is most common, but a group session with two or more PWAs is useful for discussions regarding food safety, nutritional supplements, or high calorie/protein diet suggestions. Your client should always have your department or office phone number, as well as several numbers of other team members, nurses or social workers, where he or she can get fast and reliable answers to questions. See Figures 20.1 and 20.2 for suggested outlines for individual or group instruction for HIV positive patients, and nutrition education presentation for persons with HIV/AIDS and their caretakers.

Monitor a patient initially with phone calls and home visits, if your institution allows, or refer the patient to a private practice, managed care, or community dietitian. If this is not possible, continue to provide at-home follow-up by calling the client's home caregiver or support services in addition to your calls to the patient. Home health care, particularly nutrition, is not being fully used even though the majority of clients feel they could benefit from home health services. (6)

In summary, early nutrition intervention, with a realistic and flexible nutrition care plan created with the patient's involvement are essential to overall management of AIDS.

Screening Checklist for HIV/ AIDS
Kaye Jessup, MPH, RD, LD

Nutritional status plays a major part in the health status of a person with HIV/ AIDS. It is important to identify warning signs that can lead to malnutrition and take steps to prevent it from happening. This screening form may help to identify persons with HIV or AIDS at nutritional risk in order for interventions to be implemented. See following checklist, which is available through your Ross Products representative.

HIV/AIDS Nutritional Checklist
Are you at risk?

The warning signs leading to poor nutritional health are often overlooked. Use this checklist to find out if you or someone you know is at nutritional risk.

Read the statements below. Circle the number in the "YES" column that apply to you or someone you know. For each "YES" answer, score the number in the box. Total your nutritional score.

• Without wanting to, I have lost 5 or more pounds over the last 2 months or 10 pounds or more over the last 6 months.	3
• I have 3 or more bowel movements per day that are significantly different from my usual bowel habits.	3
• I have had 2 or more unscheduled visits to my health care professional over the last 2 months due to HIV-related problems.	3
• I eat fewer than 2 meals per day.	3
• I take 3 or more different prescribed or over-the-counter drugs a day.	1
• I have had a persistent fever and/or infection for 1 week or more.	3
• I am not always able to buy food, cook or feed myself.	3
• I take 3 or more vitamin, mineral and/or herb supplements a day.	1
• I have 3 or more drinks of beer, liquor or wine almost every day.	2
• I eat very few fruits, vegetables or milk products.	2

• I have limited food intake due to:
  Nausea and/or vomiting
  Food aversions
  Chewing and/or swallowing difficulties
	2
	1
	2

Total	

Total your nutritional score.

If it's.....

0-2 **GOOD!** Recheck your nutritional score in 3 months.

3-5 **You are at moderate nutritional risk.** Talk with your doctor, dietitian, social service or other health care professional to see what can be done to improve your eating habits. You may want to use ADVERA* (2-3 cans per day), which is specifically designed to help provide effective nutritional management for people with HIV or AIDS.

6+ **You may be at high nutritional risk.** Show this checklist to your doctor, dietitian, or other qualified health or social service professional. You may want to use ADVERA (2-3 cans per day), which is specifically designed to help provide effective nutritional management for people with HIV or AIDS.

Remember, warning signs suggest risk,
but do not represent diagnosis of any condition.

A6871/SEPTEMBER 1994

© 1994 ROSS

Figure 20.1

Nutrition Education Session for the HIV Positive Individual or Group (Suggested Outline)

Nutrition Goals Include:
- Preserve and enhance weight and nutritional status
- Support medical treatments to maximize effectiveness
- Improve client's quality of life by feeling as well as possible
- Establish and build a relationship with healthcare professional

I. Obtain baseline nutritional assessment and diet history

II. Review rationale for eating well and maintaining a balanced diet

    A. Enhances nutritional status and immune system for healthier mind and body
    B.   Alleviates symptoms associated with later complications
    C. Generally improves quality of life.

III. Review basic food categories (see Food Guide Pyramid for Healthful Eating), phasize variety.

IV. Discuss individual energy, protein, nutrient and fluid requirements

    A. Calculate energy needs to maintain or gain weight if indicated
        1. Discuss need for adequate calories to maintain weight and strength
        2. Interpret into daily food intake guidelines

    B. Calculate protein requirements
        1. Interpret to patient in terms of number and size of protein food sources
        2. Discuss rationale for adequate protein

    C. Replete any nutritional deficits with increased food sources of these nutrients and/or supplements if necessary

    D. Discuss merits of multiple vitamin/mineral supplements

        1. Advise against single nutrient supplements unless indicated (e.g. calcium supplements if client does not drink milk
        2. Discuss when to take supplements, size of supplements, the need for adequate fluids; how to avoid dehydration

V. Review general considerations for immune system and HIV

    A. Encourage avoidance of fad diets

        1. Note the costs
        2. Note potential harm or interference with good nutrition

Figure 20.1 continued

HIV Positive Individual or Group (Outline continued)

        B. Discuss the nutritional supplements available commercially

                1. Consider how to *use* homemade nutritional supplements
                2. Discuss current use
                3. Discuss how to make ahead for ***possible*** future use during times of fatigue or anorexia

        C. Advise avoidance of alcohol and smoking because of potential effect of depression on immune system

        D. Discuss food safety/handling tips

                1. Discuss importance because of lowered resistance to infection
                2. Use tips in Appendix K, Food Safety at Home

        E. Advise adequate rest and *possible* relaxation techniques for times of stress

        F. Encourage patients to check with physician regarding appropriate level of exercise, weight resistance training for muscle building

        G. Provide information about local support groups, social services, *meal* delivery and food bank programs available for help now or in the future

        H. Encourage calls as desired to registered dietitian with any questions and for individual counseling for any complications such as diarrhea, swallowing difficulty, etc.

        I. Discuss potential nutritional concerns, side effects for any HIV medications

    VI.   Questions and Discussion

Note: This is only a suggested outline of nutrition information to include and is not intended to cover all possible topics for program content.

Nutrition Handbook for HIV/AIDS - 3rd Edition (Professional Page)
Copyright 1999 Carrot Top nutrition Resources, PO Box 460172, Aurora CO 80046

Figure 20.2

Nutrition Education Session for HIV/AIDS
Groups of Patients or Caretakers
(Late Stage HIV or AIDS Diagnosis)
Suggested Outline

I. Nutritional implications of HIV/AIDS

    A. How HIV/AIDS can change the way the body uses nutrients
    B. Weight Loss

        1. Discuss body composition, how different body compartments may be affected (fat stores, visceral, somatic) including possible lipodystrophy
        2. Note reasons for weight loss (decreased intake, increased energy requirements, possible Malabsorption, other)

    C. Infection and Fever
        1. Discuss effects on energy protein, fluid, and nutrient requirements
        2. Note how anti-HIV medications and medications to treat infection may affect appetite, diet tolerance, and nutrient requirements

    D. Dyspnea, Fatigue, and Pain
        Note how appetite, eating ability, and interest in eating may be affected.

    E. Gastrointestinal Tract
        1. Discuss how food consistency and composition can affect tolerance and eating ability
        2. Review possible causes of diarrhea, its effects on nutritional requirements including fluid and electrolytes

II. Nutritional Assessment

    Note types of information, measurements, and tests the dietitian may use to assess nutritional status:

Height	arm muscle circumference	food intake records
Weight	BIA	food preferences
weight history	laboratory values	medications
skinfolds	clinical appearance	physical activity
triceps	diet history	eating ability

III. Dietary Suggestions

    A. Weight Loss: the variety of causes
        1. Encourage weekly (not daily) monitoring of weight
          • Note how hydration status may affect
          • Advise to keep weight record for physician

Source: Carrot Top Nutrition Resources. Copyright 1999.

Figure 20.2

        2. Discuss pattern of eating for weight gain
- Multiple small meals, snacks
- Recommend recipes

        3. Discuss nutrient density of foods and beverages: how to increase
        4. Review role of supplements

B. Poor appetite
    1. Again note to increase calories to "make every bite count"
    2. Discuss easy-to-prepare items, keeping favorite items on hand; Display cookbooks geared for HIV positive individuals

C. Oral, Esophageal Complications
    1. Note how diet consistency and food choices can affect as does food temperature
    2. Give suggestions on soft/liquid diets
    3. Encourage supplemental beverages; refer to Carrot Top's "High Calorie Beverage Recipes," or "Soft Bland Meal and Snack Ideas."

D. Vitamins, Minerals, and Fluids
    1. Suggest balanced diet with a multiple vitamin/mineral supplement that does not exceed 100-200% of the RDA
    2. Discuss commercial nutrient-fortified supplements
    3. Discuss pros and cons of nutrient megadoses
    4. Note fluid requirements and means of fluid replacement if fever or diarrhea is present
    5. Encourage use of calorie-containing fluids over noncaloric (e.g., juice instead of tea)

E. Additional Considerations
    1. If elevated blood lipids are of concern, discuss how to modify type and amount of fat without compromising adequate calories, protein, and nutrients. Note dietary intervention not proven effective in lowering blood lipids in this group of patients.
    2. Discuss need to individualize schedule for types and timing of meals, snacks with regard to anti-HIV and other drugs.
    3. Discuss food/beverage suggestions to keep on hand, to prepare double amounts and freeze for later use.
    4. Encourage to take advantage of the times the patient feels well, to increase intake.
    5. Check into community resources, help groups, support groups, hospital social services, and local health departments for help with meal preparation, shopping, home health aides, or visiting nurses.
    6. Note food safety considerations; refer to Carrot Top's "Food Safety at Home."

Figure 20.2

7. Encourage avoidance of fad diets; note potential harm or interference with good nutrition. Research herbs and popular supplements in order to be resource of good alternative information for patients, families, and colleagues. Provide unbiased information.
8. Advise to seek counseling by Registered Dietitian, especially with any concerns such as weight loss, vomiting, diarrhea; may need eating plan modified in fiber, lactose, or fat.

IV. Questions and Discussion

Note: Add other topics that meet the needs of your patients.

To order HIV/AIDS manual contact Carrot Top Nutrition Resources, P.O. box 460172, Aurora, CO 80046-0172

ADDITIONAL RESOURCES

Hickey M S. *Handbook of Enteral, Parenteral, and ARC/AIDS Nutritional Therapy.* Stylus, MO: Mosby; 1992. For health care professionals.

National AIDS Clearing House 1-800-458-5231. For consumers and professionals.

Salomont SB, Davis M, Newman CF. *Living Well with HIV and AIDS: A Guide to Healthy Eating.* Chicago, IL: American Dietetic Association; 1993. Twenty-eight pages for consumers and professionals.

Schreiner JE. *Nutrition Handbook for AIDS, 3rd ed.; 1999.* Carrot Top Nutrition Resources, PO Box 460172, Aurora, CO 80046-0172, (303) 690-3650. For health care professionals.

References
1. Kilter DP, Tierney AR, Wang J, Pierson RN. Magnitude of body cell mass depletion and the timing of death from wasting in AIDS. *J Clin Nutr.* 1989: 50:444-447.
2. The American Dietetic Association and The Canadian Dietetic Association. Position of The ADA and The CDA: Nutrition intervention in the care of persons with human immunodeficiency virus infection. *J Am Diet Assoc.* 1994: 94:1042-1044.
3. Smith J, Birmingham CL. HIV seropositivity and deliberate weight gain. *N Eng J Med.* 1990:322:1089.
4. Schreiner JE. *Nutrition Handbook for AIDS,* 3rd ed. Aurora, CO: Carrot Top Nutrition Resources; 1999.
5. DilleyJW, Ochitill HN, Peril M, Volberding PA. Findings in psychiatric consultations with patients with acquired immune deficiency syndrome. *Am J Psych.* 1985:142:82.
6. Udine LM, Rothkopf MM. Utilization of home health care services in HIV infection: a pilot study in Ohio. *J Am Diet Assoc.1994*: 94:83-85.

Section IV

Maximizing Success

Chapter 22

Reimbursement, Documentation, and HIPAA

Bridget Klawitter, PhD, RD, FADA

After reading this chapter, the reader will be able to:
- ♦ Identify healthcare changes impacting dietetic practice.
- ♦ Connect evidence-based practice to reimbursement efforts.
- ♦ Identify different types of codes used in the billing process.
- ♦ Distinguish between Diabetes Self-Management Training (DSMT) and Medical Nutrition Therapy (MNT) codes and services.
- ♦ Understand the link between coding and documentation.
- ♦ Understand the basic implications of the Health Insurance Portability and Accountability Act (HIPPA) Introduction.

Today's dietetic practitioners are faced with many unique challenges and opportunities. The profession has grown from a primary focus on hospital-inpatient services only, to private practice, corporate wellness, publishing ventures, travel industry, and innovative technologies. As stated by Kathy King, "nutrition's window of opportunity is wide open and the field of nutrition will continue to offer new opportunities for some time." (1)

Hospitals are our roots as dietetic practitioners. Historically, hospitals and healthcare facilities were the largest single employers of registered dietitians and dietetic technicians. Recognition of our clinical expertise often became buried as clinical services became "bundled" with food service and "room and board." Dietetic practitioners were not recognized for their revenue potential and were excluded from the majority of financial arrangements.

The opportunities for reimbursement by payers for services provided by dietetic practitioners have been hit and miss at best. But in the same vein, many dietitians have provided services free or at reduced cost as a "value-added" service. Fortunately, times are changing.

HEALTHCARE IS A CHANGING BUSINESS

Historically, a clinical perspective has dominated healthcare. Services were designed to address specific diagnoses or groups of patients. Outcomes were clinical measurements of care effectiveness. Nutrition education consisted of patient-centered materials, focused teaching, and in more recent times, behavior change strategies and disease self-management. Over time, a shift to the business perspective occurred in order to survive reduced payer payments and increased costs. Dietetic practitioners need to add new skills to their repertoire such as business skills, marketing, communication, customer service, service excellence, technology, finance and budgeting, legislative savvy, and research.

Healthcare has been impacted by several changes and trends such as:
- national and local economics
- new focus on industry
- loss of autonomy (physicians and patients)
- "Patient's Rights"
- vast numbers of under- and uninsured
- focus on prevention
- increasing ambulatory and alternate site care
- advanced imaging techniques
- minimally invasive surgery

- biotechnology and advanced pharmaceutical development
- advanced information and medical record technology
- internet or e-health

It is important to understand the overall climate of healthcare in which dietetic practice must operate. As far back as the early 1980's, when Diagnosis Related Groups (DRGs) hit healthcare, inpatient days dropped significantly in just 10 years. Patients in hospitals had shorter length of stays (LOSs) and/or fewer patients entered the acute care setting. The overall shift to outpatient/ambulatory care settings impacted what dietetic practitioners did in the acute care setting. The provision of medical nutrition therapy (MNT) in the non-acute care setting became more necessary to facilitate self-management of nutrition-related illnesses and conditions.

The primary goal of successful dietetic practitioners, especially those in healthcare facilities, has shifted to increased recognition and demand for services. Successful endeavors have focused on:

- Shifting from a cost center to a revenue center.
- Promoting programs for capital gain versus financial loss.
- Designing practices as an asset versus a liability.
- Establishing a new culture of evidence-based practice.
- Educating billing and contract staffs on the services offered, and the MNT or diabetes G-codes for billing.
- Evaluating practice processes, forms, and procedures.
- Promoting services internally and externally to establish a referral base.

Disease prevention has become a goal in today's competitive healthcare environment. Now, a healthy population is more profitable than a population with high healthcare utilization. Third party payers (TPP) have taken on a variety of forms, and it is important for dietetic practitioners to understand the type of payers and their focus in order to design appropriate, marketable services. An interesting overview of payer types and definitions used in the health insurance industry can be found at www.healthsymphony.com/definitions.htm.

OUTCOMES MANAGEMENT

The concept of continuous quality improvement should no longer be foreign to nutrition practitioners. We have come a long way from the days of quality control measures and, as healthcare professionals, we now find ourselves designing outcome management initiatives to promote the value of our services. We have become aware of key quality characteristics (KQCs) of medical nutrition therapy and the need to document the effectiveness of our services. Our customers are interested in our actual performance, not just what we say we can do. Quality management projects define opportunities and problems in a measurable way, and track our efforts at improvement.

Outcomes management (showing positive results) should be the cornerstone of dietetic practice. The involvement of various disciplines in the development of practice standards serves as the foundation to measure outcomes and prove professional value. Dietetic practitioners must be willing to "get out of the box" and measure effectiveness of interventions to demonstrate the value of our services. Evidence-based Practice (EBP) demands we make practice decisions based on the strength of scientific data. Existing guides for nutrition practice vary in their level and strength of evidence. A process for the development of evidence-based guides for practice (also known as clinical practice guidelines) has been published. (2)

Table 22.1   **TOOLS FOR EVIDENCE-BASED PRACTICE**

Nutrition Practice Guidelines
- Systematically developed statements or specifications, based on scientific evidence and/or verified through rigorous field-testing, which are designed to help practitioners and clients choose appropriate nutrition care in typical settings. *
- Recommended course of action for specific condition, procedure, or patient population.
- Looks at effectiveness and appropriateness of procedures or practices.

Protocols
- Plan or set of steps that clearly define level, content, and frequency of nutrition care that is appropriate for the disease or condition. *
- May be highly organized and directive, such as an algorithm, or more general and flexible.

Standards
- A statement that defines the performance expectations, structures, or processes that must be substantially in place to enhance the quality of care. **
    - Standards of care
    - Standards of Professional Practice

Source: * American Dietetic Association
          ** Joint Commission on Accreditation for Healthcare Organizations

---

Should you use a guideline or a protocol? Often dietetic practitioners feel "usual practice" is less tedious and more within their comfort zone. The decision on whether to move towards using these tools of EBP can be determined by asking yourself, "Is the goal to provide services that:

Improve the client's health?
Reduce costs to clients or the health care system?
Reduce unexplained variation in practice?
Build the scientific bases linking nutrition to positive outcomes?
Affect policy decisions, relevant to Medicaid, Medicare, and other payers?"

If your answer is "yes" to any of these, EBP is the direction for you.

The continual use of data is the expectation for EBP to improve practice and demonstrate the cost-effectiveness of nutrition interventions and counseling. Often, dietitians have been referred to as a type of clinical case manager because the dietetic practitioner:

- Is often the provider with the most patient contact.
- Coordinates and monitors the patient's care in the clinical setting.
- Coordinates care with the primary care physician who determines the course of treatment.

In this case management approach, the process is cyclical:

A = access clients/patients
P = plan for and integrate care
D = deliver one level of care

With EBP, nutrition care is pre-planned according to diagnosis, condition, or procedure. This approach provides the setting-specific consistency needed to collect outcome data, yet individualize care as needed. The American Dietetic Association MNT protocols (3,4) and guidelines (5-8) clearly define level, content, and frequency of nutrition care that is appropriate for a disease or condition. Just recently, the American Dietetic Association's evidence-based guides have been included in the

National Guideline Clearinghouse database. The National Guideline Clearinghouse promotes widespread access to evidence-based clinical practice guidelines through an Internet database of guideline summaries. You can access the database at www.guideline.gov.

Three distinct terms are used in outcomes-focused MNT: (9)

- **Outcomes measurement**
  Systematic quantification at a single point in time of outcome indicators.
- **Outcomes monitoring**
  Repeated measurement of outcome indicators over time to deduce how outcomes produce.
- **Outcomes management**
  Use of information gained from monitoring care to achieve optimal outcomes through improved clinical decision-making and delivery of quality care.

The importance of monitoring outcomes cannot be overemphasized. Outcomes should be used to guide the treatment process and determine interventions. Collection of outcome data for a group of patients can validate practice patterns, and facilitate the role of the dietetic practitioner in achieving positive outcomes. For more guidance and examples of outcomes management, see references 10-15.

CODES, CODES, AND MORE CODES

Code selection will vary among payers and it is necessary to become proficient in working with the various codes. With increasing technology, the majority of billing is transmitted electronically; codes serve to communicate what was done, computer-to-computer!

Diagnosis codes are derived from the *International Classification of Diseases, 9th revision* and *Clinical Modification*. Commonly these codes are referred to as ICD-9 codes. Key points to be aware of regarding ICD-9 codes include:

- The category code (3 digit) is used to classify or define symptoms, conditions, diagnosis, and injuries.
- Always code to the highest level of specificity (4th or 5th digit) whenever possible.
- The billing diagnosis code should match the base code of the physician making referral.
- If no code is assigned, a claim processor may "choose" one for you.
- Coding is a method of demonstrating medical necessity.

When deciding how to code the diagnosis for billing, it is important to differentiate primary and secondary diagnosis. A primary diagnosis is the major health problem generating the referral, and is listed first on the claim. The secondary diagnoses are concurrent conditions addressed during the same encounter. The ICD-9 reference book (16) is a necessary tool, and is categorized into lists in order to facilitate diagnosis. An example of the disease tabular list includes:

- Endocrine, Nutritional and Metabolic Diseases, and Immunity Diseases (240-279)
- Mental Disorders (290-319)
- Digestive System (520-579)
- Genitourinary System (580-629)
- Complications of Pregnancy, Childbirth and the Puerperium (630-677)
- Congenital Anomalies (740-759)
- Symptoms, Signs, and Ill Defined Conditions (780-799)
- Injury and Poisoning (800-999)

An example of ICD-9 detail (coding to the 4th or 5th digit) is given for diabetes in Table 22.2.

Table 22.2

EXAMPLE OF ICD-9 DETAIL

250.40	Diabetes w/renal manifestations	Type 2 DM
250.41	Diabetes w/renal manifestations	Juvenile onset
250.42	Diabetes w/renal manifestations	Type 2 DM, uncontrolled
250.43	Diabetes w/renal manifestations	Type 1 DM, uncontrolled

V-codes are often called "enhancer" codes and can communicate special circumstances influencing the patient encounter. V-codes are factors influencing health status and contact with health services (V01-V82). They can be used to indicate a person is not currently ill, but encountering health services for a specific reason, like to receive counseling. V-codes cannot be used as a primary diagnosis or reason for encounter, but can be assigned when the patient's history, status, or problem has some significance for the episode of care. V-codes are also listed in the ICD-9 reference. (16) Some V-code examples pertinent to dietetic practice include:

- V12.1   Personal history of nutritional deficiency
- V12.71   Personal history of peptic ulcer disease
- V15.41   History of physical abuse
- V23.3   Grand multiparty
- V24.1   Lactating mother
- V41.0   Problems with sight
- V41.6   Problems with swallowing and mastication
- V44.3   Artificial opening – colostomy
- V49.7   Lower limb amputation
- V60.4   No other household member able to render care
- V65.40   Counseling NOS
- V65.41   Exercise counseling
- V65.3   Dietary surveillance and counseling

Current Procedural Terminology codes, or **CPT codes,** were developed to identify work performed by physicians. It is the most widely used coding system, required virtually by all payers. CPT codes define the different locations in which services were provided, the types of procedures or services provided, and the purpose of the services.

Evaluation and Management codes, also known as **E/M codes** or "office codes," are created and maintained by the American Medical Association. These 5-digit codes, plus modifiers, are used for reporting surgical, medical, diagnostic, evaluation, and management codes. Although developed for physicians, some payers have allowed other practitioners, including dietitians, to use these codes. However, Medicare has specifically stated that it will not accept E/M codes from dietitians. An example of what an E/M code may communicate follows:

- 1-992   Office or other outpatient
- 1-9920   New patient encounter
- 1-9921   Established, previous patient
- 1-99201   Lowest level new patient
- 1-99211   Lowest level established patient
- 1-99205   Highest level new patient
- 1-99215   Highest level established patient
- 1-99215-21 Additional time spent

HCPCS codes, derived from HCFA's Common Procedure Coding System, were developed for use by non-physicians, for products, or for services, reimbursable primarily under Medicare. The HCPCS codes are often referred to as Level II codes and reflect those items not included in the CPT codes. These codes typically start with a letter (A-V) and four numbers. The G-codes used for diabetes self-management training (DSMT) are an example of HCPCS codes.

Diabetes Self-Management Training (DSMT) Codes
The Balanced Budget Act of 1997 permits Medicare coverage of diabetes outpatient self-management training services (DSMT), when offered by a certified provider who meets certain quality standards. The training must be ordered by the patient's physician or qualified non-physician practitioner treating the diabetes, and must be recognized/certified by the American Diabetes Association.

A Medicare beneficiary is eligible to receive 10 hours of initial training within a continuous 12-month period (the 12-month period does not need to be on a calendar-year basis). Up to 9 hours of initial training may be provided in a group setting consisting of 2 to 20 individuals. One hour of training may be provided on an individual basis for the purpose of conducting an individual assessment and providing specialized training. If any special condition or circumstance exists that makes it impossible for a beneficiary to attend a group training session, that beneficiary may attend individual training, as long as the patient's physician or qualified practitioner treating the diabetes, requests it.

Medicare also covers 2 hours of follow-up DSMT training each year starting with the calendar year following the year in which the beneficiary completes the initial 10 hours of training. The 2 hours of training may be given in any combination of half-hour increments within each calendar year on either an individual or group basis without the certification of the ordering physician, if special conditions exist.

The G-codes specific for diabetes services became effective August 1, 2000 and were originally in 60-minute increments. Legislation passed on February 27, 2001 changed billing to 30-minute increments and required providers to have Recognition status with the American Diabetes Association.

Table 22.3

G-codes

G0108 One-to-one counseling in 30-minute increments
G0109 Group counseling, 2 or more individuals in 30-minute increments

---

Medical Nutrition Therapy (MNT) Codes

Effective January 1, 2001, after many years of legislative activity, three new CPT codes for MNT became available. MNT was defined in the legislation specifically as a service provided by registered dietitians. Based on scope of practice and state licensure regulations, individuals without the RD credential may not be eligible to provide MNT services to the public.

The new MNT codes are time-based codes. While each code can be used only once, dietitians may use multiple units of time for the MNT service provided. The first 2 codes, for initial and follow-up MNT service, are listed in 15-minute time increments, while the group MNT code is listed in 30-minute increments. Time prior to the visit in which you acquire clinical information, or time spent in record documentation after the patient has left cannot be part of the units of time billed for the MNT service. Only the actual time you spend in front of the patient can be counted. Physicians often save time by documenting comments in the patient's medical record while talking to their patients. If you choose to chart while the patient is present, then this time does count as face-to-face time.

Table 22.4   **MNT Codes**

97802 Medical nutrition therapy initial assessment and intervention, individual, each 15 minutes
97803 Re-assessment and intervention, individual, each 15 minutes
97804 Group - 2 or more individual(s), each 30 minutes

Usually dietetic practitioners provide MNT, however, some physicians may also perform nutrition evaluations and intervention. To avoid confusion, the American Medical Association directed physicians to use the E/M or Preventive Medicine CPT codes. This has prevented multiple uses of the MNT codes on patients receiving nutrition services.

The Medicare MNT benefit for individuals with diabetes and kidney disease became effective January 1, 2002. For diabetes, the MNT codes provide an avenue for coordination of benefits to provide supplementary education to the G-codes. For example, a Medicare beneficiary who has had his or her one hour of one-to-one education as part of DSMT may access an additional 2-3 hours of additional MNT services if deemed medically necessary by the physician. The physician must then complete a separate referral specific for MNT services.

In April 2003, two new MNT codes were added to differentiate initial visit sets from extended follow-up visits as ordered by the physician. These codes are listed in Table 5.

Table 22.5	Additional Follow-up MNT Codes
G0270: Medical Nutrition Therapy, reassessment and subsequent intervention(s) following second referral in same year for change in diagnosis, medical condition, or treatment regimen, individual, each 15 minutes	
G0271: Medical Nutrition Therapy; reassessment and subsequent intervention(s) following second referral in same year for change in diagnosis, medical condition, or treatment regimen, group (2 or more individuals), each 30 minutes	

In order to take advantage of the Medicare MNT benefit, beneficiary requirements include:
- Must have Medicare Part B benefits
- Diagnosis – Type 1, 2, or gestational diabetes; non-dialysis kidney disease (including post-transplant)
- Diagnosis criteria:
  FBG >126 mg/dl
  GFR 13-50 ml/min/1.73 m^2
  Post-kidney transplant up to 36 months

Medicare Provider Status for Dietitians

The Centers for Medicare and Medicaid Services (CMS) is the agency responsible for determining and monitoring the regulations for the Medicare MNT benefit. CMS also determines the diagnosis, eligibility criteria, practice setting, documentation, and billing procedures required for the providers of the benefit. (17) As of September 2003, nutrition professionals may not bill Medicare Part B for MNT services provided to beneficiaries for diseases *other than diabetes and pre-renal disease*. Medicare providers must accept "assignment," which is an agreement between Medicare and the practitioner to receive direct payment from the Medicare program, and accept the Medicare-approved amount as payment in full. The Medicare-approved amount is the 20% co-pay from the beneficiary and the 80% amount from the fiscal intermediary.

Provider requirements for registered dietitians include:

- Registered dietitian (RD) meeting the following requirements:
  BS degree or higher
  Program in nutrition or dietetics
  At least 900 hours of practice experience
  Licensed or certified by state
- Original legislation grandfathers in those who were licensed or certified as of December 31, 2000
- Must have a Medicare Provider Identification Number (PIN) to provide Medicare services

To become a provider for the Medicare Part B MNT benefit, dietetic practitioners can enroll at any time. The forms needed depend on your practice setting(s) and employment relationship. Once submitted, applications typically take up to 60 days for enrollment to be completed. You may start providing MNT services for the designated diagnoses from your practice location, based on the date you enter on your application, but you must hold claims until you receive your PIN number.

To obtain the Medicare PIN, you may use a person who is a credentialing specialist or who handles new physician credentials to help complete the application forms. This is especially important for dietitians working in healthcare facilities who may need to reassign their benefits so payment goes to the institution. Application forms can be downloaded from www.cms.gov.

Once you are a Medicare provider, it is critical you understand the approved benefits, covered visits, diagnostic criteria, physician referral process, billing codes, use of the MNT guides for practice, and required documentation. Once you have started seeing qualified beneficiaries, you must collect outcome data to demonstrate the effectiveness of MNT interventions.

DSMT versus MNT Codes

When implementing one or both of the Medicare-covered benefits for Diabetes Self-Management Training (DSMT) and Medical Nutrition Therapy (MNT), it is important to know the indications and limitations of coverage and/or medical necessity for each benefit. For example, DSMT and MNT services will not be reimbursed if care is provided on the same day. An excellent comparison of the two Medicare benefits is available at www.eatright.org./member/policyinitiatives/83_16691.cfm and looks at such considerations as:

- Referral requirements
- Benefit coverage
- Beneficiary requirements
- Place of service requirements
- Benefit content
- Provider qualifications
- Codes
- Claims processing forms
- Utilization guidelines

Opting Out

Opting out is a process in which an eligible Medicare provider makes a decision not to participate in the Medicare program, and officially does not seek to obtain a provider number by completing and submitting forms obtained from Medicare. In this case, a dietetic practitioner that "opts out," may charge a Medicare Part B beneficiary with diabetes or pre-renal disease their usual or customary fee through a private contract. The language of this contract is very specific and must contain the directions and language as specified by the Part B carrier. A specific affidavit with the regional Medicare carrier must also be on file within ten days of the first private contract. If the dietitian has opted out, Medigap insurance claims must not be filed. Non-Medicare secondary insurance plans may be billed.

Many dietitians in private practice have explored this route, as they feel they cannot financially support the current Medicare payment rates. If you are considering the opting out approach, it is important to have any private contracts reviewed by legal counsel. It is also important to realize that once you formally opt out, you may not change your mind and apply as a provider for two years. For some, this may have employment implications if seeking another position requiring the provider status. Additional resources on opting out and current fee schedules for MNT codes are available on the ADA website for Medicare provider information at www.eatright.org/provlinks.html.

Registered dietitians have several reasons to use the MNT codes:

MNT codes truly define nutrition services versus general office codes that have previously been used for MNT services.

MNT use of the codes allows for consistency in tracking MNT services provided. Over time, the codes can indicate the frequency of MNT services provided by dietitians.

MNT codes add credibility and recognition to dietitians. With the MNT codes, some healthcare professionals may more openly acknowledge dietitians as part of the healthcare team.

MNT codes can be used as leverage when negotiating additional MNT coverage by private insurance companies.

The Billing Process

The ability to differentiate between the three main billing forms, UB-92 (also known as the CMS-1450), CMS-1500 (formerly HCFA-1500), and superbill, is important. The choice of form is often determined by practice setting. The **UB-92** is used in hospital settings for inpatient and outpatient billing. Prior to April 1, 2003, many hospital-based dietitians were unable to participate as Medicare Part B providers, as their facilities were not equipped to submit CMS-1500 claims electronically for professional services.

The **CMS-1500** is the basic billing form prescribed by CMS for the Medicare program for billing submitted by physicians, other Medicare providers, and suppliers. It is printed in red ink to facilitate the electronic process; photocopies or fax copies are not accepted. Guidelines for dietitians to complete the CMS-1500 are available on the ADA website. See additional resources at the end of the chapter on how to obtain CMS-1500 claim forms.

The **Superbill** is a non-standardized billing form that contains information about the professional providing a service, as well as an itemized listing of codes, services, and charges. A superbill is designed so the patient can submit the bill directly to a health care insurer. If you are a Medicare provider, note that CMS will not accept non-standardized forms such as a superbill. The Pennsylvania Dietetic Association has developed a superbill specific for dietetic services, and updates it as necessary to keep it current. See Appendix 22-A for example of the Superbill claim forms. For those not in healthcare facilities, a listing of billing resources is available at www.eatright.org/Member/PolicyInitiatives/83_billresource.cfm.

The Link Between Coding and Documentation

Time spent face-to-face counseling the patient is the driving force for code choice. Third party payers may request charts for audits to determine the appropriateness or medical necessity for the counseling visit and the continuity of care. Key points when setting up a documentation system include:

- every patient needs a separate chart
- patient name, date, and identifier should be on each page
- easily recognized allergy information
- pertinent medications and labs are noted
- the record should be organized, complete, and legible
- insurance information should be copied and/or verified
- no information should be shared or released unless a formal release of information, signed by the patient, is in the chart
- data for each visit is clearly documented
- documentation supports billing
- the chart is a legal document

In the legal medical record, each visit entry should include:

- date of visit
- diagnosis (primary and secondary)
- reason for visit
- relevant history/identification and evaluation of risk factors
- assessment and rationale for treatment
- goals and patient progress towards goals
- provider signature and time spent

Specific guidelines for documentation for Medicare Part B services to facilitate reimbursement have been reviewed. (18) An overview of MNT documentation is also available at www.eatright.org/gov/mntdoc.html. See Appendix 22-B and 22-C for other sample MNT assessment and documentation forms developed by Mary Ann Hodorowicz, RD, MBA, CDE (To order these EZ Forms for the Busy RD: phone 708-361-1290 or hodorowicz@aol.com).

Links to Financial Viability

Regardless of the practice setting, the dietetic practitioner should know their financial status. Key financial indicators may include profit and loss statements, payer mix, cash flow (charged vs. received revenue), cost per unit of service (UOS), and days in accounts receivable (days in AR). For any dietetic practitioner involved in reimbursable MNT services, a good foundation in business and financial processes is useful.

To determine cost effectiveness of services, it is important to develop a well-defined budget. This includes determining the costs of providing the services and the fee schedule needed to cover these expenses. To determine a competitive price structure for your geographical area, network with colleagues and investigate what your market will bear.

Often dietetic practitioners struggle to gain the support of financial staff in healthcare facilities. A prime example was the inability of many healthcare facilities to bill MNT using the CMS-1500 claim form prior to April 1, 2003. This author has learned through experience that it is important to identify key financial decision-makers in a healthcare facility, and educate them on the following:

- what professional dietetic practitioners do
- benefits of MNT to the facility
- impact of MNT on patients

In the same vein, it is important to understand the terminology and procedures for billing and reimbursement so you can facilitate your message in terms the financial decision-makers will understand.

Optimizing Reimbursement

The first step in any reimbursement situation is to know the legislative requirements of coding for services. You should always access the legislative source documents to determine coverage requirements and billing procedures. See Additional Resources at the end of the chapter for some key source documents you should be familiar with in regards to DSMT and MNT Medicare services.

The next step is to know your organization's billing process and procedures. How is a charge master created? How are codes linked to charges? Is the billing process electronic, or are paper claims submitted? How are prices determined? Are there individual payer contracts that determine reimbursement? A review of billing guidelines for Medicare Part B MNT has been published (19) and may be helpful as you work with the set-up of billing for those services.

You should always track and investigate denials closely. A claim can be denied for a variety of reasons. You can send a letter to the payer to facilitate resolution. At times, incorrect or incomplete forms or the assignment of a wrong diagnosis code may be the culprit. Many practitioners have included writing appeal letters for patients as a value-added service (VAS) to their practice as a way to enhance patient satisfaction and increase their value and visibility to the payers.

For those dietetic practitioners in healthcare facilities, creating linkages with other departments such as Patient Accounts or Billing, Finance, Medical Records, and coding staff can save valuable time and resources. You know you have developed those linkages when you receive updates pertaining to your scope of services. We, as dietetic practitioners, do not have to be experts in all of these fields to be successful. We need to learn the art of collaboration to facilitate an understanding among others of what our services involve.

Always look for opportunities to improve practice patterns. One valuable resource available to increase your networking is the dietitians' Reimbursement listserv. The web page contains a searchable archive of messages since February 2000. The sharing of files and other reimbursement-related resources is invaluable. For information on the listserv and joining, contact reimburse@eatright.org.

HEALTH INSURANCE PORTABILITY AND ACCOUNTABILITY ACT (HIPAA)

The Health Insurance Portability and Accountability Act (HIPPA) was developed in the mid-1990's to expand privacy protections for healthcare information and records. It also addressed some of the issues regarding extended insurance coverage for those with pre-existing conditions and when employment status changed. The HIPAA privacy guidelines became effective on April 14, 2003 and included dietitians and dietetic technicians, along with other healthcare providers as covered entities.

Are you a covered entity? Rubinger and Gardner (20) provide some excellent insight into the definition of "covered entity." The bottom line is if your facility furnishes, bills, or receives payment for health care in the normal course of business, you should consider yourself a healthcare provider for the purposes of the privacy rule. If your facility transmits any of the covered transactions via electronic media, you may proceed directly into the world of HIPAA compliance!

The basic privacy rules require covered entities to:

- Distribute a privacy notice to all patients.
- Post privacy notices in public areas and offices.
- Make a good faith effort to obtain written acknowledgement from patients that they have received the notice.
- Allow patients access to their records if requested, and understand and fully implement the privacy measures in the practice setting.

For more specific HIPAA information and resources for dietetic practitioners, you can access the ADA website at www.eatright.org/gov/hipaa.html.

There are many considerations to think about when dealing with privacy protections. For acute care dietitians, it may be tray tickets left on dirty trays on top of carts in a public hallway, or tube feeding cans labeled with the patient's name and room number on a counter. For private practice dietitians, considerations may include the provision of privacy notices to clients, and how physician follow-up and billing information is transmitted. A sample privacy notice is available at www.eatright.org/images/gov/hipaa040203b.doc For hospital-based dietetic practitioners, adherence to facility policies, procedures, and education on such are key. The biggest change for patients is more papers to read and sign.

For those dietetic practitioners who communicate with patients via e-mail, it is important to know your server configuration and whether or not messages are encrypted, incoming and/or outgoing. If in doubt, or encryption is not available, the following guidelines may be helpful:

- E-mail communications are not secure once they travel outside a non-encrypted server. Messages then travel on the Internet, unprotected.
- All e-mail that travels on the Internet should be automatically stamped with a footer that is a disclaimer of liability.
- E-mail to patients should not be actively marketed unless you can guarantee privacy protection. It is recognized that many patients love using e-mail, so total discouragement may not always be feasible.
- If you decide to use e-mail with a patient, you should discuss the lack of security with the patient and document the discussion in the patient's medical record.
- When sending e-mail, do not put protected health information in the subject line; evaluate what you choose for the subject carefully. Would someone have a clue to the contents of the e-mail by the subject line?
- Whenever possible, place any individually identifiable health information in an attachment to the message, rather than the body of the message itself. Attachments are less apt to be read than are the body of the e-mail.
- After sending the e-mail, go to your "Sent" folder and print a copy of the e-mail. The copy will have the date and time sent. Also print any attachments mailed.
- File the printed copies in the patient's medical record as documentation.

Some excellent overviews of the impact of HIPAA electronic transmissions for dietetic and other healthcare practitioners have been published (21,22), as well as information that can be used for dietitians in private practice. (23)

Summary
Healthcare has been/is continuing to change. But change is difficult. It requires us to wear our clinical and business hats, and to link our clinical and business skills.

Keys to reimbursement success for dietetic practitioners include:

- Know the lingo
- Persistence is the key
- Appeal denials—be a patient advocate
- Ongoing marketing
- Track and document cost per unit of time
- Include key elements of documentation
- Be prepared for chart audits by payers by conducting your own random audits
- Develop a business plan for expanding services
- Implement effective and efficient processes
- Identify, define, and describe your services
- Establish a plan for charging for services
- Explore provider status when opportunities exist
- Obtain physician support and referrals
- Implement a nutrition counseling practice model
- Know your coding and billing processes inside out
- Document impact of MNT on client outcomes
- Track your reimbursement
- Be prepared to sell your worth to the business side
- Network with other professionals

The changing healthcare arena is rich with new rules, regulations, and reimbursement opportunities for dietetic practitioners. Explore the wealth of references and resources available and remember, if opportunity knocks at your door, be sure to be there to open it!

Learning Activities

1. Discuss the health care changes and trends, and the impact on dietetic practice in your own community.
2. Visit a local hospital and meet with the outpatient dietetics manager or staff. Discuss how billing and documentation processes are set up. What obstacles have been encountered? How is reimbursement tracked?
3. Visit a private practice dietitian. Discuss how billing and documentation processes are set up. What obstacles have been encountered? How is reimbursement tracked?
4. Review one of the ADA Guidelines for Practice packages. What implications does this have for evidence-based practice? What differences do you see between the guidelines and documentation? What have you observed in usual practice by dietitians not using the guidelines?
5. Review the general principles for HIPAA. Discuss what implications this would have for a hospital-based outpatient dietitian versus a private practice dietitian.

References
1. King K. The Entrepreneurial Nutritionist, 3rd ed. Lake Dallas TX: Helm Publishing; 2002.
2. Splett PL. *Developing and Validating Evidence-Based Guides for Practice: A Tool Kit for Dietetic Professionals.* Chicago IL: American Dietetic Association; 2000.
3. American Dietetic Association. *Hyperlipidemia medical nutrition therapy protocol.* Chicago IL: American Dietetic Association; 2001.
4. American Dietetic Association. *Chronic Kidney Disease (Nondialysis) Medical Nutrition Therapy Protocol.* Chicago IL: American Dietetic Association; 2002.

5. American Dietetic Association. *Nutrition Practice Guidelines for Type 1 and Type 2 Diabetes Mellitus.* Chicago IL: American Dietetic Association; 2001.
6. American Dietetic Association. *Nutrition practice guidelines for gestational diabetes mellitus.* Chicago IL: American Dietetic Association; 2001.
7. The American Dietetic Association and Morrison Health Care. *Medical Nutrition Therapy Across the Continuum of Care, 2nd ed.* Chicago IL: The American Dietetic Association; 1998.
8. The American Dietetic Association and Morrison Health Care. *Medical nutrition therapy across the continuum of care: supplement 1.* Chicago IL: The American Dietetic Association; 1997.
9. American Dietetic Association. *Chronic Kidney Disease (Non-dialysis) Medical Nutrition Therapy Protocol.* Chicago IL: American Dietetic Association; 2002. (Outcomes Management section)
10. Collins RW, Anderson JW. Medication cost savings associated with weight loss for obese non-insulin dependent diabetic men and women. *Preventive Medicine.* 1995; 24(4): 1018-1024.
11. Packard PT, Heaney RP. Medical nutrition therapy for patients with osteoporosis. *J Am Diet Assoc.* 1997; 97(4): 414-417.
12. Lacey K, Pritchett E. Nutrition care process and model: ADA adopts road map to quality care and outcomes management. *J Am Diet Assoc.* 2003; 103(8): 1061-72.
13. Daly A, Warshaw H, Pastors JG, Franz MJ, Arnold M. Diabetes medical nutrition therapy: practical tips to improve outcomes. *J Am Acad Nurse Pract.* 2003; 15(5): 206-11. Review.
14. Delahanty LM, Hayden D, Ammerman A, Nathan DM. Medical nutrition therapy for hypercholesterolemia positively affects patient satisfaction and quality of life outcomes. *Ann Behav Med.* 2002; 24(4): 269-78.
15. Sikand G, Kashyap ML, Wong ND, Hsu JC. Dietitian intervention improves lipid values and saves medication costs in men with combined hyperlipidemia and a history of niacin noncompliance. *J Am Diet Assoc.* 2000; 100(2): 218-24.
16. *ICD-9-CM. International classification of diseases (10th revision) 2003.* Los Angeles CA: Practice Management Information Corporation; 2002.
17. Federal Register, 42 CFR, Part 405 et al, Vol 66, No 212, November 1, 2001; *Medicare program; revisions to payment policies and five-year review of and adjustments to the Relative Value Units under the physician fee schedule for calendar year 2002:* Final rule, pages 55275-55281.
18. Michael P, ed. *Medicare MNT documentation.* The Medicare MNT Provider. 2002; 1(3): 1,3.
19. Infante M. *Correct billing for Medicare Part B MNT.* The Medicare MNT Provider 2003; 1(9): 1,3.
20. Rubinger H, Gardner R. The road to compliance: where are you? *Cont Care* 2003; 22(1): 17-19.
21. Michael P, Pritchett E. The impact of HIPAA electronic transmissions and health information privacy standards. *J Am Diet Assoc.* 2001; 101(5): 524-528.
22. Fain JA. Protecting patients' health information: overview of the health insurance portability and accountability act. *The Diabetes Educator.* 2003; 29(2): 186.
23. Price B. *HIPAA: what the driver needs to know.* Huntington Woods MI: Jump Start Consulting, 2002.

Additional Resources

CMS web page for program memorandums and original source documents
www.cms.hhs.gov/manuals/pm

American Dietetic Association legislative resources
www.eatright.org/gov/

American Dietetic Association Medicare MNT resources (many pages are member only)
www.eatright.org/member/policyinitiatives/

HIPAA – US Government sites
www.cms.hhs.gov/hipaa2/default.asp
www.hhs.gov/ocr/hipaa/

HIPAA – Searchable regulations
www.hipaadvisory.com/regs/

The Medicare MNT Provider (newsletter)
Chicago IL: The American Dietetic Association

CMS (HCFA)-1500 claim form
- Can be purchased from local office supply stores
- US Government Printing Office 1-202- 512-1800
- American Medical Association 1-800 621-8335

Articles and Books

Cross AT. Practical and legal considerations of private nutrition practice. *J Am Diet Assoc.* 1995; 95(1): 21 – 29.

Duester KJ. Building your Business-Setting Your Fees: A Cost-Based Approach. *J Am Diet Assoc.* 1997; 97(10 suppl): S129 - S130.

Hodorowicz MA. Establishing a Successful Outpatient MNT Clinic in Any Practice Setting: The Complete Manual. Palos Heights IL; 2002.

Schatz GB. Coding for nutrition services: challenges, opportunities and guidelines. *J Am Diet Assoc.* 1993; 93(4): 471-477.

Stollman L, ed. *Nutrition Entrepreneurs Guide to Reimbursement Success,* 2nd ed. Chicago IL: The American Dietetic Association; 1999.

Chapter 23

Successful Business Skills

Kathy King, RD, LD

After reading this chapter, the reader will be able to:
- ♦ Describe key marketing techniques to use in promoting your services.
- ♦ Critique the scheduling of an appointment done over the phone for effectiveness.
- ♦ List key components of the outpatient chart.
- ♦ Discuss rationale for setting fee schedules.

You can increase your chances for counseling success by improving the way you get referrals, schedule appointments, and offer small amenities to patients and clients. It is not uncommon for patients or clients to be turned off by a counselor because of what was said or omitted, while scheduling the initial appointment. Some outpatient clinics report having as many as 25-50 percent of their appointments not show. This shows something is very wrong with the way patients are referred or how they are handled upon referral.

IMPROVING HOW PATIENTS ARE REFERRED

For the purposes of this discussion assume you are a 43-year-old female office manager who just had your gallbladder removed, and you are going home. This morning your physician diagnosed high cholesterol (326 mg/dl) from your routine hospital blood work. You come from a family with bad hypertension usually controlled with drugs. You have no symptoms but have about 20 extra pounds for your height. When your physician told you about your cholesterol he or she said, "You are too young to have cholesterol this high. It has to come down. I don't want you to eat any eggs and have red meat just twice a week. If you can't bring it down with your diet, I'll give you medication. I'll make a referral to our dietitian."

What was "right" about this scenario from the physician's and your (the patient's) perspective?

1. The physician expressed concern about your cholesterol level so you would feel a need to change it.
2. The physician indicated several food guidelines to help assist lowering your cholesterol level.
3. The physician gave a backup option for cure in case the first one didn't work, so you would not worry.
4. The physician gave you a referral to the dietitian for more in-depth nutrition instruction.

Did this scenario "work" for both you and your physician? Yes, it probably did. What was "incomplete" with this scenario from the referral dietitian's point of view? Put yourself in the dietitian's role now.

1. The physician did not explain enough about the importance of lifestyle changes on the patient's prognosis, i.e., low-fat diet, exercise, and moderate weight loss. If there wasn't time for that, there should have been at least an explanation in physiologically simple terms why cholesterol is dangerous. This is especially true given her family history.
2. The physician gave incorrect and incomplete guidelines on how to eat, which will mean the dietitian has to contradict them and risk confusing the patient.

3. The physician didn't "market" the dietitian's abilities and skills. This isn't a simple referral for blood work. The physician is asking the patient to make major lifestyle changes in order to accomplish the goal of reducing her blood cholesterol level. A strong third party referral at this point is very important.

4. And finally, the physician didn't involve the patient in the discussion. Good medical practice today should involve the patient and the patient's consent for what is about to take place. The physician should have asked if she wanted a referral to the dietitian, and if so, would she rather have the consult before she leaves or on an outpatient basis after she recuperates from surgery.

It would really help if physicians made referrals differently, but who's going to change them? You do! Figure out what you want physicians and other health professionals to say when they refer their patients to you, and present the information in person at monthly hospital or clinic meetings, at their private offices, and over lunch. Have fun with it but make it short and sweet and back everything up with examples and researched information on patient compliance and behavior change.

The next time your friend Dr. Jones says, "I refer at least a half dozen patients a week to your office." You can say, "Boy, that's great. But they are getting lost somewhere. Tell me what you say when you refer them."

He or she explains what's said. You can then say, "Let me tell you how to market my services so patients will want to call for an appointment."

Give referral agents examples of short phrases to say to patients like, "Changing your diet and your weight are the most important things you can do to lower your cholesterol. Our dietitians on staff can help you fit the guidelines to your lifestyle, and work with you long-term on problems that make it difficult for you to change. They've had patients who lowered their cholesterol by _____mg/dl in six months."

Look at your long-term patients and let your referring health professionals, colleagues, and employers or consultant accounts know how well they are doing, whether you work in inpatient, clinic, or private practice settings. People refer patients to professionals they trust and respect who produce results with patients. Market your services through your patients' successful outcomes in monthly or quarterly newsletters or direct mailings, through presentations at meetings, and by writing personal letters to referral agents. *(If you don't have any successful patients, work on that situation first and foremost.)*

"Seamless" Dietitian-to-Dietitian Referrals

This discussion is not complete without mentioning that dietitians need to refer patients and clients to each other more often. In private practice when one dietitian is a specialist in allergies, vegetarian diets, or eating disorders, it is common in many cities to see referrals to each other. In private practice, having successful patient outcomes is so crucial for professional image and ultimate survival that it takes precedence over the possible loss of income from the consult. Today, dietitians in other settings are no less accountable for positive outcomes from their nutrition intervention.

Another growing opportunity for referrals among dietitians is from inpatient to outpatient clinic, home health, private practice, or long-term care and back to inpatient, if necessary, in a continuing circle. A nutrition summary or a quick call to the next practitioner should be made in order to create "seamless" dietetic care for our patients and clients. Just as your family would expect the hospital Nutrition Support dietitian, taking care of your mother on TPN, to call the Home Health dietitian or nurse who will carry on the therapy, our other patients expect that same continuity and should receive no less.

It shows professionalism and maturity on a dietitian's part to make sure patients are referred to other practitioners when they need more long-term follow-up or more specialized nutrition therapy than you can provide.

Even if a referred patient is given your name and phone number, ask your referring colleagues to send you a note or call you with the patient's name and number. In the first few days after the referral is made, you should call and introduce yourself, show interest in helping, and send a brochure. If the patient is interested in making an appointment, he or she will mention it, otherwise do not turn the call into a sales call. The brochure will reinforce your credibility and availability. This simple phone call could bring in an extra five to ten or more referrals per week.

CREATING AN EFFECTIVE OPERATION

If you work at an office, establish office hours and days, and try to follow your schedule as closely as possible to help develop an image of stability and continuity. As long as clients can leave a message for you, it is not necessary to be available in the office, in person, five days a week. When starting a new private practice at a fitness center or medical complex, try to condense your client consultations to a few days per week. The remaining days can then be used to hold down another job while you start your business, or give you time to market your business, write, take care of family, or whatever.

Telephone

Telephone coverage for your department or business is extremely important. The telephone is your clients' major link with you. During normal business hours Monday through Friday, clients should be able to either reach you by phone or leave a message with a receptionist, answering service, or voice mail machine. Messages on telephone answering recorders should be well prepared—keep trying until you record a message that people will not only listen to but also, most importantly, respond to. A higher level of service is perceived when calls are returned promptly.

Some hints that may be important to you concerning your telephone answering service or receptionist include the following:

1. Do not allow your services and fees to be given to clients unless the person is trained to properly "market" your business. Have them say, "I will be happy to take your name and number and have the nutrition therapist call you back."
2. Caution your answering service or receptionist about giving out your private home phone number and address. *Have the answering service try to reach you* instead of letting them give out your number.
3. When you are out of town, instruct your answering service to tell people that "Ms. Jones will be in the office to return your call on Monday, July 10th. Can she call you back at that time?" Or, if you have another dietitian cover your practice, you might have the answering service say, "Mary Smith, a Registered Dietitian, is covering all calls and I will have her call you if you wish." If it is an emergency in private practice, leave the number of the local hospital clinical nutrition department, or leave a number where *your answering service* can reach you or leave a message for you. In an outpatient clinic, have the receptionist call or page an inpatient clinical staff person who is covering clinic calls.

HOW TO SCHEDULE APPOINTMENTS

Worst-case scenario is when a prospective patient calls your office for an appointment, is treated as an inconvenience by you or the receptionist, and is only asked information about scheduling the appointment. Later when a prospective patient considers the cost (time and financial) of the appointment and the apparent quality of the service, it's easy to see why he or she may decide *not* to keep the appointment. Why don't patients call to cancel? Because they didn't feel anyone cared if they called in the first place.

So, how can this scenario be improved? First, there needs to be an attitude adjustment. It must be remembered who is the consumer and who is the provider. Who will continue to make a living because of the other? The dietitian, of course! The dietitian must control this situation better and institute changes that will make the potential patient feel special, nurtured, and cared for from the very beginning. That means the dietitian should take the initial contact with the client more seriously.

Philomena Koulbanis, RD, the dietitian in Chapter 1 who only had four patients not show for appointments in seven years, shared her secret. She said, *"I'm a one person office with an answering machine. I record a very pleasant message on the machine and let it take the messages when I'm with clients. I never call anyone back unless I have at least 10-15 minutes to talk. In that time I find out how they heard about my business, who their physician is, if there is a diagnosis, and most importantly, what their problems and needs are from their point of view. Then I briefly tell them what I can do for their specific problems, how I like to work long-term with clients, and that I would like to work with them. I always mention how much my services cost so they can plan better or wait to make an appointment if they can't afford it at that time."*

What we can learn from Ms. Koulbanis' strategy is that clients like to feel they are special to their therapist, their needs are her priority, and money isn't much of an issue if the perceived value is high. The initial phone call also lets the two parties involved screen each other to see if they want to work together, and to help the therapist anticipate barriers and problems better.

If you work in a clinic or office where someone else answers your phone first, you must train the office phone staff how to say one of two things: first choice) pleasantly thank the person for calling and put the person through to the dietitian or take the phone number so the dietitian can call back to schedule the appointment and answer any questions, *or if that is impossible;* second choice) she or he can pleasantly recite several sentences you wrote about your services, philosophies, the fee, and then ask questions about scheduling the appointment.

Even if you share a receptionist with other professionals or work in a busy clinic, you must become an advocate for professional treatment of your clients. You are not overstepping your boundaries to train the person(s) on the phone how to represent your practice because you are the one who ultimately will be held responsible for your productivity and the quality of patient interaction in your office. If there is an office manager, start by discussing your needs with this person and offer to *"work together to give the patients excellent care."*

Six Keys to Good Scheduling Interaction

When a prospective client calls for an appointment, there are six keys to successful phone interaction:
1. Begin to establish rapport between the client and the dietitian through showing interest, concern and undivided attention.
2. Screen each other to see if macro philosophies and expectations are compatible (this is most important in situations like when a patient is looking for a quick weight loss program that you don't offer, or he thinks you can diagnose diabetes from his symptoms). A referral to another program or professional may be in order.
3. Find an appointment time that is convenient for both of you. You don't have to accommodate your clients by being available 7am-7pm every day of the week. But for therapists who work with a high percentage of working clients, it often works well to open early one day each week and work later another day or two. To keep you healthy and happy, leave early on the days when you work early, and sleep in and go in later when you work late.
4. Make sure your client has your office phone number, address, and directions to the office, and knows where to park. This is especially important when the office is in a large medical complex. Let clients know if there is a parking fee, or a close place to park that doesn't charge a fee.
5. Ask your clients to recite all appointment arrangements, including what to bring like food records and lifestyle questionnaire, if you mail one in advance, and to give 24 hours notice if they need to cancel or reschedule.
6. You should reconfirm appointments by postcard sent at least five days in advance, or have your receptionist or another paid person (this better assures that the calls are made) call your initial appointments the day before to remind them of the visit and what to bring. By adding this step to your practice, you should save at least four or more visits each week.

Chart System

The chart system for your dietetic or private office can be as expensive as a computer system or as simple as a manila folder for each client. Because of the importance of continuity and documentation of a client's progress, it is best to have the client's nutrition chart available for all visits.

In an outpatient setting when you must generate the chart for a client, the information to include in the chart is:
- Name
- Address
- Work and home phone numbers
- Physician's name, the referring physician's name (if different)
- Copy of the diet prescription (if available)
- Pertinent lab values (if available—or call referring physician's office)

264

You will probably add to that, depending upon your practice: a diet evaluation, health risk appraisal, food records, action plan, goals, and evaluation.

Follow-up session notes should list any changes in lab values and other objective measurements, plus notations on any progress toward achieving nutritional outcomes, as well as significant quotes made by the client like: "My medicine made me sick so I stopped taking it," or "Do you have the woman's shelter number?" or "I made myself throw up every day this week." Be sure to identify clients' comments by using quotes.

Keep your remarks pertinent to the client and his or her progress instead of writing personal conjectures, like "Mother is sabotaging Johnny's weight loss efforts." Instead write what the client actually said, "My mother keeps feeding me second helpings and giving me cookies and stuff." Also, instead of writing the remark, "noncompliant," which labels the client, perhaps unfairly, write what the client did that leads you to that conclusion. For example, you might say, "Agreed to keep food records but has not kept them for five weeks; no change in high-fat noon meal; is exercising 1-hr. 2x/week." This more extensive statement states the facts as you know them, instead of subjectively drawing conclusions. It may be that the client found it easier to begin exercising first instead of changing his food habits. That's his choice, and not deserving of the label "noncompliant" or any other.

After the initial instruction and when something significant happens to a client or patient, the referring physician should be notified, and the contact documented. You can use a form letter personalized on the computer, or write a cover letter on your letterhead, and send a copy of the nutrition interview sheet.

Educational Materials

Educational materials for your clients enhance your service and reinforce what you teach. They may also improve the image of your practice. See the earlier recommendations on how to make handouts appropriate to your various markets. The typeface should be easy to read, not script; some people with poor eyesight also have trouble reading small single-spaced elite type (10 pt. on computer).

Information overload is a common problem. Avoid giving clients too many pages. Start with what each client needs or wants. Most patients and their families: 1) get confused by material that is not specifically for their diet, and 2) can only absorb a small amount of information on a new subject at any one time. Patients lose sight of the most important points of the diet when so many new points are made in the additional booklets. Save the less specific material and the larger number of booklets for the few clients who want them and will use them appropriately.

Impress your clients by using folders to hold take-home materials. Use a folder with pockets on the inside and the therapist's, department's, or company's name or logo on the outside for easy identification of the contents and for advertising purposes. Attach your business card to the folder to provide your address and phone number.

Diet manuals are readily available to all practitioners today. Pages should not be photocopied directly from a manual unless it was designed for that purpose, or you request permission from the copyright owner. If you want to be a private practitioner and are unaware of your local medical community's nutritional biases, try to purchase diet manuals from the local hospitals, or make an appointment with a hospital dietitian to discuss what she or he uses.

WHAT TO WEAR

Dress appropriate for the occasion and your patient population's expectations. People initially are more trusting of others who are like themselves. At a fitness center, that might mean warm ups, or shorts and a top. At a medical complex or outpatient clinic it will mean professional dress or more casual dress (depends on the area of the country) with or without a lab coat—whatever is your personal preference and the institution's policy. In private practice, dress code can range from men and women in fancy suits to more casual slacks and shirts or blouses. Again, lab coats are optional, but most therapists who work with the well population do not wear them.

The most important point to remember is that you should dress so that you look professional, successful, and well-groomed without distracting from the purpose of the session. The patients and clients are not coming to dwell on your appearance, so let it be a nonissue.

FEES IN OUTPATIENT SETTINGS

The most important thing to remember about fees is that the "perceived value" of your services *must be equal to or higher than the actual fees you charge in order to continue attracting clients.* Put yourself in their place: assume you are a physician talking to an overweight, 35-year-old woman with three kids and a modest income. Who would you refer her to: the local Weight Watchers group that costs $25 to join and $10 per week with a record of support and success, or the local private practice dietitian who charges $75 per hour but has a reputation for working miracles with clients using a client-centered cognitive-behavioral/fitness approach? It may be a toss-up, but without the reputation for success by the dietitian, Weight Watchers would win every time because it's perceived value is usually equal to or higher than its fees. The above example is called marketplace competition and it is moving from the private practice arena into more traditional dietetic markets.

The variables to consider when determining your fees are:

- Level of expertise your work requires
- Your reputation and image as compared to the competition
- Amount of overhead you must cover
- Amount of time needed for preparation, the consultation, and follow-up.
- What the market will bear--fees are usually lower in rural, small town, and lower income areas than in affluent metropolitan areas.

Even with all of these considerations, the one that most institutions and practitioners use is the last one: they charge what they think their clients and insurers are willing to pay. Whatever your fee strategy, choose fees that you feel comfortable with and ones that are reasonable given the going rates for psychiatric social workers and physical therapists with similar years of education and experience in your area.

You can tell your fees are low when the majority of the prospective clients who call you say, "Oh, that's not bad." Or, when physicians and colleagues say, "Can you make a living on that?" You can tell your prices are too high for your target market when the majority of people gasp when you state the fee, or they say, "Let me call you back." Another indication that your fees are higher than the perceived value of your service is when most new clients refuse to schedule a revisit, or they say, "I don't know my schedule right now, I'll have to call you back," and they never do.

When people are comfortable with your fees or committed to the program, they ask how soon they can make the appointment or schedule a revisit. These clients also will be more interested in special prepayment offers on follow-up visits like six visits for $120 or $20 per session instead of the usual $25. They don't mind the prospect of long-term commitment.

Business-wise you will come out ahead professionally and financially, if you charge fair, reasonable fees that encourage clients to return for follow-up and send their friends instead of charging the most that your market will bear, and clients only come once. If your contract accounts like HMOs and PPOs perceive that your fees are too high, they may limit the number of client visits to such a point that your services become ineffective. If you know your fees are equitable, don't be afraid to defend them and show documentation of your effectiveness.

ENDING A SESSION AND COLLECTING FEES

The end of the interview is a good time to talk about rescheduling a visit, or to discuss why it is not necessary. This is a good "ending" subject and lets the client know that the visit is over. As you are winding up, be sure to incorporate some system to collect the fee. You may simply state, "I will make out your receipt now—how do you want to pay for your instruction?" or "The fee for the initial visit is $____ and revisits are $____. I will give you an itemized receipt that you can attach to your insurance company's form along with a copy of the referral slip from your doctor. You can try to get reimbursed for our visit." If you have a secretary or receptionist, be sure to train her or him on how to collect fees.

If a patient continues to linger after the closing of the session and you have other commitments, you can either relax and take a minute longer, or you can try standing up and walking slowly toward the door to show him out and simply state, "I want to thank you very much for coming. I am sorry to rush, but I have another client waiting."

Third party reimbursement by health insurers and coverage by managed care programs for nutrition intervention are still sporadic. Every dietitian who counsels clients should be making the effort to introduce herself or himself to all the local managed care agencies and insurers. State dietetic associations should follow the lead of Georgia and market their members' services to all the major health insurers and managed care programs in the state. Nutrition departments in hospitals can work through the person(s) on staff who market the hospital to those entities.

LOCATION—LOCATION—LOCATION

In real estate, they say there are only three things to remember about what to look for in a good property: location, location, and location. Whether you work in a hospital, clinic, private practice, or home health agency, where you counsel a patient or client is very important.

In outpatient settings, the appearance of the building where you work, the actual office layout, and even the color and style of the furnishings can influence your clients' and colleagues' opinions of your services. Poor location choices can make you look less than successful. The goals are to have it clean, private, and comfortable. Make the effort to create a counseling space where you and your clients are relaxed and comfortable with some of your own personality in the decor.

The other major consideration in any setting is quiet. It is not a good idea to meet patients or their families in the corner of a hospital cafeteria, in a cubical in an open-plan office, or even in their homes when kids and pets are running through. The patient/client needs and deserves your undivided attention during the therapy session. Likewise, you will be more effective if you have the full attention of the patient or client. Close doors, turn off TVs or radios, negotiate for more private space, use a conference room if your office is too open, and turn your phone over to the answering machine or have the receptionist hold all calls.

In the patient's hospital room, pull the curtain for more privacy in a semi-private room, or schedule the consult, if you have that luxury, at a time when the roommate is out of the room. Offer patients the opportunity to put on a robe instead of assuming they want to sit in their hospital gown on the edge of the bed or in the hall lobby.

In an office, try to sit level with the client and at a reasonable distance apart. Avoid looking over a large, imposing desk where the client and his family feel like school kids on the other side. Make the chairs comfortable but sturdy, and not too soft. A heavy person or someone with back problems cannot easily get in and out of a too soft couch or chair. Some counselors and clients prefer working around a table while others prefer an office space with a homey living room atmosphere, either can be effective.

If you see clients at your home, the location should be easy to find, the pets should be outside or in a bedroom, the phone should be on an answering service, and the kids and spouse invisible. Extra time should be allotted between patients' visits so that the person who comes a little early doesn't have to wait in the kitchen.

Any location should be clean and safe out of respect for the client and to avoid hurting anyone and incurring liability. Edges of carpets should be secured and steps should be well lighted. After group meetings at night, encourage clients to walk out together or call the security guard to walk people to their cars. Do the same for yourself. When the weather is snowy, make sure the sidewalks and parking lot are accessible and sufficiently clear. If the weather and roads are icy and dangerous, stay home, and call clients to reschedule them before they risk making the trip to your office. Clients don't keep appointments well during tornado alerts, hurricanes, floods, and after earthquakes, so call to confirm or reschedule appointments.

MANNERS

Greet your patients or clients with kind words, a smile, and handshake or other appropriate gesture, being sensitive to the client's culture and personal style. As you know by now from the discussion in this book, initial impressions are extremely important to the development of rapport with the client or patient.

Years ago, a nurse friend told a story about a young physician walking into a room to do a pap smear on a middle-aged woman he had never met.

He said, *"Please put your feet up here and I'll do your exam."* The woman reached out to shake hands and said firmly, *"I'd like to introduce myself first."* The physician got the message.

A patient isn't "a hypertensive or a diabetic" as we commonly refer to them in medical care. The patient is *a person* with hypertension or diabetes. People expect respect, civility, and manners.

HERMAN

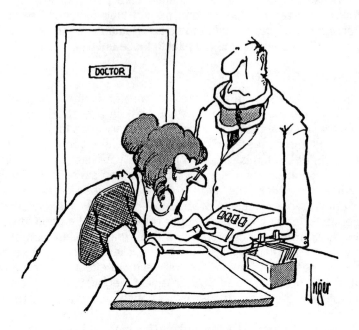

"That pain-in-the-neck's out here, doctor."

OFFER BEVERAGE OR FOOD

Consider asking your clients if they would like a beverage like coffee or tea, or a cool beverage in the summer. In a survey of her office clients several years ago, Alanna Dittoe, RD, found that the amenity the clients liked best was not her friendly manner or live receptionist, but instead it was the coffee and tea offered at the beginning of the appointment.

Another dietitian shared the secret to her success, *"'Breaking bread' with my clients. I always try to offer a beverage and some tasty low-fat muffin or cookie. My clients are very loyal, and I think its because we enjoy food together instead of taking it away as they expected."*

MAINTAINING COMMUNICATION

Therapists show consideration for their patients and clients (and good marketing savvy for their practice) through notes and phone calls. The note may be a simple summary of goals until the next visit, a note of encouragement, a note of appreciation for referring a friend for counseling, or a reminder.

The call may serve the same purposes, as well as establish two-way communication so you can get feedback on how well a patient or client is doing. More and more therapists are trying short phone calls in between visits for clients who need more support in the beginning or during crisis times. Either party usually makes the call at a designated time.

Many sports nutritionists maintain relationships with their clients by attending training sessions, or meets and games to see their clients compete. This extra effort shows interest and concern on the part of the therapist, and can be the source of great personal and professional satisfaction, especially if nutrition intervention helped the athlete perform better.

SUMMARY

There are many noncounseling elements that contribute to the success of a nutrition therapist's practice. By evaluating your present circumstances or establishing procedures to avoid problems mentioned in this chapter and others, you will increase the number of referrals who become patients or clients, lose fewer initial appointments, and keep your patients and clients coming back for more.

Learning Activities

1. With a colleague, role-play scheduling an appointment with a client over the phone. What questions will you ask? How will you identify your potential client's needs? After the role-play, critique your performance with your colleague.

2. Observe a counseling encounter with a dietetic professional. What business skills discussed in this chapter could you identify? Which ones were done well? What changes would you make to strengthen the encounter?

3. Look at the two counseling settings (one-on-one and "Mom & Me" good nutrition for kids) below in the photographs below. Critique each setting. How could you improve it?

ONE-ON-ONE COUNSELING SETTING

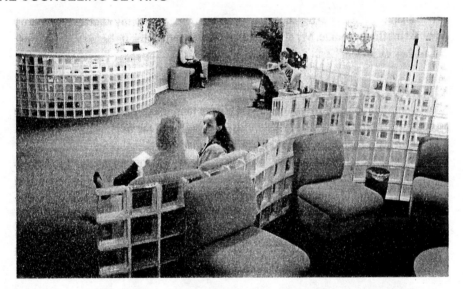

Photo courtesy of Mark Albertini. All Saints Healthcare, Racine, WI

MOM & ME GOOD NUTRITION FOR KIDS

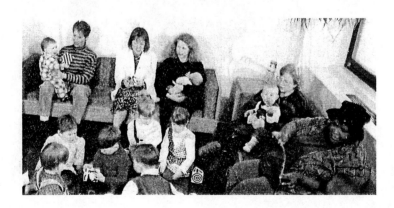

Photo courtesy of Mark Albertini. All Saints Healthcare, Racine, WI

The National Certified Counselor (NCC) Credential

Alison Murray, EdD, NCC, CCMHC, LMHC, RD

The National Board for Certified Counselors (NBCC), a nonprofit organization formed in 1982 and accredited in 1985, functions with three purposes. The NBCC monitors national certification procedures, and represents and maintains a current register of counselors. NBCC also administers the National Counselor Exam (NCE), which is used by licensing boards in approximately thirty states.

National Certified Counselor (NCC) certification may be achieved by successfully completing graduate-level course work, a counseling practicum, the NCE, and 2,000 hours of postgraduate counseling, supervised experience. Prior to sitting for the exam, one must complete a minimum of 32 hours of graduate-level course work in eight of ten subject areas, two of which are required. Required courses include counseling theory and practice, and a supervised counseling practicum. The remaining six courses may be selected from human growth and development, social and cultural foundations of counseling, the helping relationship, group dynamics, processing and counseling, lifestyle and career development, psychological testing, research and evaluation in social sciences, and/or a professional orientation/ethics course.

The counseling practicum, a component of required course work must be completed during the graduate degree program. Students gain up to 500 hours of practical counseling experience in a variety of mental health settings including school guidance clinics, career counseling centers, community mental health centers, drug abuse clinics, acute psychiatric hospitals, and/or ambulatory psychiatric clinics. All counseling is performed under the supervision of a licensed professional from a related mental health discipline, i.e. clinical social worker, psychologist, psychiatrist, marriage and family therapist, or a licensed mental health counselor.

The National Counselor Exam is a two hundred item, multiple-choice test offered in the spring and fall of each year. The exam assesses one's *knowledge* of counseling theory and practice, and covers the course work areas described above. Thus, the test assesses the degree to which a counselor possesses information, which should be known by all counselors, regardless of specialty. Many state level licensing boards use the NCE as a regulatory requirement.

The final component of the NCC package is completing an approved and supervised counseling work experience. The minimum required hours are 2,000. The supervisor, as described above, notifies the board in writing that the counseling experience was completed. This requirement must be met no later than two years after completing the NCE.

After certification is obtained, it is maintained by completing 100 hours of continuing education every five years. The NBCC publishes a list of approved providers of continuing education. Continuing education records are maintained by each counselor, and are subject to auditing every five years. The cost of certification is currently $ 25.00 annually. The NCC certification is useful in that it provides the dietitian an opportunity to perform advanced level counseling. The NCC is also a basic requirement for licensure as a counselor in approximately 30 states. Licensure may require additional education and training in one of four specialty areas including National Certified Career Counselor (NCCC), National Certified Guidance Counselor (NCGC), National Certified School Counselor (NCSC), and/or Certified Clinical Mental Health Counselor (CCMHC).

For more information contact:

National Board for Certified Counselors
3-D Terrace Way
Greensboro, NC 27403
(910) 547-0607

Becoming A Licensed Psychotherapist

*Lisa Dorfman, MS, RD, LMHC, Athlete, Lecturer, and Licensed Mental
Health Counselor/Licensed Nutritionist, Food Fitness International, Inc.*

Although practicing "Nutrition Therapy" appears a great deal more glamorous than "doing a diet consult," it takes several years of education and training to be qualified to be a Licensed Mental Health Counselor (LMHC) and provide psychotherapy. I became interested in this area of expertise in 1983, when I graduated from Florida International University with a B.S. in Dietetics and Nutrition and a minor in Psychology. Since I loved to work with people diagnosed with eating disorders and mental health issues, I began to pursue the licensure requirements for mental health counseling. I chose these credentials because it was broad enough to allow me to work with many populations.

Being a Licensed Mental Health Counselor means incorporating the use of scientific and behavioral science theories, methods, and techniques for the purpose of describing, preventing, and treating undesired behavior and enhancing mental health and human development. Mental Health Counseling includes, but is not limited to counseling, psychotherapy, behavior modification, hypnotherapy, sex therapy, consultation, client advocacy, crisis intervention, and/or providing needed information and education to clients. The counseling can be given to groups, families, individuals, couples, organizations and/or communities.

Although the terminology for the title may vary between states, the license requirements are similar. In the state of Florida, "Psychotherapist" can also be used in place of Licensed Mental Health Counselor, Clinical Social Worker, or Marriage and Family Therapist. Check with your state Mental Health Licensing organization for requirements in your state.

The preparation for the licensing credential, L.M.H.C., includes a Master's Degree from a fully accredited university; 32 hours of graduate course work in counseling theories and practice, human development theories, personality theory, psychopathology, human sexuality, group theories and practice, ethics, and individual evaluation and assessment; 3 years clinical experience in mental health counseling, (2 years at the postmasters level under the supervision of a LMHC or the equivalent) and a passing grade on the state examination. After the completion of these requirements and a successful examination grade, a LMHC must take a 3-hour state approved HIV course, and maintain 30 CEU hours every 2 years.

In addition to being a member of the national and local Mental Health Counselors Association, I belong to the American Psychological Association and North American Association of Master's in Psychology. I've been a Licensed Mental Health Counselor for 5 years now, and I am very satisfied with my credentials because it allows me to practice both diet and mental health counseling, charge higher fees for my expanded expertise, secure third party reimbursement for mental health issues which affect eating, and maintain a practice that never has a dull moment.

SAMPLE—Have your legal counselor evaluate before using.

West Side Nutrition Clinic

Nutrition Therapist—Patient Agreement

Welcome to Our Clinic

The purpose of this agreement is to allow us to serve you more completely and to help you get the best results. It is our experience that those patients who adhere to the following agreements are more satisfied. We are here to help you make healthy lifestyle changes, and to guide and support you as you learn new habits and new ways of thinking.

Appointments

Please arrive on time for your appointment. We will make every effort to see you at the scheduled appointment time. If you must change your appointment, please give at least 24-hours notice; we charge $35 for missed or cancelled appointments without adequate notice.

Weighing

We do not normally weigh patients because we believe in the nondiet approach to lifestyle change. We also may have other routines or therapies that are unfamiliar to you. We will make every effort to explain things thoroughly as we go. If you want to be weighed or you have other requests that are important to you, please just ask.

Confidentiality

We will not share your personal information or conversations without your written consent, except with your referring physician for your benefit. You will be asked to sign a Privacy document.

Financial Agreements

Payment is expected at the time of the visit. We will give you a bill showing our services rendered and proof of your payment for you to file a claim with your insurance company. We are a Preferred Provider for American Mutual PPO and will accept the co-payment from policyholders of that company. We are a Medicare Provider for diabetes and renal Medical Nutrition Therapy consultations. We will bill Medicare for the services we provide to you.

I have read the above and I understand and agree to these office policies.

_____   _____
Patient Signature   Date

_____   _____
Dietitian's Signature   Date

SAMPLE—Have your legal counselor evaluate before using.

Informed Consent to Medical Nutrition Therapy

       I hereby request and consent to Medical Nutrition Therapy by the dietitians at West Side Nutrition Clinic. The services may include nutrition assessment of my eating behaviors and beliefs, strategies to overcome barriers to change, suggestions for moderate physical activity (within the limits set by my physician), use of counseling therapies, routine follow-up, and re-evaluation as I practice new lifestyle choices.

       I have had an opportunity to discuss the nature and purpose of Medical Nutrition Therapy with the dietitian. I understand that results are not guaranteed, and that the final choices and decisions are mine. I also understand that treatments and advice will be made in my best interest, using information I provide, as well as current laboratory values, if available. The dietitian will exercise judgment based upon current scientific research and my unique physical and psychological characteristics.

       I understand that the nutrition guidance and printed nutrition materials I am provided are solely for my use.

       By signing below, I agree to the above named services. I intend this consent form to cover the entire course of treatment, for any future conditions for which I seek treatment, and for maintenance follow-up.

Print patient's name_____

Patient's signature_____

Date signed_____

All Saints Healthcare, Racine WI

OUTPATIENT COUNSELING PEER REVIEW CRITERIA

Counselor:_____ Peer Reviewer: _____

Date: _____ Topic/Order: _____

COUNSELING SKILL	POSITIVE DEMONSTRATION	AREA FOR IMPROVEMENT
Non Verbal Attending Skills: • Good eye contact • Tone of voice (inflection and volume) • Positive body language		
Active Listening Skills: • Reflective responses • Non-judgmental responses • Develop rapport/empathy		
Verbal Leading Skills: • Questions used to gather additional information • Appropriate use of open questions • Appropriate use of closed questions • Appropriate use of "why" questions • Limited use of confrontation responses • Limited use of advice versus client development of actions		
Self-Referent Skills: • Appropriate use of self-involving responses. • Avoidance of self-disclosure in counseling session		
Goal Identification: • Achievable client goals are positive, specific, and under client control • Evidence of client empowerment • Goals involve client behavior, not actions of someone else • Goals distinguished from results		
Identification of Goal Barriers: • Lack of client knowledge • Lack of client skills • Lack of client ability to change or take risks • Lack of social support		
Clinical Integrity: • Information is clinically accurate and up-to-date • Information is appropriate given the age of the client • Appropriate education materials are used		

6/97, Revised 1/02
Bridget Klawitter, PhD, RD, CD, FADA

Becoming a Certified Lactation Consultant
Robin Blocker, MA, RD, IBCLC

Dietitians should consider becoming a certified lactation consultant if you are currently involved in, or are interested in, lactation counseling. Through the process of studying for certification, you will concentrate on the entire subject of lactation including anatomy, physiology, and the vast number of circumstances that complicate breastfeeding success. Many well-paying jobs are available in public health and health education for Certified Lactation Consultants.

Certification validates special knowledge and skills. The International Board of Lactation Consultant Examiners, Inc. (IBLCE) administers the certification exam and will send you a brochure containing detailed information on how to apply. A fee is required to take the exam.

All Registered Dietitians with experience counseling breastfeeding mothers can qualify to take the exam, which consists of two components, a didactic section (of about 150 multiple choice questions) and a clinical component with 35-50 multiple choice questions on clinical problem identification photographs. In order to pass the test, it helps to have experience working with many different breastfeeding problems.

Once the exam is passed, the lactation consultant is certified for five years and must maintain certification through continuing education. At the end of five years, there are two options: submit 75 Continuing Education Recognition Points (CERPS), or successfully complete the IBLCE certification exam. The person must retake of the exam at least once every ten years to maintain certification status. The IBLCE will provide a list of suggested resources to read to stay current or to study for the exam. Many certified lactation consultants become members of the International Lactation Consultant Association (ILCA) and receive the Journal of Human Lactation (a quarterly publication).

New mothers who want to breastfeed their children are anxious for information. With the growing body of research in breastfeeding and its known benefits for health of the infant, this area of practice will continue to be a growing career option.

Write to:

The International Board of
Lactation Consultant Examiners
P.O. Box 2348
Falls Church, VA. 22042

Dietitian as Team Leader in Caring for a Child with a Feeding Disability

Harriet H. Cloud, MS, RD

Increasing numbers of children are referred to dietitians for feeding disabilities. Often the child may be classified as "failure to thrive" (FTT), which is a syndrome of growth failure due to inadequate intake, retention or utilization of nutrients to allow normal growth for age. (1) Feeding disabilities often result in FTT or growth failure. Traditionally the causes have been classified as organic, stemming from a medical condition, or nonorganic implying a social, emotional or behavioral factor. (2) In actuality, the cause of FTT or growth failure may include a combination of organic or nonorganic factors. (3)

Identification of the cause of the feeding disability is essential when counseling the child's family in a counseling mode. It requires careful assessment of the clinical history of the child and is best served when that assessment is provided in a team setting. (4) The team often includes an occupational therapist, physical therapist, social worker, nurse, psychologist and dietitian/nutritionist. Team makeup can vary and also may include a speech therapist, special educator, dentist and physician. Understanding the role or contribution of each discipline is important for good team interaction. Training in working with children and adults with developmental disabilities and interdisciplinary teams may be required for dietitians wishing to provide counseling and nutrition intervention. Training programs exist in University Affiliated Programs in almost every state.

Following is an overview of the principles involved in caring for a child in this setting.

Assessment

The team assessment should include a review of medical records, socioeconomic status, and nutrition assessment to determine height, weight, head circumference, fat fold measures, usual food intake, an oral motor assessment, positioning, and developmental evaluation. Watching the child eat or be fed by a parent or caregiver is necessary for adequate determination of any problems that exist. (4)

Intervention

Once a list of problems and family strengths is generated, the team in concern with the parents will prioritize the various problems to solve. Including the parent in problem selection and intervention also reflects the legislative language for children with disabilities, which recommends, "all services be comprehensive, family centered, culturally appropriate and community based." (5)

If the child is enrolled in a state funded" early intervention" or school program, the strategies selected for intervention should be included in the child's Individualized Education Program (IEP). This increases the possibility of intervention occurring both in the home and in the school. The following case study is an example of the principles just outlined.

CASE STUDY

Sarah is a two-year-old girl with a diagnosis of spastic quadriplegia (Cerebral Palsy), hydrocephalus and esotropia (eyes don't focus). She receives ongoing health care from the Children's Rehabilitation Service. Her problems include developmental delays, inability to walk, shunting for hydrocephalus secondary to intraventricular hemorrhage, visual problems for which glasses were prescribed, and since birth inadequate nutritional intake leading to growth failure.

History

Sarah had a birth weight of four pounds and a gestational age of 30 weeks. Her feeding was difficult due to her weak suck and poor tolerance of milk-based formula. The mother is a single parent with three other children. Sarah is receiving S.S.I. benefits, and the mother receives Aid to Dependent Children and Food Stamps, but Sarah was not on the WIC program.

Nutrition Information

On Sarah's first visit to the nutritionist, anthropometric measurements were taken: length was 29 1/8", weight 14 1/2 lbs, both below the 5%tile. Her mother reported an intake of 12 small jars of baby food mixed with six ounces of infant formula, given in a 24-hour period (mostly at night from the "infa-feeder," which totaled approximately 540 calories/ day). Vomiting was reported if milk was given in a cup or bottle. She never slept through the night, but took naps throughout the day. Following her first visit, the dietitian referred Sarah to the feeding clinic where occupational and physical therapy, and social work services were provided through Children's Rehabilitation Services, a state agency. The dietitian served as the team coordinator for Sarah's care.

Feeding Evaluations

During these evaluations it was determined that Sarah was attending a program for children with disabilities, but no feeding intervention had occurred since birth. Positioning while feeding was identified as a problem since she was held in her mother's lap for feeding or was fed lying down in bed. At school Sarah was fed sitting in a wheel chair. Her oral motor problems were multiple: immature sucking from the "infa-feeder," difficulty swallowing liquids, and resistance in the form of crying when a therapist tried to evaluate her oral-motor skills. She appeared to have resistance to tactile stimulation inside her mouth, but less resistance around her mouth. Although she could move her tongue laterally, spoon-feeding caused her great distress. All of this resulted in inadequate energy, nutrient, and fluid intake. Sarah was video taped while she ate in order to be evaluated at a parent/ team meeting, which enabled collaboration in problem identification and selection.

Recommendations

1. Gradually discontinue the use of the infa-feeder.
2. Feed in her wheel chair at all feeding times.
3. Thicken fruit juice and lactose-free milk to increase calories and enhance swallowing.
4. Feed blended table foods, gradually added to baby foods.
5. Introduce a high calorie, lactose-free commercial beverage to replace the food given in the infa-feeder as the transition to spoon-feeding is made.
6. Regular follow-up visits through school, Children's Rehabilitation Services, and the feeding clinic.

Follow-up

All of the recommendations were acceptable to the mother; however she elected starting with feeding in the wheel chair as her first priority. She was willing to thicken beverages and utilize the high calorie, lactose-free beverage. The Department of Human Resources provided a homemaker to give support in the home and the school reinforced all of the feeding recommendations. The nutritionist also accessed WIC to cover the cost of the supplemental beverage. The health department monitored Sarah's growth and she returned for feeding clinic evaluations every 4-6 weeks. At the end of a year, her weight gain had improved, she was fed in her wheel chair, and she was eating by spoon.

For this example of nutrition therapy, the nutritionist/dietitian was the coordinator of the team assessment and follow-up. The multifactoral nature of Sarah's problems made the need for a team approach imperative. This represents the type of counseling and intervention frequently required for successful management of children with feeding disabilities.

REFERENCES
1. Ramsay M, Gisel EG, Boultry M. Nonorganic failure to thrive: growth failure secondary to feeding skills disorder. *Develop Med &Child Neurol.* 1993; 35:285-297.
2. Bithoney WO, Dubowitz H, Egan H. Failure to thrive/Growth deficiency. *Pediatr in Rev.* 1992; 13:453-459.
3. Bithoney WG, Dubowitz H. Organic concomitants of nonorganic failure to thrive: Implications for research. In: Drotar D, ed. *New Directions in Failure to Thrive.* New York, NY: Plenum Press; 1985: 47-68.
4. Lane SJ, Cloud HH. Feeding problems and intervention: an interdisciplinary approach. *Topics Clin Nutr.* 1988; 3:23-32.
5. Lichtnwalter 1,Freeman R, Lee M, Cialone J. Providing nutrition services to children with special needs in a community setting. *Topics Clin Nutr.* 1993; 4:75-78.

ACTION WORDS

These types of action verbs may be useful for developing competency statements.

Accelerate	Collect	Differentiate	Fix
Accomplish	Combine	Direct	Focus
Achieve	Communicate	Discover	Formulate
Activate	Compare	Discriminate	Found
Adapt	Compile	Discuss	Fund
Address	Complete	Disperse	Gather
Administer	Compose	Display	Generalize
Advise	Comprehend	Dissect	Generate
Advocate	Compute	Distinguish	Give
Allocate	Conceive	Distribute	Grab
Alter	Conceptualize	Document	Grasp
Analyze	Conclude	Draft	Guard
Apply	Conduct	Draw	Guide
Appoint	Consolidate	Earn	Handle
Appraise	Construct	Edit	Help
Appreciate	Consult	Educate	Hire
Approve	Contrast	Effect	Identify
Arbitrate	Contribute	Eliminate	Illustrate
Arrange	Control	Enable	Implement
Assemble	Convert	Encourage	Improve
Assess	Coordinate	Enforce	Improvise
Ask	Copy	Engage	Include
Assign	Correct	Engineer	Increase
Assist	Counsel	Enhance	Indicate
Attain	Create	Ensure	Induce
Attend	Criticize	Equip	Infer
Audit	Debate	Establish	Influence
Balance	Decide	Estimate	Inform
Budget	Decrease	Evaluate	Initiate
Build	Deduce	Examine	Inspect
Calculate	Defend	Exceed	Inspire
Capture	Define	Execute	Install
Carry	Delegate	Exercise	Institute
Categorize	Demonstrate	Exhibit	Instruct
Chair	Describe	Expand	Integrate
Change	Design	Expedite	Interpret
Choose	Designate	Experiment	Interview
Choreograph	Detail	Explain	Introduce
Clarify	Detect	Express	Invent
Classify	Determine	Facilitate	Investigate
Clean	Develop	Fasten	Involve
Code	Devise	File	Isolate
Collaborate	Diagnose	Find	Join
Collate	Diagram	Finish	

ACTION WORDS

Launch	Predict	Repair	Support
Learn	Prepare	Rephrase	Surpass
Lecture	Present	Replace	Survey
Led	Preserve	Report	Synthesize
Lift	Prioritize	Represent	Systematize
List	Process	Reproduce	Tabulate
Listen	Procure	Research	Tailor
Lobby	Produce	Restate	Take
Locate	Program	Restore	Taught
Maintain	Project	Restructure	Terminate
Manage	Promote	Revamp	Testify
Map	Proofread	Review	Train
Market	Propose	Revise	Transform
Master	Prove	Revitalize	Translate
Match	Provide	Rewrite	Transport
Maximize	Publicize	Save	Travel
Measure	Publish	Schedule	Update
Mediate	Pull	Screen	Use
Mobilize	Purchase	Sculpt	Utilize
Moderate	Push	Select	Validate
Modify	Qualify	Sell	Vary
Monitor	Question	Separate	Verify
Motivate	Raise	Serve	Visualize
Name	Reason	Service	Wash
Negotiate	Rearrange	Set up	Weigh
Nominate	Reassemble	Shape	Won
Observe	Recall	Simplify	Wrote
Obtain	Receive	Solicit	Xray
Omit	Recognize	Solve	
Operate	Recombine	Speak	
Order	Recommend	Staff	
Organize	Reconstruct	Stage	
Originate	Record	Start	
Outline	Reconcile	State	
Package	Recruit	Stimulate	
Paraphrase	Redesign	Stock	
Participate	Reduce	Streamline	
Pass Test	Reevaluate	Strengthen	
Perceive	Refer	Structure	
Perform	Refine	Study	
Persuade	Regroup	Submit	
Photograph	Relate	Substitute	
Pick	Rename	Succeed	
Place	Renegotiate	suggerst	
Plan	Reorganize	Summarize	
Point (out)	Reorder	Supervise	

Reviewed: August 19, 2002, CCT

All Saints Healthcare
Competency & Validation Tool – Online Form

Competency ID #:
Categories:
Competency Title:

References and Learning Resources:
- ◆
- ◆
- ◆

Validation Frequency:
- ☐ Orientation Period
- ☐ Annual
- ☐ Other:

Factors:
- ☐ Risk H ☐
  -    L ☐
- ☐ Volume H ☐
  -    L ☐
- ☐ Problem Prone
- ☐ Performance Improvement
- ☐ Process Improvement

Age Specific:
- ☐ Not Applicable
- ☐ Birth to 1 Month
- ☐ 1 Month to 1 Year
- ☐ 1 Year to 3 Years
- ☐ 3 Years to 6 Years
- ☐ 6 Years to 12 Years
- ☐ 12 Years to 18 Years
- ☐ 18 Years to 65 Years
- ☐ 65 Years +

Competency Statement:

Behavioral Criteria (knowledge, skill, critical decision-making)	Validation Method *	Validator's Initials	Date

* Validation Method (when "or" used, circle method used)

Date Initiated: _____ Successful Completion of Competency Date: _____

Employee Name:_____   Validator(s) Name:_____
Position #:_____ **Department #:**_____   _____
Hire Date:_____   _____

Formulated By:
Date Approved:
Date Revised:

---

* **Validation Method:**

O = Direct Observation
RD = Return Demonstration
WT = Written Test/Quiz
V = Verbal Testing/Interview/Feedback
Other = Write In

D = Documentation/Anecdotal Recording/Chart Review
CD = Computer Demonstration/Simulation
RP/RR = Role Play/Role Reversal
CS = Case Study/Scenario/Competency Station

281

All Saints Healthcare System, Inc.
Competency & Validation Tool – Online Form

Competency ID #: 103557
Categories: Cross-Departmental
Competency Title: Patient Education, Basic Skills

References and Learning Resources:
- ASHS policies and procedures
- Disease- or condition specific information
- Department specific policies and procedures
- Micromedex modules
- Department patient education materials
- Age specific learning modules

Validation Frequency:
- ☒ Orientation Period
- ☐ Annual
- ☐ Other:

Factors:
- ☐ Risk H ☐
-         L ☐
- ☒ Volume H ☒
-         L ☐
- ☒ Problem Prone
- ☐ Performance Improvement
- ☐ Process Improvement

Age Specific:
- ☐ Not Applicable
- ☐ Birth to 1 Month
- ☒ 1 Month to 1 Year
- ☒ 1 Year to 3 Years
- ☒ 3 Years to 6 Years
- ☒ 6 Years to 12 Years
- ☒ 12 Years to 18 Years
- ☒ 18 Years to 65 Years
- ☒ 65 Years +

Competency Statement: Provides patient and family education.

Behavioral Criteria (knowledge, skill, critical decision-making)	Validation Method *	Validator's Initials	Date
Assesses patient/family knowledge regarding topic.	O or V, D		
Identifies religious, cultural, motivational, physical or other barriers that may impact learning experience.	O, D		
Addresses age-specific learning needs -1 month to 3 years	O or V, D		
-3 years to 6 years	O or V, D		
-6 years to 12 years	O or V, D		
-12 years to 18 years	O or V, D		
-18 years to 65 years	O or V, D		
-65 years +	O or V, D		
Identifies and utilizes organizational resources (ie. interpreters, specialized materials, educational devices).	V or O		
Involves patient in determining education goals.	O, D		
Selects and/or adapts education methods, techniques and activities appropriate to the learning needs of the patient and desired outcomes.	O, V, D		
Assesses comprehension/motivation of patient and/or family.	O or V, D		
Develops individualized teaching plan and goals.	O, D, V		
Involves family/significant others in teaching as appropriate.	O, D		
Completes referrals/communicates to other disciplines as appropriate.	O or D or V		
Documents teachings, patient comprehension and likelihood of adherence using documentation policies and procedures.	D		
Ensures patient confidentiality to enhance teaching experience.	O		
Provides patient with additional resources as requested.	O, D		
Applies learning principles to promote an environment conducive to learning.	O, V		

* Validation Method (when "or" used, circle method used)

Date Initiated: _____ Successful Completion of Competency Date: _____

Employee Name:_____ **Validator(s) Name:**_____

Position #:_____ **Department #:**_____ _____ _____

Hire Date:_____ _____ _____

Formulated By: Bridget Klawitter, Director, Medical Nutrition Therapy and Diabetes Services and Karen Peterson, Patient Education Coordinator, Education Resources

Date Approved: 8/9/00, Core Competency Team

Date Revised: 3/7/01, Core Competency Team

* Validation Method:

O = Direct Observation
RD = Return Demonstration
WT = Written Test/Quiz
V = Verbal Testing/Interview/Feedback
Other = Write In

D = Documentation/Anecdotal Recording/Chart Review
CD = Computer Demonstration/Simulation
RP/RR = Role Play/Role Reversal
CS = Case Study/Scenario/Competency Station

Appendix 6-B

All Saints Healthcare System, Inc.
Competency & Validation Tool – Online Form

Competency ID #: 103354
Categories: Departmental
Competency Title: Nutrition Evaluation: Clinical Dietetics

References and Learning Resources:
- Department Policies and Procedures
- Department Acuity List for Nutrition Risk
- Computrition NutraCom User Manual
- Preferred Process (1999)

Validation Frequency:
- ☒ Orientation Period
- ☐ Annual
- ☐ Other:

Factors:
- ☐ Risk H ☐
- L ☐
- ☒ Volume H ☒
- L ☐
- ☒ Problem Prone
- ☐ Performance Improvement
- ☐ Process Improvement

Age Specific:
- ☐ Not Applicable
- ☐ Birth to 1 Month
- ☒ 1 Month to 1 Year
- ☒ 1 Year to 3 Years
- ☒ 3 Years to 6 Years
- ☒ 6 Years to 12 Years
- ☒ 12 Years to 18 Years
- ☒ 18 Years to 65 Years
- ☒ 65 Years +

Competency Statement: Evaluates clients for nutritional risk.

Behavioral Criteria (knowledge, skill, critical decision-making)	Validation Method *	Validator's Initials	Date
Performs nutrition evaluation using department criteria to identify patients at nutrition risk	D		
Assesses patients' learning needs barriers to learning and educational level and provides education accordingly.	O, D		
- 1 month to 3 years			
- 3 years to 6 years			
- 6 years to 12 years			
- 12 years to 18 years			
- 18 years to 65 + years			
Identifies need for nutrition supplementation for patients with compromised eating patterns.	D		
Identifies potential food-drug interactions according to system policy and provides education	D		
Collects, reviews and evaluates data to determine nutrition needs of patients	D		
Refers patients appropriately based on department criteria	V, D		
Develops measurable goals as part of nutrition plan of care.	D		
Documents nutrition evaluation using department format.	D		
Enters visit information into Computrition	CD, D		

* Validation Method (when "or" used, circle method used)

Date Initiated: _____ Successful Completion of Competency Date: _____

Employee Name:_____ Validator(s) Name:_____

Position #:_____ Department #:_____ _____ _____
Hire Date:_____ _____ _____

Formulated By: Bridget Klawitter, Manager, Medical Nutrition Therapy and Diabetes Services
Date Approved: 7/19/00, Core Competency Team
Date Revised: 6/14/01, Core Competency Team

* Validation Method:
O = Direct Observation
RD = Return Demonstration
WT = Written Test/Quiz
V = Verbal Testing/Interview/Feedback
Other = Write In

D = Documentation/Anecdotal Recording/Chart Review
CD = Computer Demonstration/Simulation
RP/RR = Role Play/Role Reversal
CS = Case Study/Scenario/Competency Station

Pediatric Nutrition Assessment (Birth to 36 months)

Children's Hospital Medical Center

Diagnosis: _____

Growth History: Previous Weights   Previous Heights   Growth Velocity: _____
date kg %ile   date cm %ile

Date					NUTRITIONAL RISK CRITERIA
Age					
Weight (kg)					< 5th %ile
%ile					
Length (cm)					< 5th %ile suggests growth retardation
%ile					
Head Circumference					< 5th %ile
%ile					
Ideal Weight for Length					
Weight/Length Index (actual weight - ideal weight for length)					80% to 90%; Mild PEM* 70% to 80%; Moderate PEM* <70%; Severe PEM*
Height/Age Index (actual HT - ideal HT for age)					90% to 95%; Mild Chronic Malnu. 85% to 90%; Mod. Chronic Malnu. <85%; Severe Chronic Malnu.
Arm Circumference/ Head Circumference Ratio					.28 to .31; Mild PEM* .25 to .28; Moderate PEM* <.25; Severe PEM*
Arm Circumference (cm)					
%ile					< 5th %ile
Arm Muscle Circumference (mm)					< 5th %ile
%ile					
Arm Muscle Area (mm²)					< 5th %ile
%ile					
Tricep Skinfold (mm)					< 5th %ile
%ile					
Subscapular Skinfold (mm)					< 5th %ile
%ile					

*PEM: Protein Energy Malnutrition

Date					NUTRITIONAL RISK CRITERIA
Albumin					0-6 mo <2.9 gm/dl 6mo-3yr <3.5 gm/dl
Transferrin					<200 mg/dl
Pre Albumin					
Retinol Binding Protein					
Total Lymphocyte Count					< 1500 mm³

Intake
Dates _____
Kcal/Kg _____
gm pro/kg _____

Oxygen consumption: Date ____ REE = _____ RQ = ____   Maintenance _____ Kcal/day
Catch Up _____ Kcal/day

NUTRITIONAL NEEDS+ ____ Kcal/Kg ____ gm pro/kg

based on _____
(+energy needs increase 7% per degree F.)

Expected rate of weight gain for size: _____

Comments: _____
_____
_____
_____

CHMC NS #1029 5,

Pediatric Nutrition Assessment (3-18 yrs.)

NUTRITION ASSESSMENT
(3 to 18 years)

Diagnosis: _____

Growth History: Previous Weights
date kg %ile

Previous Heights
date cm %ile

Previous Growth Velocity: _____

Date						NUTRITIONAL RISK CRITERIA
Age						
Weight (kg)						< 5th %ile
%ile						
Height (cm)						< 5th %ile suggests growth retardation
%ile						
Ideal Weight for Height						
Weight/Height Index (actual weight - ideal weight for height)						80% to 90%; Mild PEM* 70% to 80%; Moderate PEM* <70%; Severe PEM*
Height/Age Index (actual HT - ideal HT for age)						90% to 95%; Mild Chronic Malnu. 85% to 90%; Mod. Chronic Malnu. <85%; Severe Chronic Malnu.
Arm Circumference (cm)						< 5th %ile
%ile						
Arm Muscle Circumference (mm)						< 5th %ile
%ile						
Arm Muscle Area (mm²)						< 5th %ile
%ile						
Tricep Skinfold (mm)						< 5th %ile
%ile						
Subscapular Skinfold (mm)						< 5th %ile
%ile						

*PEM: Protein Energy Malnutrition

Date				NUTRITIONAL RISK CRITERIA
Albumin				<3.5 gm/dl
Transferrin				<200 mg/dl
Pre Albumin				
Retinol Binding Protein				
Total Lymphocyte Count				< 1500 mm³
Intake Dates				
Kcal/Kg				
gm pro/kg				

Oxygen consumption: Date _____ REE = _____ RQ = _____

NUTRITIONAL NEEDS+ based on _____ Kcal/Kg _____ gm pro/kg

Maintenance _____ Kcal/day

Catch Up _____ Kcal/day

Expected rate of weight gain for size: _____

Comments:

(+energy needs increase 7% per degree F.)

CHMC NS #1150 5/90

Name: _____   MRN: _____

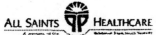

DEPARTMENT OF CLINICAL DIETETICS
PEDIATRIC OUTPATIENT NUTRITION ASSESSMENT PROFILE
PRESCHOOL (Age 1 to 6 years)

Name: _____   Date _____

DOB: _____ MRN: _____ Diet Prescribed: _____

Referring Physician: _____

	Potential or ↑ Risk for Problem	Impaired Nutrition Management Remarks
MANAGEMENT PLANNING		

Health Education Barriers to Learning ☐ No
  ☐ child
  ☐ parent/caretaker
	☐ Yes
	  ☐ Dyslexia ☐ Reading
	  ☐ Language ☐ Vision
	  ☐ Hearing ☐ Other
		Who present for appointment?

CLINICAL FINDINGS		

• **Anthropometrics**
   • weight: _____
   • length/ht: _____
   • head circ: _____
   • BMI: _____
	☐ >95th%ile wt for age
	☐ >95th%ile ht for age
	☐ >95th%ile wt for ht
	☐ <5th%ile wt for age
	☐ <5th%ile ht for age
	☐ <5th%ile wt for ht
		Growth Issues:

• **Pertinent nutrition labs** ☐ WNL	☐ Abnormal findings	
MEDICAL HISTORY		

• **Family History**
   • Diabetes   ☐ No
   • Heart Disease   ☐ No
   • Hypertension   ☐ No
• **Medical Conditions**
   • Cardiac   ☐ No
   • Hypertension   ☐ No
   • Thyroid   ☐ No
   • Obesity   ☐ No
   • Renal   ☐ No
   • GI Disorders   ☐ No
   • Post Natal   ☐ No
   • Prenatal problems ☐ No
   • Recent surgery ☐ No
   • Recent acute illness ☐ No
   • Diabetes   ☐ No
   • Other: _____ ☐ No
	☐ Yes
	☐ Yes
	☐ Yes
	
	☐ Yes
	☐ Yes
	☐ Yes
	☐ Yes
	☐ Yes
	☐ Yes
	☐ Yes
	☐ Yes
	☐ Yes
	☐ Yes
	☐ Yes
	☐ Yes	

Hx chronic illness/disorders ☐ No	☐ Yes (describe/list)	

Name: _____   MRN: _____

		Potential or ↑ Risk for Problem	Impaired Nutrition Management Remarks

Feeding Ability Issues	☐ No	☐ Yes
		  ☐ developmental delay
		  ☐ poor suck/swallow
		  ☐ problems chewing
		  ☐ coordination problems
		  ☐ extended periods to feed
		  ☐ oral hypersensitivity
		  ☐ negative oral experience
		  ☐ dental problems
		  ☐ other _____	

Intake Difficulties	☐ No	☐ Yes
		  ☐ stomach aches
		  ☐ chronic diarrhea
		  ☐ chronic constipation
		  ☐ nausea and/or vomiting
		  ☐ reflux/spitting up
		  ☐ poor appetite/food refusal
		  ☐ enteral nutrition
		  ☐ other: _____	

PHYSICAL APPEARANCE			
• skin	☐ No	☐ Yes (dry, scaling, rash) (↓ subQ fat, pale, bruising)	
• hair	☐ No	☐ Yes (dull, thin, easily pluck)	
• nails	☐ No	☐ Yes (thin, spoon-shaped) (brittle, ridged)	
• mouth/lips	☐ No	☐ Yes (inflammed, cracked) (sores)	
• tongue	☐ No	☐ Yes (inflammed, swollen) (sores)	
• gums	☐ No	☐ Yes (spongy, bleeding)	
• eyes	☐ No	☐ Yes (pale, drainage)	
• teeth	☐ No	☐ Yes (missing, caries, braces)	
• muscle tone	☐ No	☐ Yes (spastic, wasting, ↓ tone)	
• extremities	☐ No	☐ Yes (edema)	
• other:	☐ No	☐ Yes (delayed healing) (dehydration)	
MEDICATIONS			
Medications ☐ No _____ _____ _____ _____		☐ Potential for Drug-Nutrient Interaction	
Vitamins/Supplements ☐ Yes _____ _____ _____ _____ _____		☐ Potential for Drug-Nutrient or Nutrient-Nutrient Interaction	

Name: _____   MRN: _____

	Potential or ↑ Risk for Problem	Impaired Nutrition Management Remarks
LIFESTYLE HABITS		
• coffee/tea/caffeine beverages ☐ No	☐ Yes type _____ _____ amt _____ _____ how often _____ _____	
• drug exposure (if pertinent)　☐ No	☐ Yes	
EXERCISE/ACTIVITY BEHAVIOR		
Activity/Development Pattern ☐ WNL • Type _____ _____ • may refuse foods/appetite declines • increased self feeding • plays with foods • hold cup and/or by handle • verbalize food preferences • unwrap foods • holds spoon • uses fork • pours foods • may refuse many foods • food jags • shows independence w/ feeding • resists help • likes to plan meals	☐ Abnormal	
Activity level changed over last 　　12 months	☐ decreased ☐ increased ☐ no change	
Preschool Activities (play, games, etc)	☐ none participated in	
After school activity (bike, run, etc)	☐ none (mainly sedentary)	
Physical ailments limit activity　☐ No	☐ Yes	
DIET BEHAVIOR		
Food Allergies or Intolerances: ☐ No	☐ Yes:	

Name: _____   MRN: _____

	Potential or ↑ Risk for Problem	Impaired Nutrition Management Remarks
Currently on a special diet ☐ No	☐ Yes	
Formula Used ☐ No	☐ Yes	
• limits fat ☐ Yes • limits sugar ☐ Yes • limits salt ☐ Yes • increases fiber ☐ Yes • other _____ ☐ Yes	☐ No ☐ No ☐ No ☐ No ☐ No	

Experiencing problems with feeding ☐ No
 	
• Eating 3 meals/day ☐ Yes
• Snacks _____
    _____
    _____
 	
• Eating pattern changes on
    weekends ☐ No
• School/daycare meals ☐ No
• Who does grocery shopping?
    _____
 	
• Limited finances ☐ No
 	
• Frequency of eating out
    ☐ never   ☐ 1-2 times/month
    ☐ 3-4 times/month
    ☐ 1-2 times/week
	☐ Yes
	
	☐ No
	
	☐ Yes
	☐ Yes
	
	☐ Yes
	☐ WIC
	☐ Other:
	
	☐ 3-4 times/week
	☐ daily
		Feeding Issues:

PAIN/DISCOMFORT:

• Does your child seem to have pain now? ☐ No	☐ Yes	☐ Provide general pain information
• Does the pain affect your child's ability to function? ☐ No	☐ Yes	☐ Provided information on Pain Program for unrelieved chronic pain issues
• **IF NO TO BOTH QUESTIONS, GO TO THE NEXT SECTION**	Where is the pain? What does pain feel/look like?	☐ Forwarded pain issues/concerns to physician ☐ other
• **IF YES, GET PAIN DETAIL & LOG ON CLINICAL FINDINGS SHEET**	How long does pain last?	
How would you rate pain?	• (0-10): _____ • What makes pain worse? • What makes pain better?	☐ **PEEP Scale** ☐ **Pediatric Faces Pain Rating Scale** ☐ **0-10 Pain Rating Scale**

OP-PRESC.DOC
3/2/98 revised 9/21/98, 10/12/01

Registered Dietitian

DEPARTMENT OF CLINICAL DIETETICS
OUTPATIENT NUTRITION ASSESSMENT PROFILE-ADULT/OLDER ADULT

Name: _____   Date _____

DOB: _____ MRN: _____ Diet Prescribed: _____

Referring Physician: _____

	Potential or ↑ Risk for Problem	Impaired Nutrition Management Remarks
DEMOGRAPHICS		
Sex ☐ Female ☐ Male Race ☐ Non-Hispanic White ☐ Hispanic American ☐ African American ☐ Asian ☐ Other		
MANAGEMENT PLANNING		
Health Education Barriers to Learning ☐ No	☐ Yes ☐ Dyslexia ☐ Reading ☐ Language ☐ Vision ☐ Hearing ☐ Other	
CLINICAL FINDINGS		
• Weight History • height: _____ • weight: _____ • UBW: _____ • IBW: _____ • BMI: _____ • Pertinent nutrition labs ☐ WNL • Blood pressure ☐ WNL	☐ >120% UBW ☐ <80% UBW ☐ >120% IBW ☐ <80% IBW ☐ BMI >27 ☐ Abnormal findings ☐ Abnormal findings	
MEDICAL HISTORY		
• Family History • Diabetes ☐ No • Heart Disease ☐ No • Hypertension ☐ No • Medical Conditions • Cardiac ☐ No • Hypertension ☐ No • Thyroid ☐ No • Obesity ☐ No • Renal ☐ No • GI Disorders ☐ No • Pregnancy ☐ No • Other: _____ ☐ No • Diabetes ☐ No	☐ Yes ☐ Yes ☐ Yes ☐ Yes ☐ Yes ☐ Yes ☐ Yes ☐ Yes ☐ Yes ☐ Yes ☐ Yes ☐ Yes ☐ Type 1 ☐ Gestational ☐ Type 2 ☐ Secondary/Other ☐ IGT	

Patient _____   MRN _____

	Potential or ↑ Risk for Problem	Impaired Nutrition Management Remarks
MEDICATIONS		
Medications ☐ No _____ _____ _____ _____	☐ Potential for Drug-Nutrient Interaction	
Vitamins/Supplements/Herbals ☐ Yes _____ _____ _____ _____ _____	☐ Potential for Drug-Nutrient or Nutrient-Nutrient Interaction	
Lifestyle Habits		

• smoker ☐ No
 • alcohol ☐ No
 	
 • drugs (if pertinent) ☐ No
	☐ Yes amt per day _____
	 ☐ Yes
	    type _____
	       _____
	    amt _____
	       _____
	    how often _____
	       _____
	 ☐ Yes	

FAMILY VIOLENCE SCREEN Because of the prevalence of violence within our community, we at All Saints are concerned about your safety and we are asking all of our patients: *Have you ever been shoved, hit, kicked, controlled or made to feel afraid within the last year?* ☐ No	**Do not ask if patient accompanied by someone.** **Ask only for age 18 and above.** ☐ Yes	☐ If yes, given resource information.
EXERCISE/ACTIVITY BEHAVIOR		

Exercise/Activity ☐ Yes
 • Type _____
   _____
 • Frequency
   ☐ daily   ☐ 4-5 times/week
   ☐ 2-3 times/week
 • Duration
   ☐ 45-60 minutes/session
   ☐ 30-45 minutes/session
   ☐ 15-30 minutes/session
 Activity level changed over last 12 months
	☐ No
	
	 ☐ < 2 times/week
	
	 ☐ < 15 minutes/session
	
	 ☐ decreased
	 ☐ increased
	 ☐ no change	

Physical ailments limit activity ☐ No	☐ Yes	

All Saints Healthcare Racine WI

Patient _____   MRN _____

	Potential or ↑ Risk for Problem	Impaired Nutrition Management Remarks
DIET HISTORY		
• up @ _____ Breakfast:		
• a.m. snack @ _____		
• Lunch @ _____		
• p.m. snack @ _____		
• Dinner @ _____		
• Before bed @ _____		
• Go to bed @ _____		

OP St. Luke's - /6/98 revised 2/11/98, 3/10/01, 9/11/01, 11/10/01

Patient _____   MRN _____

	Potential or ↑ Risk for Problem	Impaired Nutrition Management Remarks
PAIN/DISCOMFORT		
• Do you have pain now? ☐ No	☐ Yes	☐ provided general pain information
• Does pain affect your ability to ☐ No function?	☐ Yes	☐ provided information on Pain Program for unrelieved chronic pain issues
• **IF NO TO BOTH QUESTIONS, GO TO THE NEXT SECTION**	Where is your pain?	☐ forwarded pain issues/concerns to physician
• **IF YES, GET PAIN DETAIL & LOG ON CLINICAL FINDINGS SHEET**	What does pain feel like? How long does pain last?	☐ other
How would you rate pain?	• (0-10): _____ • What makes pain worse? • What makes pain better?	☐ 0-10 Pain Rating Scale ☐ Faces Pain Rating Scale ☐ Pain/Discomfort Behavioral Scale
Food Allergies or Intolerances: ☐ No • Currently follows a special diet	☐ Yes	
☐ No	☐ Yes	
• limits fat ☐ No	☐ Yes	
• limits sugar ☐ No	☐ Yes	
• limits salt ☐ No	☐ Yes	
• increases fiber ☐ No	☐ Yes	
• other ☐ No	☐ Yes	
• Experiencing problems following special diet ☐ No	☐ Yes	
DIET BEHAVIOR		
Eating 3 meals/day ☐ Yes	☐ No	
• Eating pattern changes on weekends ☐ No	☐ Yes	
• Eating patterns altered due to work schedule ☐ No	☐ Yes	
• Prepares own meals ☐ Yes	☐ No	
• Who does grocery shopping? _____		
• Limited finances ☐ No	☐ Yes	
• Frequency of eating out ☐ never ☐ 1-2 times/month ☐ 3-4 times/month ☐ 1-2 times/week	☐ 3-4 times/week ☐ daily	
• Difficulty eating/oral health issues ☐ No	☐ Yes ☐ chewing ☐ swallowing ☐ ill-fit dentures	

If you had to make changes in your diet or activity pattern, what would you see as the most challenging or difficult?

1. _____

2. _____

_____
Registered Dietitian

All Saints Healthcare Racine WI

Determine Your Nutritional Health

DETERMINE YOUR NUTRITIONAL HEALTH

The Warning Signs of poor nutritional health are often overlooked. Use this checklist to find out if you or someone you know is at nutritional risk.

Read the statements below. Circle the number in the yes column for those that apply to you or someone you know. For each yes answer, score the number in the box. Total your nutritional score.

	YES
I have an illness or condition that made me change the kind and/or amount of food I eat.	2
I eat fewer than 2 meals per day.	3
I eat few fruits or vegetables, or milk products.	2
I have 3 or more drinks of beer, liquor or wine almost every day.	2
I have tooth or mouth problems that make it hard for me to eat.	2
I don't always have enough money to buy the food I need.	4
I eat alone most of the time.	1
I take 3 or more different prescribed or over-the-counter drugs a day.	1
Without wanting to, I have lost or gained 10 pounds in the last 6 months.	2
I am not always physically able to shop, cook and/or feed myself.	2
TOTAL	

Referral services (linked to statements):

- Nutrition Education & Counseling, Nutrition Support
- Social Services, Nutrition Education & Counseling
- Nutrition Education & Counseling, Nutrition Support
- Nutrition Education & Counseling, Mental Health, Medications Use
- Oral Health, Nutrition Education & Counseling, Nutrition Support
- Social Services
- Social Services, Mental Health
- Medications Use
- Nutrition Education & Counseling, Nutrition Support, Medications Use
- Social Services, Nutrition Support

Total Your Nutritional Score. If it's —

0-2 **Good!** Recheck your nutritional score in 6 months.

3-5 **You are at moderate nutritional risk.** See what can be done to improve your eating habits and lifestyle. Your office on aging, senior nutrition program, senior citizens center or health department can help. Recheck your nutritional score in 3 months.

6 or more **You are at high nutritional risk.** Bring this checklist the next time you see your doctor, dietitian or other qualified health or social service professional. Talk with them about any problems you may have. Ask for help to improve your nutritional health.

These materials developed and distributed by the Nutrition Screening Initiative, a project of:

AMERICAN ACADEMY OF FAMILY PHYSICIANS

THE AMERICAN DIETETIC ASSOCIATION

NATIONAL COUNCIL ON THE AGING

Remember that warning signs suggest risk, but do not represent diagnosis of any condition. Turn the page to learn more about the Warning Signs of poor nutritional health.

Nutrition
FACT SHEET

Weight Loss Readiness Quiz

Are you ready to lose weight? Your attitude about weight loss affects your ability to succeed. Take this Readiness Quiz to learn if you need to make any attitude adjustments before you begin. Mark each item true or false. Be honest! It's important that these answers reflect the way you really are, not how you would like to be. A method for interpreting your readiness for weight loss follows:

1.___I have thought a lot about my eating habits and physical activities to pinpoint what I need to change.

2.___I have accepted the idea that I need to make permanent, not temporary, changes in my eating and activities to be successful.

3.___I will only feel successful if I lose a lot of weight.

4.___I accept the idea that it's best if I lose weight slowly.

5.___I'm thinking of losing weight now because I really want to, not because someone else thinks I should.

6.___I think losing weight will solve other problems in my life.

7.___I am willing and able to increase my regular physical activity.

8.___I can lose weight successfully if I have no "slip-ups."

9.___I am ready to commit some time and effort each week to organizing and planning my food and activity programs.

10.___Once I lose some initial weight, I usually lose the motivation to keep going until I reach my goal.

11.___I want to start a weight loss program, even though my life is unusually stressful right now.

Scoring the weight loss readiness quiz. To score the quiz, look at your answers to items 1, 2, 4, 5, 7, 9. Score "1" if you answered "true" and "0" if you answered "false."
. For items 3, 6, 8,10, 11, score "0" for each true answer and "1" for each false answer. To get your total score, add the scores for all questions.

No one score indicates for sure whether you are ready or not to start losing weight. However, the higher your total score, the more characteristics you have that contribute to success. As a rough guide, consider the following recommendations: 1) If you scored 8 or higher, you probably have good reasons for wanting to lose weight now and a good understanding of the steps needed to succeed. Still, you might want to learn more about the areas where you scored a "0" (see "Interpretation of Quiz Items" below). 2) If you scored 5 to 7, you may need to reevaluate your reasons for losing weight and the methods you would use to do so. To get a start, read the advice below for those quiz items where you received a score of "0."

3) If you scored 4 or less, now may not be the right time for you to lose weight. While you might be successful in losing weight initially, your answers suggest that you are unlikely to sustain sufficient effort to lose all the weight you want or to keep off the weight that you do lose. You need to reconsider your weight loss motivations and methods and perhaps learn more about the pros and cons of different approaches to reducing. To do so, read the advice below for those quiz items where you marked "0."

Interpretation of Quiz Items. Your answers to the Quiz can clue you in to potential stumbling blocks to your weight loss success. Any item score of "0" indicates a misconception about weight loss, or a potential problem area. While no individual items score of "0" is important enough to scuttle your weight loss plans, we suggest that you consider the meaning of those items so you can best prepare yourself for the challenges ahead.

1. It has been said that you can't change what you don't understand. You might benefit from keeping records for a week to help pinpoint when, what, why, and how much you eat. This tool is also useful in identifying obstacles to regular physical activity.

Typical Nutrition Section of Health Risk Appraisal

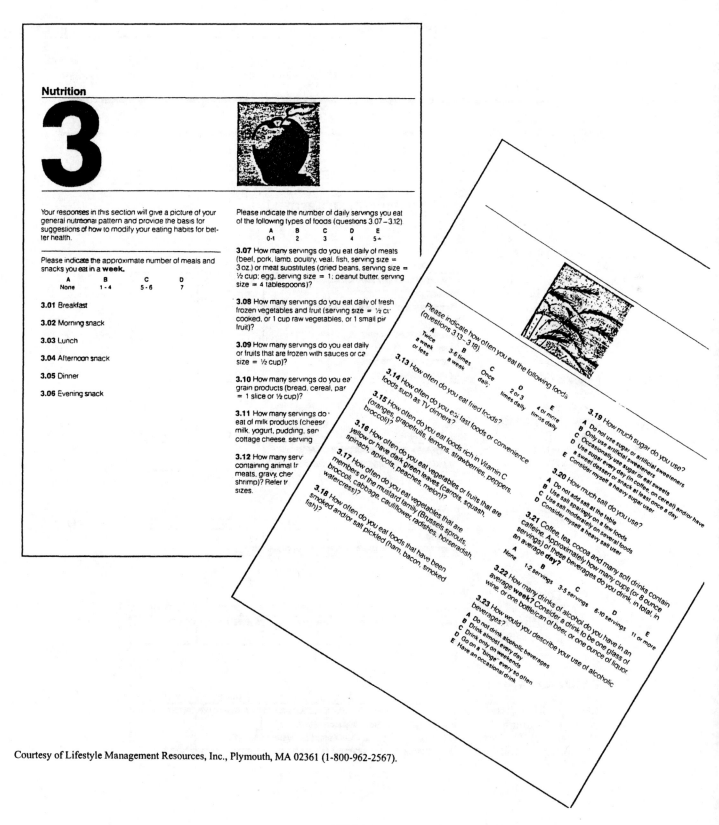

Nutrition

3

Your responses in this section will give a picture of your general nutritional pattern and provide the basis for suggestions of how to modify your eating habits for better health.

Please indicate the approximate number of meals and snacks you eat in a **week.**

A	B	C	D
None	1 - 4	5 - 6	7

3.01 Breakfast

3.02 Morning snack

3.03 Lunch

3.04 Afternoon snack

3.05 Dinner

3.06 Evening snack

Please indicate the number of daily servings you eat of the following types of foods (questions 3.07 – 3.12).

A	B	C	D	E
0-1	2	3	4	5+

3.07 How many servings do you eat daily of meats (beef, pork, lamb, poultry, veal, fish, serving size = 3 oz.) or meat substitutes (dried beans, serving size = ½ cup; egg, serving size = 1; peanut butter, serving size = 4 tablespoons)?

3.08 How many servings do you eat daily of fresh frozen vegetables and fruit (serving size = ½ cup cooked, or 1 cup raw vegetables, or 1 small piece fruit)?

3.09 How many servings do you eat daily or fruits that are frozen with sauces or ca size = ½ cup)?

3.10 How many servings do you eat grain products (bread, cereal, pa = 1 slice or ½ cup)?

3.11 How many servings do eat of milk products (cheese milk, yogurt, pudding, ser cottage cheese, serving

3.12 How many serv containing animal f meats, gravy, che shrimp)? Refer t sizes.

Please indicate how often you eat the following foods (questions 3.13 – 3.18)

A	B	C	D	E
Twice a week or less	3-5 times a week	Once daily	2 or 3 times daily	4 or more times daily

3.13 How often do you eat fried foods?

3.14 How often do you eat fast foods or convenience foods such as TV dinners?

3.15 How often do you eat foods rich in Vitamin C (oranges, grapefruits, lemons, strawberries, peppers, broccoli)?

3.16 How often do you eat vegetables or fruits that are yellow or have dark green leaves (carrots, squash, spinach, apricots, peaches, melon)?

3.17 How often do you eat vegetables that are members of the mustard family (Brussels sprouts, broccoli, cabbage, cauliflower, radishes, horseradish, watercress)?

3.18 How often do you eat foods that have been smoked and/or salt pickled (ham, bacon, smoked fish)?

3.19 How much sugar do you use?
A Do not use sugar, or artificial sweeteners
B Only use artificial sweeteners
C Occasionally use sugar or eat sweets
D Use sugar every day (in coffee, on cereal) and/or have a sweet dessert or snack at least once a day
E Consider myself a heavy sugar user

3.20 How much salt do you use?
A Do not add salt at the table
B Use salt sparingly on a few foods
C Use salt moderately on several foods
D Consider myself a heavy salt user

3.21 Coffee, tea, cocoa and many soft drinks contain caffeine. Approximately how many cups (or 8 ounce servings) of these beverages do you drink, in total, on an average **day?**

A	B	C	D	E
None	1-2 servings	3-5 servings	6-10 servings	11 or more

3.22 How many drinks of alcohol do you have in an average **week?** Consider a drink to be one glass of wine, or one bottle/can of beer, or one ounce of liquor.

3.23 How would you describe your use of alcoholic beverages?
A Do not drink alcoholic beverages
B Drink almost every day
C Drink only on weekends
D Go on a "binge" every so often
E Have an occasional drink

U. LOVELY **BIOMETRIC PROFILE SERIES 150-HR** 012-31-2231

December 2, 1994 Age: 24 Sex: m

HEALTH ALERT

Blood Pressure

BIOMETRIC PROFILE

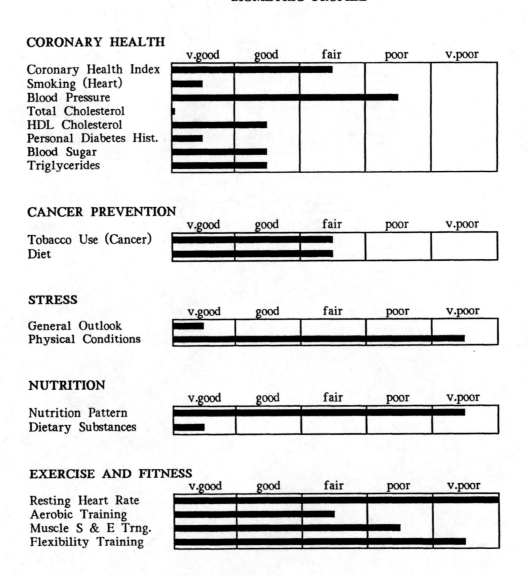

CORONARY HEALTH

	v.good	good	fair	poor	v.poor
Coronary Health Index					
Smoking (Heart)					
Blood Pressure					
Total Cholesterol					
HDL Cholesterol					
Personal Diabetes Hist.					
Blood Sugar					
Triglycerides					

CANCER PREVENTION

	v.good	good	fair	poor	v.poor
Tobacco Use (Cancer)					
Diet					

STRESS

	v.good	good	fair	poor	v.poor
General Outlook					
Physical Conditions					

NUTRITION

	v.good	good	fair	poor	v.poor
Nutrition Pattern					
Dietary Substances					

EXERCISE AND FITNESS

	v.good	good	fair	poor	v.poor
Resting Heart Rate					
Aerobic Training					
Muscle S & E Trng.					
Flexibility Training					

298

Counselor Evaluation System

PART 1 EVALUATING WHAT YOU SAY

A. Counselor's Verbatim Record of Responses. From an audio or video recording write out your responses verbatim including mmhmm's, uh-huh's, etc. Use as many sheets of paper as necessary. Number each response and catagorize it: mmhmm; reflective response; open question; closed question; why question; advice-giving; information-giving; self-disclosure, and other. Rate the responses as good or effective, neutral, negative or ineffective. Responses/ Category/Rating (+,0,-)

B. Counselor's Behavior

    1. Nonverbal Behavior: Summarize your notable nonverbal behaviors. What impact did your nonverbal behaviors have on the client? Be specific.

    2. Verbal Behavior

        a. Total number of responses made:_____

        b. Percentage in each category:

            Mmhmm_____   Advice-giving_____

            Reflective_____   Information-giving_____

            Open question_____   Self-disclosure_____

            Closed question_____   Why question_____

C. Self-assessment of Verbal Responses

    1. What responses could have been better phrased? Exactly how would you re-state them?

    2. Which responses could or should have been omitted? Why?

PART 2 UNDERSTANDING THE CLIENT

A. List the most important specific topics discussed by the client.

B. What feelings does the client have about each topic?

C. Describe how these topics are related to each other.

D. Describe how the topics relate to what you know about the client; in other words, connect the client to the problem.

E. Based on the information above, what is your understanding of the client's concern?

PART 3 GOAL SETTING GUIDE

A. Goal Identification

    1. Using the client's concern/problem identified above, describe it as a positive and specific goal that the client has expressed an interest in attaining.

        a. Is the goal described stated positively? Positively stated goals describe some action the client wants to take. He/she can create a picture in his/her mind of what it is he/she wants to have happen rather than something he/she doesn't want to have happen.

        b. Is this goal stated specifically? When a client makes a specifically stated goal he/she knows when it is attained. With general goals a client may have trouble knowing when he/she has reached it; they often use words like "good," "better," "more" or "less."

        c. Is the goal under the client's control? When a client selects a goal that requires the actions of someone else rather than the client, the client does not have control over whether the goal is attained. Setting goals such as "being successful," "winning" or "being happy" are really results, not goals. Goals are the actions a client can take to reach these results.

    2. Describe the dimensions of the goal:

        a. How long has the client wanted to achieve this goal?

        b. What, if anything, has the client tried to reach the goal?

        c. Describe the specific situation in which the client came closest to reaching the goal.

        d. Describe the specific situation in which the client felt farthest from the goal.

        e. Why is it important to the client to reach this goal now?

    3. Restate the goal, if necessary.

B. Determining Goal Importance

    1. What makes the goal important to the client? Is it more important to the client than to other people in the client's life?

    2. Is the goal something the client wants to accomplish or feels he/she should or ought to accomplish?

3. From your perspective, is it worthwhile for the client to achieve the goal? Why?

4. What does the client gain by reaching the goal?

5. What does the client gain by not reaching the goal?

6. How likely is it that the client can reach the goal?

C. Roadblocks to Goal Attainment: Why has the client been unable to reach the goal?

1. Is it lack of knowledge? If so, what knowledge is needed to reach the goal?

2. Is it lack of skills? If so, what does the client need to know how to do?

3. Is it the inability to take risks? If so, what would assist the client in overcoming the fear of taking the risk?

4. Is it a lack of social support? If so, what support does the client need and who can provide it?

PART 4 IF YOU COULD. . .

A. If you could do this session over again, given your understanding of the client's concerns/problems/ goals, how would you approach the session differently, if at all, and why? Be specific.

B. What issues would you like to explore with the client in a next session? How would you pursue this direction?

C. Things I will work on related to my counseling skills:

NUTRITION COUNSELING TREATMENT PLAN

Patient Name:_____

Date:_____

Objectives of Treatment:

1._____

2._____

3._____

4._____

Problematic Behaviors	*Target Strategy*	*Estimated Date of Meeting Goal*
1._____	_____	_____
_____	_____	_____
2._____	_____	_____
_____	_____	_____
3._____	_____	_____
_____	_____	_____
4._____	_____	_____
_____	_____	_____

_____   _____
Client's Signature   Dietitian's Signature

SELF MONITORING FORM

Time	Food	Amount	With Who	Activity	How Fast?	Mood

MOOD ADJECTIVE LIST

loving - friendly - thankful		**happy**	**hurt - frustrated**	
adaptable	affectionate	accepted	awful	bothered
agreeable	amorous	at ease	clumsy	crabby
caring	empathic	cheerful	sore	threatened
forgiving	generous	glad	harassed	imprisoned
genuine	giving	joyous	mistreated	perturbed
grateful	longing for	lighthearted	pressured	restless
mindful	optimistic	magnificent	rotten	sore
passionate	patient	peaceful	strained	swamped
sensitive	sincere	poised	terrible	threatened
tender	tolerant	refreshed	uneasy	unhappy
trustful	understanding	relaxed	unsatisfied	wounded

ashamed - guilty - embarrassed		**confused**	**sad - depressed - gloomy**	
awkward	blamed	baffled	disappointed	discouraged
cheapened	condemned	dismayed	falling apart	grief stricken
degraded	disgraced	disorganized	hopeless	let down
dishonored	doomed	distracted	mournful	pained
exposed	foolish	forgetful	pessimistic	sad
humiliated	punished	overwhelmed	serious	solemn
regretful	ridiculous	puzzled	sorrowful	tearful
shamed	silly	tricked	troubled	weary
		uncertain		

energetic		**worried**	**weak - defeated - shy**	
active	agile	alarmed	disheartened	helpless
alert	animated	anxious	impotent	inadequate
attentive	busy	concerned	incompetent	inferior
daring	diligent	disturbed	intimidated	insecure
eager	encouraged	fearful	needy	neglected
enthusiastic	excited	hesitant	powerless	self-conscious
hardworking	interested	nervous	stifled	timid
lively	resourceful	panicky	troubled	unable
self-confident	spirited	restless	unqualified	unstable
tireless	vital	unsettled	vulnerable	worthless

angry - aggravated		**content - comfortable**		**lonely - forgotten**	
agitated	annoyed	agreeable	bright	abandoned	betrayed
bitter	cranky	cheerful	easy going	empty	ignored
enraged	furious	gratified	pleased	isolated	rejected
infuriated	resentful	secure safe	supported	stranded	unimportant

PHYSICAL MOOD ADJECTIVE LIST

energetic - alert

active agile	alive	
animated	attentive	
capable	fresh	
lively	peppy	
powerful	quick	
rested	strong	
sturdy	tireless	
vivacious	wakeful	

lethargic - fatigued - sleepy

dazed	debilitated	disabled
drained	drowsy	exhausted
feeble	fragile	frazzled
inert	inactive	limp
listless	nodding	run down
sleepy	sluggish	tired
weary	worn	yawning
	unstable	

painful - hurt -sore

abrasion	ache
acute	bruised
chronic	crampy
discomfort	distress
inflamed	injured
piercing	stabbing
suffering	swelling
tender	wounded

well - healthy

comfortable	healing
fit	flexible
fresh	hearty
good	invigorated
refreshed	restful
robust	relaxed
stimulated	strong
tranquil	trim

restless - jumpy

agitated	fidgety
jittery	quiver
nervous	shaky
shiver	sleepless
spasmodic	tingling
trembling	twitching
unsettled	unsteady
unstable	wobbly

ill - sick

chills	diarrhea
dizzy	faint
feverish	flushed
infected	lousy
nauseated	queasy
unwell	vomit

hot

boiling
burning
heated
sweating
warm

cold

chilly
frigid
frozen
icy
numb

hungry

devouring
famished
gluttonous
insatiable
ravenous
starved
voracious

full

bloated
bursting
content
comfortable
gorged
satisfied
satiated

slender - thin

bony	emaciated
gaunt	lean
lanky	scrawny
skinny	slim

heavy - fat

chubby	flabby
fleshy	hefty
huge	massive
plump	portly
stout	weighty

STIMULUS CONTROL

Trigger	Strategy
1	a. b. c. d. e.
2	a. b. c. d. e.
3	a. b. c. d. e.
4	a. b. c. d. e.
5	a. b. c. d. e.

COGNITIVE
IRRATIONAL BELIEFS FORM

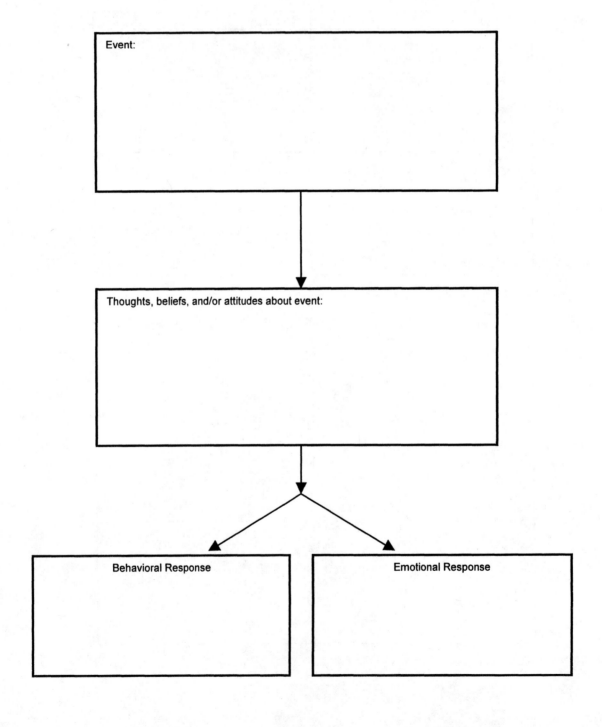

IRRATIONAL BELIEFS DAILY LOG

Event	Thoughts about Event	Emotional Response	Behavioral Response

MEDICAL NUTRITION THERAPY - INITIAL EVALUATION

Date: _____ Time: _____

Diagnosis: _____

Medical History: _____

Ht ____ in.   Admit Wt. ____ lbs.   BMI: ____ Wt. Eval/Hx: _____

Diet order: _____

Food allergies/intolerances: _____ □ NKA-foods

Oral/nutrition intake: □ >75%   □ 50-75%   □ 25-50%   □ <25%   _____

Religious/cultural/ethnic requests: _____

Trigger nutrient/drug interactions: _____

Alteration in nutritional status related to:

□ below acceptable body wt/BMI<19
□ above acceptable body wt/BMI>30
□ moderate/excess wt gain (_____)
□ moderate/severe wt loss (_____)
□ surgery/wound healing
□ impaired skin integrity (stage:_____)
□ multiple trauma
□ therapeutic diet during hospitalization
□ s/s disordered eating patterns

□ nausea/vomiting
□ poor dentition/problem chewing
□ inadequate nutrient intake
□ dysphagia/swallowing difficulty
□ feeding issues
□ constipation/diarrhea
□ infection
□ alcohol/drug abuse

□ knowledge deficit related to: _____
□ communication/learning barriers: _____
□ herbal/vitamin supplement intake: _____
□ altered nutritional labs: _____
□ other: _____
□ no significant nutrition risk factors noted at this time

Nutrition Plan of Care

□ current diet appropriate for diagnosis/condition
□ continue to provide routine medical nutrition therapy services
□ inappropriate for diet instruction/counseling due to:_____
□ see Physicians Orders for supplemental feedings/Communication Orders
□ see Patient Care Plan for individualized goals and medical nutrition therapy interventions
□ see Patient Education Record for counseling on:_____
□ see Interdisciplinary Patient Progress Notes for goals/progress toward goals
□ see Interdisciplinary Patient Progress Notes for recommendations
□ Estimated Needs: _____
_____

□ other: _____
□ other: _____

Dietetic Practitioner: _____

DISCHARGE SUMMARY FORM

Name_____   Discharge date_____

Hospital Number_____   Admission date_____

Age _____   Sex _____   Diagnosis_____

Anthropometrics: Ht._____   Wt.:_____   Admit Wt.:_____   DC Wt.:_____

            Usual Wt.:_____   Activity level_____

Laboratory: Albumin_____   Prealbumin_____   Date assessed_____

        Other:

Diet: Estimated needs   _____Kcal   _____gm protein

                         _____Kcal/ kg   _____gm/ kg

      Diet order:

      Nutritional supplements:

Pertinent medications:

Major nutritional problems: On-going

                                    Resolved

Interventions / Outcomes

Education / Expected progress

Recommendations

Continuum of care

Other team members advised?

HABIT INVENTORY

Put the corresponding number on the blank line next to the answer. Answer each of the questions based on your normal eating habits (not when you are trying to diet). For each question, answer "often," "sometimes," or "rarely." The answer has a number correspondent with it; put the number on the line and total the numbers.

Example: I consume bread at snacks and/or meals

	Often	2
___	Sometimes	1
___	Rarely	0
Total ___		

Starch Intake

1. I consume bread at snacks and/or meals

___	Often	2
___	Sometimes	1
___	Rarely	0

2. I consume starches at dinner like potatoes, rice, noodles, and corn, etc.

___	Often	2
___	Sometimes	1
___	Rarely	0

3. I snack on crackers, fruit, bread, pretzels, or cereal.

___	Often	2
___	Sometimes	1
___	Rarely	0

4. I eat more starch at dinner than I do the main entrée.

___	Often	2
___	Sometimes	1
___	Rarely	0

Total ___

Fat Intake

1. I eat proteins like beef, hamburgers, and red meat at lunch or dinner.

___	Often	2
___	Sometimes	1
___	Rarely	0

2. I snack on cheese, nuts, chips, peanut butter, candy bars, chocolate, and leftovers from dinner.

___	Often	2
___	Sometimes	1
___	Rarely	0

3. I consume fast foods like fries, onion rings, fried chicken, milkshakes, burritos, or hot dogs.

___	Often	2
___	Sometimes	1
___	Rarely	0

4. I use oils, margarine, butter, sauces, salad dressing on foods.

___	Often	2
___	Sometimes	1
___	Rarely	0

Total ___

Approach to Weight Loss

When trying to lose weight, I:

1. eliminate sweets, desserts and treats.

___ Often	2
___ Sometimes	1
___ Rarely	0

2. eliminate bread, rice, noodles, potatoes, and other starches.

___ Often	2
___ Sometimes	1
___ Rarely	0

3. include my favorite food.

___ Often	2
___ Sometimes	1
___ Rarely	0

4. choose high protein foods like meat, cheese, and poultry.

___ Often	2
___ Sometimes	1
___ Rarely	0

Total ___

Sugar and Alcohol Intake

1. I consume alcoholic beverages.

___ Often	2
___ Sometimes	1
___ Rarely	0

2. I drink Coke, lemonade, or other soda-type drinks.

___ Often	2
___ Sometimes	1
___ Rarely	0

3. I consume fruit packed in syrup or pancake syrup.

___ Often	2
___ Sometimes	1
___ Rarely	0

4. I consume sweets like donuts, pies, and hard candy.

___ Often	2
___ Sometimes	1
___ Rarely	0

Total ___

Eating When Not Hungry

1. I eat when I am bored.

___ Often	2
___ Sometimes	1
___ Rarely	0

2. I eat when I am under stress.

___ Often	2
___ Sometimes	1
___ Rarely	0

3. I eat when I am depressed or unhappy.

___ Often	2
___ Sometimes	1
___ Rarely	0

4. I eat when I am tired.

___ Often	2
___ Sometimes	1
___ Rarely	0

Total ___

Assertiveness as it Relates to Eating

1. I eat when people offer food.

    ___ Often   2
    ___ Sometimes   1
    ___ Rarely   0

2. I find it difficult to say no when people push food on me.

    ___ Often   2
    ___ Sometimes   1
    ___ Rarely   0

3. I speak up to family, friends, and co-workers about my feelings.

    ___ Often   2
    ___ Sometimes   1
    ___ Rarely   0

4. I have difficulty asking for help.

    ___ Often   2
    ___ Sometimes   1
    ___ Rarely   0

Total ___

Motivation for Losing Weight

1. I want to lose weight for myself.

    ___ Often   2
    ___ Sometimes   1
    ___ Rarely   0

2. I want to lose weight because my family, friends, or physician think it's important.

    ___ Often   2
    ___ Sometimes   1
    ___ Rarely   0

3. My family, friends, and/or physician have stronger feelings than I to lose weight.

    ___ Often   2
    ___ Sometimes   1
    ___ Rarely   0

4. I want to lose weight because I am concerned about my health..

    ___ Often   2
    ___ Sometimes   1
    ___ Rarely   0

Total ___

My Attitudes Towards Losing Weight

1. I feel my friends or relatives eat more than I do to maintain or lose weight.

    ___ Often   2
    ___ Sometimes   1
    ___ Rarely   0

2. I resent the fact that my friends or relatives can eat more than I do to maintain or lose weight.

    ___ Often   2
    ___ Sometimes   1
    ___ Rarely   0

3. I find the resentment prevents me from helping myself lose weight.

    ___ Often   2
    ___ Sometimes   1
    ___ Rarely   0

4. I resent not being able to eat anything or at anytime.

    ___ Often   2
    ___ Sometimes   1
    ___ Rarely   0

Total ___

Activity Levels

1. I have a regular exercise program.

    ___ Often   2
    ___ Sometimes   1
    ___ Rarely   0

2. I spend my days sitting down.

    ___ Often   2
    ___ Sometimes   1
    ___ Rarely   0

3. I spend my evenings sitting down.

    ___ Often   2
    ___ Sometimes   1
    ___ Rarely   0

4. I sit around on weekends or my days off.

    ___ Often   2
    ___ Sometimes   1
    ___ Rarely   0

Total ___

Attitudes Towards Exercise

1. I find exercise boring.

    ___ Often   2
    ___ Sometimes   1
    ___ Rarely   0

2. I feel I have no energy to exercise.

    ___ Often   2
    ___ Sometimes   1
    ___ Rarely   0

3. I do not feel I have time to exercise.

    ___ Often   2
    ___ Sometimes   1
    ___ Rarely   0

4. I feel that exercise does not help me lose weight..

    ___ Often   2
    ___ Sometimes   1
    ___ Rarely   0

Total ___

Organization Goals

1. I set specific goals and objectives for myself on a regular basis (i.e. weekly, monthly, yearly).

    ___ Often   2
    ___ Sometimes   1
    ___ Rarely   0

2. I feel that I have a variety of work, interests, and hobbies.

    ___ Often   2
    ___ Sometimes   1
    ___ Rarely   0

3. I organize my time to do my favorite activities (e.g. shopping, sports, social activities, reading).

    ___ Often   2
    ___ Sometimes   1
    ___ Rarely   0

4. I organize my time to spend the least amount of time to do chores and tasks that I consider unpleasant.

    ___ Often   2
    ___ Sometimes   1
    ___ Rarely   0

Total ___

313

Eating Style

1. I eat slowly and take small bites of food.

   ___ Often   2
   ___ Sometimes   1
   ___ Rarely   0

2. I sit down when I eat snacks and meals.

   ___ Often   2
   ___ Sometimes   1
   ___ Rarely   0

3. I set the table with utensils, plate, napkin and beverage when I eat snacks and meals.

   ___ Often   2
   ___ Sometimes   1
   ___ Rarely   0

4. I usually watch TV, read books, magazines or newspapers or do something else while eating.

   ___ Often   2
   ___ Sometimes   1
   ___ Rarely   0

          Total   ___

Salt

1. I consume cured meats like bacon, salami, ham or cheese.

   ___ Often   2
   ___ Sometimes   1
   ___ Rarely   0

2. I snack on chips, salted crackers, pretzels, or salted peanuts.

   ___ Often   2
   ___ Sometimes   1
   ___ Rarely   0

3. I consume fast foods like pizza, cheeseburgers, fried chicken, fries, onion rings, frozen items like TV dinners, prepared entrees; canned items like vegetables, tomato sauce, spaghetti, etc.

   ___ Often   2
   ___ Sometimes   1
   ___ Rarely   0

4. I use the following: salt shaker, onion or garlic salt, barbecue sauce, teriyaki sauce, salad dressing and meat tenderizer.

   ___ Often   2
   ___ Sometimes   1
   ___ Rarely   0

          Total   ___

Caffeine Intake

1. I consume diet sodas or soft drinks.

   ___ Often   2
   ___ Sometimes   1
   ___ Rarely   0

2. I consume regular coffee or iced coffees.

   ___ Often   2
   ___ Sometimes   1
   ___ Rarely   0

3. I consume tea or iced tea.

   ___ Often   2
   ___ Sometimes   1
   ___ Rarely   0

4. I consume chocolate drinks, chocolate candy, chocolate cake or cookies.

   ___ Often   2
   ___ Sometimes   1
   ___ Rarely   0

          Total   ___

314

Meal Frequency

1. I skip breakfast or lunch to save calories.

___ Often   2
___ Sometimes   1
___ Rarely   0

2. I become so hungry sometimes that it results in overeating.

___ Often   2
___ Sometimes   1
___ Rarely   0

3. I keep nibbling on food.

___ Often   2
___ Sometimes   1
___ Rarely   0

4. I snack while preparing food.

___ Often   2
___ Sometimes   1
___ Rarely   0

Total ___

Quantity

1. I have second helpings of food.

___ Often   2
___ Sometimes   1
___ Rarely   0

2. I eat a lot when I snack.

___ Often   2
___ Sometimes   1
___ Rarely   0

3. I have large portions of food.

___ Often   2
___ Sometimes   1
___ Rarely   0

4. I There are times that I knew I could not get by with eating less.

___ Often   2
___ Sometimes   1
___ Rarely   0

Total ___

Sensitivity to Hunger and Satiety

1. I find myself eating because it is "lunch time" or "dinner time".

___ Often   2
___ Sometimes   1
___ Rarely   0

2. I eat when I am not hungry.

___ Often   2
___ Sometimes   1
___ Rarely   0

3. I find myself eating when I am stuffed.

___ Often   2
___ Sometimes   1
___ Rarely   0

4. I notice that I eat until I am just satisfied.

___ Often   2
___ Sometimes   1
___ Rarely   0

Total ___

Gross Obesity: from a Recovered Patient's Perspective

Bob Wilson, BS, DTR, Weight Counselor, Kaiser Permanente and Private Wellness Practice, Portland, OR
(Adapted from his presentations to obese clients about his experiences and successful program)

ROOTS PARABLE

From our earliest experiences after birth, we are conditioned to have certain thoughts, attitudes, emotional response patterns and learned coping behaviors. These conditioned responses form our inner unconscious "computer program" from which we create our lives and evaluate input from our environment.

Getting to the "root" causes of a specific behavior pattern or symptom (for example, being overweight) is quite a challenge. Frequently, there are many "tangled roots" that are all knotted together. You can cover up the problem by keeping the tops trimmed and neat so other people are not aware that such deep roots and problems exist. It may take many years and lots of soul-searching hard work to get to and change root causes of problems. Examples of common root problems include the need to please everyone else in order to feel self-worth (being yourself isn't enough), feeling shame or low self-esteem (which may stem from comments someone once made to you), or experiencing relationship, drug, or alcohol addiction. To change, you must learn to become a "healthy caretaker" to your inner emotional self. You must learn how to nurture yourself.

To begin the process of taking care of yourself, it is important to evaluate the relationships in your life: family, work, friends, material things, your feelings about yourself, and see how these things effect your relationship with food. Seek support from a nutrition therapist, mental health counselor, or support group like the 12-step program, which provides terrific support in the evaluation process. If you are depressed, having difficulty relating to people, or feel manipulated and unable to cope, psychotherapy can be invaluable.

I found that as I honestly looked into each of these areas and made plans to change each area of imbalance, my relationship with food became healthier and healthier. My relationship with myself also improved. I've come from a space of total self-hatred and disgust with myself, to a place of being a loving compassionate friend to me! I've come to accept me for who I am and who I am not. I've let the child in me have fun again. It has been a very gradual process as I've pruned and nurtured my roots as I untangled them and released their influence on my life.

MY BACKGROUND

I weighed somewhere between 320-400 pounds in the eighth grade. There were cruel jokes and mockery of my body size and me. I believed them all. I came from what would be called a dysfunctional family with multiple addictions. I was a lover, not a fighter. I wanted everyone to be happy, so I tried to take care of everyone's needs. I thought that would make me a "good person."

Food was my outlet for stress and coping. I followed the "see-food diet." Whenever I saw food, I ate! I ate lots of fast foods, convenience foods, huge portions, lots of candy, pastries, ice cream and sweets. I never preplanned any meals or snacks. My exercise was watching TV and playing the stereo.

> **I did not associate food with my problems; it was my friend and the only comfort I had in life.**

Psychologically, I hated and loathed myself. I believed I was worth nothing.

Finally, in 1972 when I was 21 years old, I decided I was tired of being fat and out of control. I wanted to make a permanent change in my life. I accomplished it through the support of Weight Watchers, a 12-step program, psychotherapy, and extensive reading, gut-wrenching soul searching and work on my part. I lost over 200 pounds, which I have maintained at about 153 pounds for over 30 years.

I discovered that weight management requires developing a comprehensive set of life skills that perhaps others learn as they grow up, but they were new to me. Even today, I find it is difficult to be healthy in our culture because of the availability of high calorie foods. It requires thought and planning to maintain my present weight.

What Worked For Me

Following is a listing of what has made my weight loss permanent. It helps to know the crucial pieces that fit to make a person whole and healthy when he or she comes from a background and weight as mine. Of course, everyone is an individual, but this is a frame of reference.

- Basic nutrition for my needs and where to get it; I had to learn how to feed myself "right."
- How to cut back on calories and fat, yet still have enough volume of food and calories to feel mentally and physically satisfied.
- I learned to plan menus, shop for healthier foods, and the art of simple cooking with tasty substitutes for many of my favorite foods.
- How to get rid of temptations in my home and work environment to help me out, rather than hinder me; I wasn't *that* strong, especially when I was stressed.
- Self-management and new ways of problem-solving; I couldn't rely on "will power." I had to make major changes in how I handled life and its choices.
- Keeping food records so I could practice problem-solving and benefit from each experience; plus the records reminded me how well I had done in the past.
- To become a compassionate observer of my lifestyle patterns, and acknowledge which ones worked and those that didn't; I learned to evaluate without flogging myself with guilt.
- To discover "healthy movement" or exercise; I found ways to make it enjoyable and at an appropriate level for my abilities at the time.
- How to set up a support network that provides encouragement and constructive feedback instead of the negative reinforcement of my youth.
- Patience. Patience. Patience. Practice. Practice. Persistence. The process of change goes *much slower* than I wanted it to go; I had to give it time.
- And finally, the most difficult thing to learn and change was my relationship with myself. Initially, the tone of my relationship was one of self-disgust and disrespect. To change my self-image required extensive work as mentioned earlier.

Today, I love myself and take very good care of me. I apply developmental and life skills. I find ways to nurture myself like gardening, hiking, entertaining friends, and so on. I learned to set boundaries and limit my care taking of others, which caused me some guilt. But I had to realize that I was not responsible for other adults in my life, just me. I learned to separate their needs and problems from my own. I channeled my energy into more constructive relationships and ventures.

My Approach As A Weight Loss Counselor

From the depth of my personal transformation, I share practical, positive, and permanent solutions with all my clients. I use an eclectic approach--many parts of this and that: humor, positive feedback and encouragement, role playing, visual aids, relaxation, self-nurturing techniques, nutrition concepts, menu planning, food tasting and more. Whatever the client and I think will work for his or her particular situation. I see myself as a trainer and guide.

I try to convey to my clients an overall way of viewing and relating to themselves--one which focuses on compassion rather than contempt. I learned another approach from Stephen Schwartz in *The Compassionate Presence.* (2)

To step beyond the examination of patterns, we must begin to notice the tone of our relationship to ourselves. We begin to notice the feeling tone in which we approach our own lives. Every experience that we meet is a proposition. "Which way am I going to experience it? Which way am I going to greet it?" All of this has to do with the tone of our relationship to ourself. "How do I greet myself each day? Am I afraid of this being? Do I belittle this being? Do I call it names? Do I wish it were some other way? Do I have plans for it that involve manipulation and control? Do I motivate myself out of punishment, fear, and rewards by belittling myself? Or is my motivation an impulse of respect that comes from the depth of my heart..."

We each create our lives differently, so just watch and observe the results of the way YOU do it. Learn the skill of compassionate observation. Become more aware of how your body, mind, and emotions respond to the way YOU CHOOSE to create your life. Do your choices bring you towards greater peace and harmony? Balance? Health? Or toward dis-ease? Just notice. (See handout: "82 Ideas for Self-Nurturing Activities")

I mention to my clients that, "If you continue to do what you've always done, you'll continue to get what you've always gotten!" This is why so many people are unsuccessful. They don't realize they can't continue to do the same thing and get different results. If you want different results, then you must be willing to do something different!

Permanent weight management requires lifestyle adjustment:

If you keep the same commitments,
the same relationships,
the same thought patterns,
the same food,
the same ways of nurturing yourself,
you'll get the same RESULTS!

The key to simplifying your life is to S...L...O...W... it down.

1. **Observe** what you do. Use recordkeeping and mental awareness.
2. **Evaluate** what you are presently doing (or not doing) and how it contributes to overweight, peace of mind, compulsive patterns, etc.
3. **Make Plans** and alter your present actions. Plan different actions and DO them! Make changes "big enough to matter, but small enough to achieve." (3) From what you learn about yourself, modify your plans.
4. **Practice New Actions.** Practice doesn't make "perfection," it makes "permanent."

> **Don't just try harder or push harder trying to out run your human limitations. What your life might be need is *pruning*.**

A major obstacle to success is being over-busy, over commitment to others and under commitment to your self (codependency). The result? No time or energy to care for yourself. I mention to clients "don't just try harder or push harder trying to out run your human limitations. What your life might be need is *pruning*."

It's essential to discover when helping you is hurting me. Notice when your commitments push you out of your zone of being healthy. Not just occasionally, but on a chronic basis. There is an excellent book and workbook by Carmen Berry that deals with this topic, *When Helping You Is Hurting Me: Escaping the Messiah Trap*. (4)

I know that each of us is committed to many very important relationships and "things" in our lives. Even too much of really good things...is...still...too much! *Balance in life is achieved by pruning commitments.*

The whole focus of my counseling is on self-empowerment. Empowerment is defined as "a process by which people gain mastery over their affairs. In this model, patients are seen as experts on their own lives...The role of the patient is to be well-informed, equal, and active partner in the treatment program." (1)

References
1. Funnell M, Anderson R, Arnold M. Empowerment A Winning Model for Diabetes Care. *Practical Diabetology*. May/June 1991; 15-18.
2. Schwartz S. *The Compassionate Presence*. Piermont, NY: River Run Press; 1988.
3. Kaiser Permanente weight loss program, Freedom From Fat.
4. Berry CR. *When Helping You Is Hurting Me: Escaping the Messiah Trap*. New York: Harper & Row; 2003.

Other Helpful Books

Hay, Louise L. *You Can Heal Your Life*. Santa Monica, CA: Hay House; 1999.
Helmstetter, Shad. *What to Say When You Talk to Yourself*. New York: Pocket Books; 1990.
Hendricks, Gay. *Learning to Love Yourself*. New York: Prentice-Hall Press; 1987.
Hollis, Judy. *Fat Is A Family Affair*. San Francisco, CA: Hazelton Foundation; 1996.
Munter, Carol and Hirschmann, Jane. *Overcoming Overeating*. New York: Ballantine Books; 1988.
Roth, Geneen. *Breaking Free From Compulsive Eating*. Riverside, NJ: Bobbs-Merrill Co/ McMillin; 2002.

82 Ideas For Self-Nurturing Activities

Listen to favorite music
Enjoy a long, warm bubble bath
Go for a walk
Share a hug with a loved one
Relax outside
Physical activity (of my choice)
Say or read a spiritual prayer
Attend a caring support group
Practice deep breathing
Do stretching exercises
Reflect on positive qualities "I am..."
Write my thoughts and feelings in a
    personal journal
Laugh
Concentrate on a relaxing scene
Create a collage representing the "real me"
Receive a massage
Reflect on "I appreciate..."
Watch the sunrise or sunset
Attend a favorite athletic event
Do something adventurous
Read a special book or magazine
Sing, hum, whistle a happy tune
Go dancing
Play a musical instrument
Meditate
Garden and work with plants
Learn a new skill
See a special play, movie or concert
Work out with weights or small hand weights
Ride a bicycle
Make myself a nutritious meal
Draw or paint a picture
Swim and relax at the beach or pool
Do aerobics to neat music
Visit a special place I enjoy
Smile and say "I love myself"
Take time to smell the flowers
Go horseback riding
Sit in front of a fireplace and watch the fire
Read a cartoon or joke book
Listen to my favorite kind of music
Reflect on "My most enjoyable memories"

Enjoy a relaxing nap
Visit a museum or art gallery
Practice yoga
Relax in a whirlpool or sauna
Enjoy a cool, refreshing glass of water
Count my blessings "I am thankful for.."
Enjoy the beauty of nature
Play as I did as a child
Star gaze
Window shop
Daydream
Tell myself the loving words I want to
    hear from others
Attend a special workshop
Go sailing or paddleboating
Reward myself with a gift I can afford
Take myself on vacation
Create with clay or pottery
Practice positive affirmations
Pet an animal
Watch my favorite TV show
Reflect on my successes "I can..."
Write a poem
Make a bouquet of flowers
Watch the clouds
Make myself something nice
Visit a park, woods, forest
Call an old friend
Read positive, motivational literature
Reflect on "What I value most in life."
Go on a picnic in a beautiful setting
Enjoy a cup of herbal tea/ decaf coffee
Participate in a favorite card game
Practice relaxation exercises
Practice the art of forgiveness
Treat myself to a nutritious meal at a
    favorite restaurant
Enjoy a my favorite hobby
Walk in the warm rain
Watch snowflakes fall or rain drops
Put out wild bird seed and watch the
    birds
Create my own list of self-nurturing activities

by Bob Wilson, DTR

319

ANOREXIA / BULIMIA NERVOSA
Expected Outcomes from Medical Nutrition Therapy

Optimal Nutrition   Consumption of adequate amounts and types of fat, protein, carbohydrate, fiber, sodium, and micronutrients

KCaloric Intake   Adequate intake of kcalories for reasonable body weight

Weight   Maintenance of reasonable body weight:

If weight gain desired: 1 to 2 pounds weekly, based on goals
If weight loss desired: 1 to 2 pounds weekly, based on goals

BIOCHEMICAL INDICES OF NUTRITION DEPLETION

Optimal Outcomes: Normal blood levels* of the following nutritional depletion indices
(ADA Manual of Clinical Dietetics)
> Hemoglobin
> Hematocrit
> Total Iron-Binding Capacity
> Serum Albumin
> Total Lymphocyte Count
> Transferrin
> Creatinine Height Index
> Electrolytes

* Laboratory values may vary from one laboratory to another. Check to see what is considered the normal ranges at laboratory used by client.

ANTHROPOMETRIC MEASUREMENTS

Outcomes:	Optimum	Acceptable
Tri-ceps Skinfold (TSF)	> 15th percentile	≥ 5th percentile
Midarm Circumference (MAC)	> 15th percentile	≥ 5th percentile
Midarm Muscle Circumference (MAMC)	> 15th percentile	≥ 5th percentile
Midarm Fat Area (MAFA)	> 15th percentile	≥ 5th percentile

Below 5th percentile may be considered malnourished
Between 5th and 15th percentile may be at risk for malnutrition (Zeman, 1991)

SKILL LEVELS ATTAINED BY CLIENT   Identifies basic nutrition principles and how they relate to eating disorders
Adheres to acceptable nutritional intake 75% or more of the time
Selects and consumes an acceptable variety of foods
Makes appropriate food selections from restaurant menus
Adheres to regular exercise schedule 75% or more of the time
Identifies inappropiate food behaviors utilized

NUTRITION RELATED COMPLICATIONS   Such complications prevented, delayed or treated

QUALITY OF LIFE   Improvement of overall health and quality of life

SATISFACTION WITH SERVICES OF DIETITIAN   Dietitian's services rated by client as 3.0 or higher on a rating instrument with a 5.0 for highest degree of satisfaction

MEDICAL CONSEQUENCES OF ANOREXIA NERVOSA (13,14,15)

Cardiovascular Changes
- heart muscle shrinking
- bradycardia (pulse less than 60)
- irregular heart beat; hypotension (systolic under 90 mm/Hg)
- electrolyte imbalance
- congestive heart failure

Hematologic Changes:
- mild anemia,
- leukopenia,
- thrombocytopenia

Endocrine Changes:
- amenorrhea: the cessation of menstruation
- hypothyroid
- hypercortisolism and increased CRH (cortical releasing hormone)
- hypoestrogenemia and decreased FSH (follicle stimulating hormone) and LH (leutinizing hormone)
- ovarian cysts

Renal Function Changes:
- elevated BUN (Blood Urea Nitrogen)
- dehydration
- kidney stones
- kidney failure

Lanugo hair: Fine body hair can develop on the body, often seen on the arms and face.
Muscle Atrophy: Skeletal muscle loss
Brain Changes: Changes of gray/white matter on MRI (16)
Metabolic Abnormalities
- hypercholesterolemia
- hypercarotenemia
- low plasma zinc

Gastric Problems:
- delayed gastric emptying
- bowel irritation
- constipation

Osteoporosis: due to low weight, low calcium, amenorrhea (occurs even when supplemented with birth control pills)
Dental Problems: if purging, stomach acid in vomit can erode tooth enamel
- throat/esophagus/stomach: if vomiting, irritation and tears in the lining

Laxative dependence: If purging, laxative abuse can result in the inability to have normal bowel movements
Emetic Toxicity: abuse of emetics such as Ipecac can lead to toxicity, heart failure and death
Swollen Glands: vomiting results in the swelling of the glands around the neck and face
Peripheral edema: particularly when purging and with refeeding

ANOREXIA / BULIMIA NERVOSA
MEDICAL NUTRITION THERAPY OUTCOMES REPORT

INTERVENTION DATA / GOAL ACHIEVEMENT

ASSESSMENT FACTORS	GOALS	INITIAL VISIT Date:	4 WEEKS Date:	8 WEEKS Date:	12 WEEKS Date:	16 WEEKS Date:
Optimal Nutrition						
Kcaloric Intake						
Weight						
Tri-cepSkinfold						
Midarm Circum						
MAMC						
Midarm Fat						
HGB / HCT						
Total Iron Bind						
Serum Albumin						
TLC						
Transferrin						
Creatinine / Ht						
Electrolytes						
Client Rated Quality of Life Scale 1 - 10 (10 = highest)						

NUTRITION RELATED COMPLICATIONS PREVENTED, DELAYED, OR TREATED

Prevent Hospitalization						

SKILL LEVELS ATTAINED　　　　　　　　　　　　　　　　　　　　　　　　**DATE ATTAINED**

Identifies basic nutrition principles and how they relate to eating disorders.　　　_____

Adheres to acceptable nutritional intake 75% or more of the time.　　　　　　_____

Selects and consumes an acceptable variety of foods.　　　　　　　　　　　_____

Makes appropriate food selections from restaurant menus.　　　　　　　　　_____

Adheres to regular exercise schedule 75% or more of the time.　　　　　　　_____

Identifies inappropriate food behaviors utilized.　　　　　　　　　　　　　_____

CLIENT SATISFACTION RATING　　　Scale 1(lowest) -5 (highest) _____　　Date Evaluated _____
COST EFFECTIVENESS　　　(RD to base cost effectiveness on individual measures such as medication reduction, prevention of complications requiring hospitalization, etc.)

Used by permission.

PROTOCOL FLOW CHART OF MNT FOR ANOREXIA / BULIMIA NERVOSA

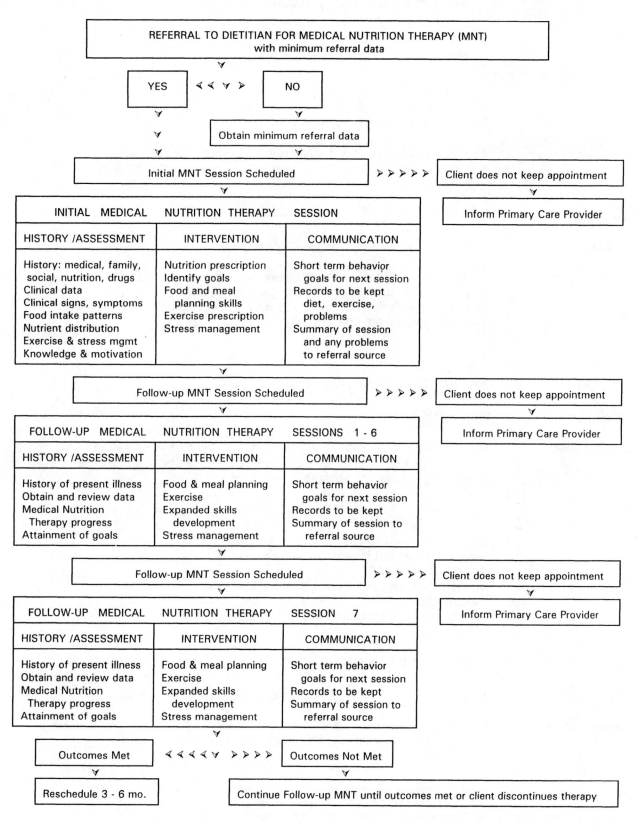

Used by permission.

ANOREXIA/BULIMIA NERVOSA
Drug/Nutrient Interactions

ANTIANXIETY AGENTS

Examples: Ativan, Buspar, Dulmane, Diazepam, Halcon, Librium, Lorazepam, Restoril, Serex, Triazolam, Valium, Xanax

Drug/ Nutrient   Avoid alcohol. Limit caffeine. Take with food. May cause drowsiness, anorexia, constipation, diarrhea, dry mouth, increase or decrease in weight. Adequate fluid intake needed.

ANTIDEPRESSANTS

Examples: Elavil, Pamelor, Prozac, Sinequan, Triavil, Zoloft

Drug/Nutrient   Avoid alcohol. Increases sun sensitivity, use sunscreen. Take with food. May cause dry mouth, weight loss or gain, diarrhea, taste changes, weakness, headache, insomnia, and anxiety. Fluoxetine products may seriously increase the effect of the drug.

ANTIDEPRESSANTS - MONAMINE OXIDASE INHIBITORS

Examples   Marplan, Nardil, Parnate

Drug/Nutrient   Avoid tyramine containing foods. Avoid alcohol. Avoid St. John's Wort. Limit caffeine. May cause dry mouth, constipation, insomnia, and weight increase from increased appetite.

LITHIUM AGENTS

Examples: Eskalith, Lithonate, Lithobid

Drug/Nutrient   Maintain balanced diet. Take with meal. May cause sodium depletion and weight gain. Drink 2-3 L fluid/day. Avoid iodine supplements. Limit caffeine. Needs consistent sodium level to stabilize drug level.

SELECTIVE SEROTONIN REUPTAKE INHIBITORS- SSRIs

Examples: Traodone, Fluroamine, Sertraline, Fluoxetine, Paroxetine (Paxil)

Drug/Nutrient   Avoid alcohol. May cause dry mouth, constipation, nausea, flatulence, and increased or decreased appetite. Adequate fluids and fiber needed.

Appendix 17-E
From: *Winning the War Within*

Mean Measurements During the Refeeding Protocol

Measurement *	Phase 1 (1,200 kcal/day)	Phase 2 (+300 kcal/d)	Phase 3 (3,600 kcal/day)	Phase 4 (Maintenance)
Number of patients	10	10	10	6
Weight (kg)	39.1 +4.1	42.4+5.3	45.6 ± 3.5	51.4+2.5
Body water (%)	70.0+5.0	72+5.0	68.0+4.0	64.0+4.0
Respiratory Quotient **	0.94+0.20	1.12+0.31	1.19+0.23	1.04 ±0.16
REE per 24 hr (kcal)	1,166+210	1,409+351	1,769 + 363	1,738 ± 149
REE/ kg body weight (kcal)***	30.0+6.4	33.5+6.7	37.3 ± 6.6	34.5 ± 4.4

*   Data for Phases 1-3 are for 10 patients; data for Phase 4 are for 6 patients who completed the weight stabilization phase.
**   Mean figures for phase refeeding; measurements were obtained daily.
*** Mean values, but calculated 3 times per week.

Nutritional Handbook for HIV/AIDS - 3rd Edition (Professional Page)

Nutritional Assessment Form

Patient Stamp/ID here

Name_____Sex_____Age_____

HIV Status (circle one): + or - Stage (circle one): Asymptomatic Early Middle Late
When diagnosed HIV+? _____ Admitting illness/conditions: _____
_____

Any concurrent illness, opportunistic conditions? (note these - include any infection, draining wounds, esophageal lesions, oral lesions) _____

Lipodystrophy present or evident? _____
_____

Wasting present? (defined as 5% decrease in ubw over 4-6 months or <95% of ibw or BMI)_____
_____
_____

Ht.(in)_____ Frame Size: (circle one) S M L Present wt. (lb):_____
Ideal wt. _____ Usual wt. _____

Wt. History if available: 1 yr ago: _____ 6 mo ago: _____ 1 mo ago: _____
BMI (kg/m squared) = _____

Triceps Skinfold: (TSF)mm   Mid-Arm Cir (MAC)   Mid-Arm Muscle Cir (MAMC)cm2
        Date: _____   _____   _____
        Date: _____   _____   _____

BIA Results: 1) BCM (kg)_____ 2) ECM (kg)_____ 3) TBF (kg)_____
Malabsorption Tests?_____ Results?_____
_____

HIV Medications: _____
Notes, dosing schedule: _____
_____

Other Medications: _____

Vitamin and Mineral supplements (Note if prescribed or patient's choice) _____
_____

Oral Liquid Nutritional Supplements _____
Other OTC supplements, herbal, etc: _____

Diet (Type and consistency, any prescribed restrictions) _____
Nourishments: _____
Enteral: _____
Parenteral (PPN or TPN): _____
_____

Support services involved in care (OT, PT, Social Services, others) _____
_____

Nutritional Assessment Data Tracking Form

DATE:					
Current wt. (lb)					
% UBW (See Appendix B to calc)					
% IBW (See Appendix B to calc)					
Wt.↓ in past Week? (Y or N)					
Wt.↑ in past week? (Y or N)					
Febrile? (Y or N)					
Albumin g/dL					
Prealbumin					
Transferrin mg/dL					
TIBC μg/dL					
Transf = (0.8 X TIBC) - 43					
Hgb. g/dL					
Hct. %					
Urinary Creatinine mg					
CHI*					
24 hour UUN (g)					
Nitrogen Balance NB = Protein $\frac{\text{Intake} - (\text{UUN}+4)}{6.25}$					
Glucose mg/dL					
HbA1c%					
CD4 cells/cubic mm					
Triglycerides mg/dL					
Cholesterol mg/dL					
HIV RNA/ml					
Testosterone					
Other:					

Diet History Check List

Yes No N/A

☐ ☐ ☐ Diarrhea? Type, duration, and/or probable cause _____

☐ ☐ ☐ Prescribed treatment for diarrhea? If yes, meds, diet, other? _____

☐ ☐ ☐ Nausea/Vomiting? (circle if applies) Worse with eating? Ongoing? Meds related?

☐ ☐ ☐ Prescribed treatment (diet or meds) for nausea, vomiting? Type_____

☐ ☐ ☐ Food Allergies? If yes, describe: _____

☐ ☐ ☐ Dysphagia? Taste changes?_____

☐ ☐ ☐ Dental Caries? Severity:_____

☐ ☐ ☐ Special dietary concerns, practices, needs? Describe: _____

☐ ☐ ☐ Appetite changes? (circle one) Increase or Decrease

☐ ☐ ☐ Fatigue? If yes, describe:_____

☐ ☐ ☐ Knowledgeable, interested in nutrition?_____

☐ ☐ ☐ Adequate food supplies? If no, make note to include in teaching plan for patient, family, caregivers.

☐ ☐ ☐ Alcohol? If yes, note type and frequency:_____

☐ ☐ ☐ Coffee, tea, colas, OTC medications with caffeine? Specify: _____

☐ ☐ ☐ Number of meals eaten away from home? _____ Type of meals, place? _____

☐ ☐ ☐ Aware of safe eating practices away from home? If no, make note to include in teaching plan for patient, family, caregivers.

☐ ☐ ☐ Receiving meals on wheels, other food program? Specify: _____

☐ ☐ ☐ Belongs to support group organization(s) _____

☐ ☐ ☐ Alternative therapies? Describe:_____
_____

☐ ☐ ☐ Monitors blood glucose? If yes, (circle if applies) diabetic? hyperglycemia? On Protease Inhibitors? On diabetic diet? Specify:_____

Typical foods for Morning:

Typical foods in Afternoon:

Usual number of meals: _____ Number and type of snacks:

Usual diet likely to meet 100% RDA for nutrients, calories, protein? Yes or No

Probable dietary shortfalls if any:

Describe usual activities, exercise (e.g. aerobic, endurance, muscle-enhancing, etc.)

Patient's perception of health:

To order up-to-date copies of this Superbill in quantity, please contact the Pennsylvania Dietetic Association at www.eatrightPA.org.

Sample Superbill

MEDICAL NUTRITION THERAPY STATEMENT

SUBSCRIBER'S NAME _____ DATE _____ __

PATIENT'S NAME _____ PATIENT'S DATE OF BIRTH _____ __

ADDRESS _____ __

INSURANCE CO. _____ POLICY NO. _____ GROUP NO. _____ __

ICD-9 Codes

☐ 783.1	Abnormal Weight Gain	☐ 722.6	Deg. Disc Disease	☐ 558.9	Gastroenteritis	☐ 627.2	Menopausal Syndrome
☐ 783.2	Abnormal Weight Loss	☐ 715.90	Deg. Joint Disease	☐ 530.81	Gastroesophageal Reflux	☐ 412	Myocardial Infection
☐ 285.9	Anemia, Unspecified	☐ 648.8	Diabetes, Gestational	☐ 271.3	Glucose Intolerance	☐ 278.0	Obesity
☐ 307.1	Anorexia Nervosa	☐ 250.01	Diabetes, Type 1	☐ 579.0	Gluten Sensitive Enteropathy	☐ 733.00	Osteoporosis
☐ 716.90	Arthritis	☐ 250.00	Diabetes, Type 2	☐ 274.9	Gout	☐ 332.0	Parkinsonism
☐ 493.90	Asthma	☐ 648.0	Diabetes with Pregnancy	☐ 042.0	HIV Infection	☐ 533.0	Peptic Ulcer Disease
☐ 414.0	Arteriosclerotic Heart	☐ 250.4	Diabetic Nephropathy		w/ Specified Infections	☐ 270.1	PKU
	Disorder (ASHD)	☐ 558.9	Diarrhea	☐ 272.2	Hyperlipidemia	☐ 564.2	Post Gastrectomy Syndrome
☐ 564.1	Bowel, Irritable Syndrome	☐ 562.11	Diverticulitis	☐ 401.9	Hypertension, Essential	☐ V22.2	Pregnancy, Normal
☐ 307.51	Bulimia	☐ 562.10	Diverticulosis	☐ 242.9	Hyperthyroidism	☐ 593.9	Renal Disease
☐ 574.20	Cholelithiasis	☐ 787.2	Dysphagia	☐ 251.2	Hypoglycemia	☐ 780.5	Sleep Apnea
☐ 585	Chronic Renal Failure	☐ 307.5	Eating Disorder, Unspecified	☐ 244.9	Hypothyroidism	☐ 556.9	Ulcerative Colitis
☐ 749.2	Cleft Palate with Cleft Lip	☐ 646.1	Excess Weight Gain,	☐ 646.8	Insufficient Weight Gain,	☐ 269.2	Vitamin Deficiency
☐ 428.0	Congestive Heart Failure		Pregnancy		Pregnancy	☐	Other _____
☐ 564.0	Constipation	☐ 783.4	Failure to Thrive/	☐ 271.3	Lactose Intolerance		_____
☐ 555.9	Crohn's Disease		Physical Retardation	☐ 263.9	Malnutrition		_____
☐ 277.00	Cystic Fibrosis	☐ 693.1	Food Allergy				_____
		☐ 535.4	Gastritis				_____

Services

MNT CPT Codes, if applicable

☐ 97802 Initial assessment & intervention, individual, face-to-face

Each unit = 15 minutes _____ Units

☐ 97803 Re-assessment & intervention, individual, face-to-face

Each unit = 15 minutes _____ Units

☐ 97804 Group (2 or more), each 30 minutes _____ Units

Other CPT Code, if applicable _____

☐ _____ Initial Eval. & Consultation

☐ _____ Follow-Up Consultation ____

☐ _____ Nutr. Assess, Comprehensive ____

☐ _____ Phone Consultation ____

☐ _____ Instructional Material ____

☐ _____ Diet Instructions ____

☐ _____ Other: ____

Total Charge _____

Amount Paid _____

Balance Due _____

RD Name _____ RD Signature _____ Date _____ __

RD # _____ Provider # _____ Phone # _____ __

Address _____ __

WHITE - Office Copy   YELLOW - Insurance Copy   PINK - Patient Copy

DATE:	1ˢᵗ Visit Assessment Values	DATE: (Outcomes)

DATE: 1ˢᵗ **Visit Assessment Values**   **DATE:**   **(Outcomes)**

Year diabetes diagnosed:_____   Medical history (previous, current co-morbidities):

NUTRITION HISTORY   Code: none=0   low=1   moderate=2   high=3   very high=4

Previous restricted diets/foods

Eating times: *B:*   *Sn:*   *L:*   *Sn:*   *D:*   *Sn:*

Usual food choices/intake:
Starches: _____ code	*Starches:* _____ code
Fruits: _____	*Fruits:* _____
Vegetables: _____	*Vegetables:* _____
Milk, yogurt: _____	*Milk, yogurt:* _____
Protein, meat: _____	*Protein, meat:* _____
Fats: _____	*Fats:* _____
Sugar, sweets: _____	*Sugar, sweets:* _____

Portion control: ☐ poor ☐ fair ☐ good ☐ very good

Person responsible for food purchasing/~~preparation~~

Adequacy of cooking facilities: ☐ poor

Calorie (energy) intake/day: ☐ estimate ~~☐ actual~~ =

Macro-nutrient intake and/or composition/day: ☐ estimate ☐ actual
CHO: _____ code	CHO: _____ code
PRO: _____	PRO: _____
FAT: _____	FAT: _____

Appetite: ☐ poor ☐ fair ☐ good ☐ very good

Digestive and/or elimination problems

Types of restaurant meals and frequency: _____ code

Alcohol intake: about _____ drinks per ☐ day   ☐ week   ☐ month   ∧ year
Type:

Vitamin / mineral use

Supplement / dietary herb use

Cholesterol intake: _____ code   Primary source =   _____ code

Sodium intake: _____ code   Primary source =   _____ code

PSYCHO–SOCIAL, ECONOMIC   Code: none=0   low=1   moderate=2   high=3   very high=4

No. visits in last year: PCP:_____   Podiatrist:_____   Dentist:_____   RD:_____
Other:

Sample

MNT ASSESSMENT and OUTCOMES FOR: ⎣ **DIABETES TYPE 1** ⎣ **DIABETES TYPE 2**

PATIENT:	∧ M ∧ F DOB:	AGE:	PHYSICIAN:
ADDRESS:			TELEPHONE:
ID NUMBER:	PREVIOUS MNT (NO. HRS):		__MEDICARE B __NON-MEDICARE

DATE: 1st Visit Assessment Values	GOALS	DATE:_____ (3 - 12 Month Follow-Up MNT Outcomes)
Labs: A1C		
FBG		
Pre-Meal BG		
Post-Meal BG		
Total cholesterol		
LDL-cholesterol		
HDL-cholesterol		
Triglycerides		
Ht: Wt: BMI: ~nt Δ:		
Blood pressure		

Tobacco use: type, frequency: about _____ . ~igars ∧ pipes per ∧ day ∧ year	
Exercise: Medical clearance ∧ yes ∧ no Limitations: ∧ per physician ∧ per patient :	
Food-drug interactions: ⎣ potential ⎣ actual	
Physical signs and symptoms	
Medications (both RX and OTC) that affect MNT	

Sample

OVER